Health and Healing in the Middle Ages
Volume 4

Death and Disease in the Medieval and Early Modern World

YORK MEDIEVAL PRESS

York Medieval Press is published by the University of York's Centre for Medieval Studies in association with Boydell & Brewer Limited. Our objective is the promotion of innovative scholarship and fresh criticism on medieval culture. We have a special commitment to interdisciplinary study, in line with the Centre's belief that the future of Medieval Studies lies in those areas in which its major constituent disciplines at once inform and challenge each other.

All enquiries of an editorial kind, including suggestions for monographs and essay collections, should be addressed to: The Academic Editor, York Medieval Press, Department of History, University of York, Heslington, York, YO10 5DD (E-mail: pete.biller@york.ac.uk)

Details of other York Medieval Press volumes are available from Boydell & Brewer Ltd.

Health and Healing in the Middle Ages

The subject matter of this series is interpreted broadly, from studies of health or palaeopathology at one end of the spectrum to a medical humanities approach to the history of healing at the other. It welcomes both monographs and focussed edited collections written in English, covering any centuries or geographical areas to which the term 'medieval' can be productively applied.

Enquiries about the series may be sent to Peregrine Horden (peregrine.horden@all-souls.ox.ac.uk), Sara Ritchey (sritchey@utk.edu) and Linda Voigts (voigtsl@umkc.edu). Book proposals should be supported by a one-page prospectus, a brief chapter outline and a one-page curriculum vitae.

A full list of titles in the series is given at the end of the volume.

Death and Disease in the Medieval and Early Modern World

Perspectives from across the Mediterranean and Beyond

Edited by Lori Jones and Nükhet Varlık

THE UNIVERSITY *of York*
YORK MEDIEVAL PRESS

First published 2022

A York Medieval Press publication
in association with The Boydell Press
an imprint of Boydell & Brewer Ltd
PO Box 9, Woodbridge, Suffolk IP12 3DF, UK
and of Boydell & Brewer Inc.
668 Mt Hope Avenue, Rochester, NY 14620–2731, USA
website: www.boydellandbrewer.com
and with the
Centre for Medieval Studies, University of York

ISBN 978 1 914049 09 5

A CIP catalogue record for this book is available from the British Library

This publication is printed on acid-free paper

MIX
Paper from
responsible sources
FSC® C013056

Printed and bound in Great Britain by
TJ Books Limited, Padstow, Cornwall

To Ann G. Carmichael, a dear friend, colleague, mentor, role model and inspiration to so many of us.

Contents

Illustrations

Acknowledgements

This volume was first conceptualised as a follow-up to two special panels entitled 'Between Death and Disease' and a subsequent round table session at the 90th annual meeting of the American Association for the History of Medicine (AAHM) in 2017. The majority of the chapters in this volume evolved from presentations made at one of the special panels or the round table; others were added as the volume was being developed. We thank our fellow contributors, both those who have been with us since the AAHM meeting and those who joined mid-stream, for their patience, collegiality and eagerness to be part of this special project. We are so pleased to have been able to include all of their work here. A few people involved in the AAHM sessions were unable to contribute to the volume, however, and they also deserve special recognition and thanks here. Monica H. Green was a driving force behind the idea to organise the special sessions and the subsequent volume. She has been a staunch cheerleader of the project from the beginning and we owe her our gratitude for her support. Sara Ritchey was a key contributor to several aspects of the volume until she unfortunately had to withdraw due to other commitments; her hand can still be felt in the Introduction, however, and we are very appreciative of her early work on the book. Winston Black has likewise been a major player and positive force in this volume, from its initial conception until the final touches were made. We are grateful for his contributions to the introductory chapter and for his review of several chapters in the volume. A number of other scholars also made valuable contributions to this volume by providing detailed reviews of and comments on individual chapters; they are recognised by name in the respective chapters and we would like to add our appreciation for their involvement here.

We would also like to express our gratitude for the generous support we have received from Peregrine Horden, Linda Ehrsam Voigts and Sara Ritchey. As series editors of York Medieval Press's *Health and Healing* series, they encouraged and guided us throughout the processes of putting together the proposal, and then preparing the volume itself. They have been patient as we, and our authors, experienced delays during the COVID-19 pandemic and always provided sound advice for any issues that arose along the way. Peter Biller, General Editor at York Medieval Press, and Caroline Palmer, Editorial Director at Boydell & Brewer, have likewise been supportive of our project from the beginning and we are thankful for their ongoing assistance. We also would like to acknowledge the friendly support we have received from staff at Boydell & Brewer, especially Elizabeth McDonald, who patiently shepherded us through the early processes of production, including the smart cover design; Judith Oppenheimer, whose copy-editing process was so straighforward; and Nick Bingham, who took the reins and led us to the end.

Ann G. Carmichael: An Appreciation

The AAHM panels and special session noted in the Acknowledgements were organised in 2017 to honour Ann G. Carmichael, a pioneering researcher in the history of infectious diseases, an inspirational mentor of younger scholars and a teacher dedicated to carrying forward to new generations the stories of humankind's struggles with health and disease. Ann's innovative studies have been many. From her work on classifying the dead and on delving into Milan's *Books of the Dead*, to her multiple explorations of plague in Florence and Milan, her hypothesis about virulent smallpox being an early modern disease, her assessments of nutrition and earthquakes and, yes, even to her proposition that alpine marmots could be at least partially responsible for plague persistence in Western Europe: all of her work has transformed the kinds of questions we ask about the history of death and disease. All of it crosses boundaries and blends conceptual and methodological categories by examining hitherto unseen connections: between medicine and religion, between disease patterns and ecology, between death records and legal justice and so on. Her ongoing collaborations with scientists and her forays into the genetics and archaeology of plague are likewise fostering consilience between two larger fields of study that have, until recent years, been approached in isolation. Through her work, Ann has nurtured a generation of scholars as inventive in their approaches as they are rigorous in their methods.

'I don't do texts' is what Ann has told us so many times. In spite of that disclaimer, she has profoundly influenced and affected the work of those of us who do base our research on texts. Her years of patiently and diligently combing through the archives have brought to life incredible amounts of raw data, information that has both enlightened and redirected historical analyses of both disease and death. In a way, then, Ann does do texts; perhaps she would be more amenable to admitting that, at the least, she does so vicariously through the rest of us. We are all better for having her in our lives, and hope that this collection of texts initially conceived in her honour demonstrates the value and long-term impact of the thought-provoking research – and the heartfelt mentoring – that she has done over the years. This collection is meant to be both a reflection of those impacts and a step towards the future of the research that Ann has inspired amongst her 'tribe'.

Contributors

NICOLE ARCHAMBEAU is an Associate Professor of History at Colorado State University. Her numerous publications uncover medieval understandings of sickness, remedy and healing practitioners. Her recent book *Souls under Siege: Stories of War, Plague, and Confession in Fourteenth-Century Provence* (New York, 2021) explores the sufferers' point of view of catastrophe through canonisation inquest narratives.

ANDREW BERNS is Associate Professor of History at the University of South Carolina. His research investigates the intellectual and cultural history of Jews in the medieval and early modern Mediterranean, especially Italy and Spain. He is the author of *The Bible and Natural Philosophy in Renaissance Italy: Jewish and Christian Physicians in Search of Truth* (Cambridge, 2015) and *The Land is Mine: Sephardi Jews, Land Use, and Bible Commentary in the Renaissance* (Philadelphia, 2022).

WINSTON BLACK holds the Gatto Chair of Christian Studies at St. Francis Xavier University. He studies the intersections of learned medicine and scholastic theology in High Medieval Europe. His publications include an edition and translation of Henry of Huntingdon, *Anglicanus Ortus: A Verse Herbal of the Twelfth Century* (Toronto, 2012) as well as the essays 'Animated Corpses and Bodies with Power in the Scholastic Age', in J. Rollo-Koster, ed., *Death in Medieval Europe: Death Scripted and Death Choreographed* (New York, 2017) and 'William of Auvergne on the Dangers of Paradise: Biblical Exegesis between Natural Philosophy and Anti-Islamic Polemic', *Traditio* 68 (2013).

ANN G. CARMICHAEL is emerita in the History Department at Indiana University. Her most recent publications focus on the ecological parameters of Western Europe's recurring plague outbreaks and on fifteenth- and sixteenth-century Milanese civic mortality registers, including 'Pesthouse Imaginaries', in C. Lynteris, ed., *Plague Image and Imagination from Medieval to Modern Times* (Cham, 2021), 'Registering Deaths and Causes of Death in Late Medieval Milan', in J. Rollo-Koster, ed., *Death in Medieval Europe: Death Scripted and Death Choreographed* (New York, 2017) and 'Plague Persistence in Western Europe: A Hypothesis', in M. H. Green, ed., *Pandemic Disease in the Medieval World: Rethinking the Black Death* (Kalamazoo, 2014).

FABIAN CRESPO is an Associate Professor in the Department of Anthropology, University of Louisville, where he studies how different forces (especially infectious diseases) have shaped inflammatory responses and overall immune competence in different human populations. His methodology to reconstruct immune competence in past populations considers a biosocial approach that integrates experimental immunology, bioarchaeology and history.

JENNIFER C. EDWARDS is Professor and Chair of History at Manhattan College in the Bronx, New York. Her research focuses on medieval religion, power, women and gender, with interest in monasticism and saints' cults. She is the author of *Superior Women: Medieval Female Authority in Poitiers' Abbey of Sainte-Croix* (Oxford, 2019).

NAHYAN FANCY is a Professor of History at DePauw University. A historian of science by training, he focuses on the intersections of medicine, philosophy and religion in pre-modern Islamic societies. He is the author of *Science and Religion in Mamluk Egypt: Ibn al-Nafīs, Pulmonary Transit and Bodily Resurrection* (Abingdon, 2013).

NICHOLA E. HARRIS is Associate Professor of European History at the State University of New York (SUNY) Ulster, where she teaches Roman and medieval history. Her research focuses on medicine and popular culture in medieval and early modern England, particularly relating to the theory and practical application of lapidary medicine and pharmacology. She is currently working on a comprehensive study of lapidary theory and practice entitled 'The Virtue of Stones: A Natural History of Lapidary Medicine from the Ancient World to the Present'. She most recently contributed to *The Sacred and the Secular in Medieval Healing: Sites, Objects, and Texts* (New York, 2016).

LORI JONES is a historian of medieval and early modern medicine at Carleton University and the University of Ottawa. Her research focuses on plague texts and images and on early modern medical manuscripts. She is the author of *Patterns of Plague: Changing Ideas about Plague in England and France, 1348–1750* (Montreal, 2022) and editor of *Disease and the Environment in the Medieval and Early Modern Worlds* (London, 2022). She has also published several book chapters and journal articles on plague treatises and images.

JENNI KUULIALA is a senior research fellow at the Centre of Excellence in the History of Experiences, Tampere University, Finland. Her research focuses on the social history of medicine in the late medieval and early modern periods, with a particular focus on lived religion and disability. She is the author of *Childhood Disability and Social Integration in the Middle Ages: Constructions of Impairments in Thirteenth- and Fourteenth-Century Canonization Processes* (Turnhout, 2016) and *Saints, Infirmity, and Community in the Late Middle Ages* (Amsterdam, 2020).

HENDRIK N. POINAR is a professor of Anthropology and Biochemisty at McMaster University and director of the McMaster Ancient DNA Centre. He likes to spend most of his time in the interstitial spaces of the overlapping fields of molecular and evolutionary genetics, history, archaeology, biochemistry and palaeontology. His laboratory's most recent works focus on two very divergent themes, plague evolutionary genetics and megafaunal extinctions.

ELAINE STRATTON HILD serves as an editor with *Corpus monodicum*, a long-term research and publication project housed at the Universität Würzburg (Germany). Her research on medieval plainchant has been supported by the University of Notre Dame Institute for Advanced Study, the DAAD (Deutscher Akademischer Austauschdienst) and the Fulbright Foundation. She is the editor of *Tropen zu den Antiphonen der Messe aus Quellen französischer Herkunft* (Basel, 2016).

NÜKHET VARLIK is Associate Professor of History at Rutgers University–Newark. She is a historian of the Ottoman Empire interested in disease, medicine and public health. She is the author of *Plague and Empire in the Early Modern Mediterranean World: The Ottoman Experience, 1347–1600* (Cambridge, 2015) and editor of *Plague and Contagion in the Islamic Mediterranean* (Kalamazoo, 2017).

Note on Translation and Transliteration

The volume draws from a rich body of source materials (published and unpublished) in multiple languages including Middle English, Latin, Arabic, Hebrew, French, Italian and Ottoman Turkish. Original text is given alongside the modern translation, either in the text following the translation or in the footnotes. Except where noted, all translations belong to the author of the respective chapter. Because the volume uses sources in multiple languages, there is no single convention for transliteration. The transliterations followed for terminology, book titles, place names and names of individuals loosely follow the conventions of the respective field of the author, while preserving the preferences of each author. See individual chapters for the method of transliteration used by their author.

Intersections: Disease and Death, Medicine and Religion, Medieval and Early Modern

LORI JONES, NÜKHET VARLIK AND WINSTON BLACK

Introduction and historiographical overview

On Tuesday, 1 April 1483, Sister Eufemia dei Magni, aged 27 years, died in south-west Milan, at the monastery of Santa Maria Maddalena al Cerchio in the Porta Ticinese district.[1] The district was named after one of the city's medieval gates, part of the twelfth-century wall system built after the city had been destroyed by Holy Roman Emperor Frederick I Barbarossa. Beyond the gates ran the Naviglio Grande, a purpose-built canal that moved people and goods in a constant motion between the city and the Ticino River, located some fifty kilometres south-west of the city. Porta Ticinese was a busy, boisterous and densely settled district. Alongside the monastery and the ancient Basilica of San Lorenzo Maggiore with its Colonne di San Lorenzo, it housed the Cittadella – like the walls and the early canal system, constructed for the medieval defence of the city against Barbarossa and his allies. Here too was located much of the city's industrial and artisanal production. A short distance away, the waters of the outer and inner canals mixed with river water, creating an ever-changing combination of clean and dirty water that both removed waste and powered the city's economic development and dominance – but also sometimes, like the by-products of the numerous commercial enterprises, gave rise to local concern about corruption and disease. Noise permeated the air, as did the fetid miasma arising from the many bodies working in the April sun in the mills and warehouses, at the workshops and on the nearby wharves. Within her darkened cell, however,

1 A brief post-mortem account of Sister Eufemia's death appears in Archivio di Stato, Milano, Atti di Governo, Fondo Popolazione, parte antiqua, cartella 76. We thank Ann G. Carmichael for generously sharing the account and her translation of it; the larger story here is a plausible historical fiction and not present in the source. Rather, it is our interpretation of what might have transpired and any errors in that interpretation are our own. Ann's more extensive examination and interpretation of Milanese post-mortem records, on which we rely, is found in chapter 2 in this volume, as well as in 'Registering Deaths and Causes of Death in Late Medieval Milan', in *Death in Medieval Europe: Death Scripted and Death Choreographed*, ed. J. Rollo-Koster (London, 2017), pp. 223–50 and 'Epidemics and State Medicine in Fifteenth-Century Milan' in *Medicine from the Black Death to the French Disease*, ed. R. French, J. Arrizabalaga, A. Cunningham and L. García-Ballester (Aldershot, 1998), pp. 221–47. Some aspects of this account also rely on G. Geltner, *Roads to Health: Infrastructure and Urban Wellbeing in Later Medieval Italy* (Philadelphia, 2019); A. Gamberini, ed., *A Companion to Late Medieval and Early Modern Milan: The Distinctive Features of an Italian State* (Leiden, 2014) and P. Boucheron, 'Water and Power in Milan, c. 1200–1500', *Urban History* 28 (2001), 180–93.

Eufemia died quietly; the sisters' desperate fluttering of care and uncertainties about how to stay well themselves passed unheard and unseen outside the monastery's thick walls.

Sister Eufemia died in the early months of a catastrophic outbreak of plague that ravaged Milan between 1483 and 1486.[2] The streets were not yet empty of people fearing the disease and, despite several possible plague deaths in the district already, life was carrying on largely as normal. Eufemia had fallen ill on the previous Thursday morning while distributing alms to the local poor. Described in her post-mortem record as 'strenuous and burdensome' ('forti et honeroso'), Eufemia's almsgiving brought her into direct physical contact with the district's most desperate residents, many of whom were ill, injured or otherwise incapacitated, hoping not only for the worldly relief that the alms offered but also some spiritual assistance as well. The district's commercial success evidently had not trickled down to all who lived there.

Feeling feverish and nauseous, Eufemia carried on as best she could as the day went on. She may have visited the monastery's infirmarian at some point, seeking medicinal relief for her symptoms: an anti-plague drink made from the herbs in the monastery's own garden and perhaps a bloodletting to rebalance her humours, she thought, should work. By Friday evening, however, she was so ill that she had to take to her bed. She declined rapidly; her fellow sisters checked in on her regularly, putting a cooling cloth infused with herbs to her feverish forehead, offering her some tried-and-true remedies and adding their prayers for her recovery alongside Eufemia's own desperate prayers. They might have sought the infirmarian's advice or sent for a university-trained physician, one with the accumulated knowledge of disease learned from the Ancients. They may have placed a textual or lapidary amulet on the sick woman's body to help cure her illness. They perhaps even requested a saintly miracle as the young nun took a drastic turn for the worse and seemed to slip from life several times. The sisters might have turned to Milan's patron saints, Gervasius and Protasius, or to its early bishop, Saint Ambrose; it is more likely in this case, though, that they would have invoked Saint Sebastian, long associated with plague, or one of the holy women known to have healing powers, such as a member of the Humiliati – their own order.[3]

It was all to no avail, however: passing in and out of consciousness for several days, delirious from a fever that never abated and her body wracked from days of violent vomiting and diarrhoea, the Last Rites performed, Eufemia finally died shortly before midnight as Tuesday became Wednesday. The sisters attending her bedside, now her deathbed, did

2 On this and other plague outbreaks in fifteenth- and early sixteenth-century Milan, see S. K. Cohn and G. Alfani, 'Households and Plague in Early Modern Italy', *Journal of Interdisciplinary History* 38 (2007), 177–205; A. G. Carmichael, 'Contagion Theory and Contagion Practice in Fifteenth-Century Milan', *Renaissance Quarterly* 44 (1991), 213–56.

3 On Saint Sebastian, see S. Barker, 'The Making of a Plague Saint: Saint Sebastian's Imagery and Cult before the Counter-Reformation', in *Piety and Plague from Byzantium to the Baroque*, ed. F. Mormando and T. Worcester (Kirksville, 2007), pp. 90–131. On women affiliated with the Humiliati, see S. M. Brasher, *Women of the Humiliati: A Lay Religious Order in Medieval Civic Life* (London, 2003).

what they could to continue easing her soul into the next life, perhaps singing softly as they awaited the arrival of the officials who would pronounce Eufemia's cause of death.

Two Milanese Health Office physicians – Catelano and Dyonisio – examined Sister Eufemia's corpse on Wednesday 2 April. A few months earlier, they had discounted acute deaths much like Eufemia's as possible cases of plague, especially in the absence of a suggestive 'dragonzello' or bubo.[4] As the case numbers started to climb throughout the city, however, they became more circumspect in their diagnosis. Seen post-mortem, Eufemia's body still offered nothing obvious to allow the physicians to make a firm diagnosis of plague: there were no colourful swellings on her groin or in her armpit, none of the typical blue-green, red, black or purple markers or tokens of the disease. However, she had had a continuous fever, followed by the appearance of worms in her vomit as well as 'passione colerica' ('choleric affliction'); because all of these symptoms were acute, taken together they presented a warning.

Catelano and Dyonisio considered Eufemia's circumstances with great caution, ultimately judging it to be a plague case. Catelano, at least, had seen plague epidemics before during his long career and thus recognised the danger that the impending outbreak – and especially mis- or undiagnosed cases – posed to the city's residents and its leaders. The sisters were called back to prepare Eufemia's body for a quick burial, the normal funerary rites afforded to the deceased sisters bypassed in an effort to remove from the monastery the threat of disease that a plague victim's corpse was believed to pose. That they were successful in containing the disease is unlikely, and those living in the monastery were probably ordered to quarantine. Catalano and his fellow physicians were likewise set apart: their distinctive over-robes – signs of their office – made it clear that they might have come into contact with diagnosed plague victims and that they too might be a source of contamination.

From our perspective more than five centuries later, a diagnosis of plague – or not – might seem obvious. Yet the distinction between what was plague and what was some other affliction was not always so clear to the doctors from the Milanese Health Office. They recognised that buboes were the most definitive sign of plague, but not the only one according to their models of disease aetiology and diagnosis. Many other illnesses, some with similar symptoms, also circulated regularly in the city and had to be considered. Since Eufemia died during the early months of a plague outbreak, however, they could tentatively and out of an abundance of caution allow that her symptoms were indicative of plague, despite the absence of buboes. Even as modern historians and scientists become ever surer that medieval and early modern plagues were caused, primarily, by the bacterium *Yersinia pestis*, we need to be reminded that this certainty does not help us to explain premodern approaches to the disease and to death more broadly. Sister Eufemia fell sick and died within a religious institution that had developed elaborate rituals and institutions of

4 For 'dragonzello', see ASMi, Pop. p.a., c. 76, 18 February 1483, cited in Ann G. Carmichael's chapter 2 in this volume, as well as her 'Universal and Particular: The Language of Plague, 1348–1350', in *Pestilential Complexities: Understanding Medieval Plague*, ed. V. Nutton (London, 2008), pp. 17–52 and 'Epidemics and State Medicine', p. 227.

healing, both spiritual and physical, to relieve her suffering and to explain her death. Even in the brief account of her death recorded in the Milanese registry, Eufemia's passing is framed in terms of one of the monastery's most important religious and socio-economic functions: the collection and distribution of alms. Her disease is implicitly blamed on the strenuous and burdensome activity that brought her into contact with the district's other potential source of pollution – its poor and its homeless – but that nonetheless also suggests the holiness and worthiness of her life and death.

Sister Eufemia's disease and death reveal voices of past human experiences that we may not have been so prepared to hear just a few decades ago. Medieval and early modern people quite concretely saw the living and the dead still in ongoing dialogue, with obligations one to another.[5] Eufemia's experience with disease and with death was a matter of concern for numerous parties beyond herself: the poor and needy of the Porta Ticenese district, her sisters and superiors at Santa Maria Maddalena al Cerchio, the physicians of the Health Office and the government of the duchy of Milan. Each group possessed different reasons for and multiple means of identifying and explaining her disease, as well as for marking the exact point and significance of her death. The implications of Eufemia's sudden illness and passing likewise differed for each group. The recipients of her alms would have noticed her absence and, if another sister did not immediately fill her empty post, they might have gone hungry, left to fend for themselves. Some among them doubtless carried the same pathogen in their own bodies but, without the institutional and healing support that the monastery offered Eufemia, they more likely died alone on the street or in an overcrowded, temporary lazaretto far from home.

For Eufemia's fellow sisters at the monastery, the suddenness and violence of her symptoms would have been frightening. They coped by tending to her as best as they could, drawing on centuries of secular and divine healing practices, all the while trying to keep their alarm and fear of plague to a minimum. The Health Office physicians Catalano and Dyonisio perhaps approached Eufemia's corpse with a more detached manner, looking for the signs that would confirm for them whether this case warranted the judgement that accompanied plague deaths and that, in turn, would set in motion a series of bureaucratic practices intended to halt the further spread of the disease. For the city's governing elite, the record of Eufemia's death soon became one among many, so many that they ultimately ordered the construction of a new, permanent lazaretto, or plague hospital. Some decades earlier, during another disastrous outbreak – and considering plague to be an environmental problem that could be cleansed and contained – they had first shipped plague victims and their families out of the city before hastily building temporary quarantine spaces along the city's perimeter. Work on the new and monumental lazaretto, the Lazzaretto di Milano, intended since 1468, finally began in earnest to the east of the city shortly after this latest outbreak was over.

5 On these obligations and interactions between the living and the dead, see P. J. Geary, *Living with the Dead in the Middle Ages* (Ithaca, 1994).

Eufemia's narrative offers historians a window into a tangle of intersecting approaches to death and disease that juxtapose and interlace varied historiographies and timelines. A previous generation of historians, informed by the enchanting rhetoric of the prolific Dutch medievalist, Johan Huizinga, might gather from this account a sense of the nuns' and the doctors' macabre fascination with the putridity of the dying. Or, following the conservative French historian Philippe Ariès, they might regard Eufemia's death as a slow process of anatomised dying: various members of her community might have momentarily interrupted her solitary repose with medicine, food and prayer, but at the heart of it all she lay alone until, finally, a saintly spectre from the past was invoked in an ultimately unsuccessful attempt to save her. Perhaps these two readings would have been brought together by an art historian such as Erwin Panofsky, who could see the Health Office record itself as a kind of transi tomb, portraying the deceased in both life and death – one layer sketches Eufemia's painful decay while the other reimagines her lively engagement with the downtrodden of Milan. For these twentieth-century historians of Europe, patently different approaches to, and understanding of, death and disease highlighted the human mechanics that separated contemporaries from their premodern subjects of study.[6]

More recent approaches to death and disease take a different, multi-lensed approach. Eufemia's story can, in fact, be seen to engage with a number of the organisational themes found in this volume: experiencing, diagnosing and explaining disease; observing and recording death; coping with the uncertainties and realities of disease and death; the inseparability of, or at least significant overlap between, secular and religious healing; the complexities of comorbidities and syndemics; the continuation of medical analysis and reinterpretation of evidence after death; and finally, the long continuities in knowledge and practice across geographies and faiths that obscure the modern tendency to separate medieval from early modern. Indeed, as the volume's twelve chapters illustrate, current scholarship on death and disease in the long Middle Ages (a historical period encompassing the Middle Ages of c. 500–1500 CE as well as the period c. 1500–1700 CE) stress human continuity over distant chronologies, interdisciplinarity over boundaried fields of study. As one historian remarked some decades ago, no clear lines exist between retrospectively created historical periods to denote that 'a narrow strait has been crossed and a new continent entered';[7] as the chapters in this volume show, the same thinking now applies to explorations of disease and death in the past. The volume thus approaches death and disease across this wide time span as universal human experiences, while also underscoring in its various chapters the historicity of those experiences in specific historical contexts.

6 J. Huizinga, *Herfsttij der Middeleeuwen* (Leiden, 1919); P. Ariès, *L'homme devant la mort* (Paris, 1977) and *Essais sur l'histoire de la mort en Occident: du Moyen Âge à nos jours* (Paris, 1975); E. Panofsky, *Tomb Sculpture: Four Lectures on Its Changing Aspects from Ancient Egypt to Bernini* (New York, 1964).

7 L. García-Ballester, 'Academicism versus Empiricism in Practical Medicine in Sixteenth-Century Spain with Regard to Morisco Practitioners', in *The Medical Renaissance of the Sixteenth Century*, ed. A. Wear, R. K. French and I. M. Lonie (Cambridge, 1985), pp. 246–70 (p. 249).

In a similar manner, studies of death and disease of the long Middle Ages traditionally have had an overwhelmingly Western European focus. This is not entirely surprising, given that the Europeanist historiography in death studies, the history of disease and related fields – supported by a larger number of researchers, better accessibility of sources and greater professional opportunities – is more developed than its sister fields. Recent scholarship on the Islamicate world, Africa, Asia and the early Americas presents valuable new research, however, adding new questions and offering comparative insights that are fundamental to moving beyond a Eurocentric focus. New historiographical interventions in medieval and early modern studies (e.g., scholarship informed by legacies of colonialism and imperialism), the promise to open the field to global perspectives (e.g., the recent emphasis on 'Global Middle Ages') and the recent proliferation of studies focusing on other regions of the world should make it possible to do better justice to the study of disease and death – a singularly universal theme.[8]

[8] See, for example, chapters on perspectives and practices concerning death and the afterlife in Islam, pre-Christian Viking lands, the fourteenth- and fifteenth-century Inca Empire and sixteenth-century Vietnam in C. K. Cann, *The Routledge Handbook of Death and the Afterlife* (Abingdon, 2018). Among others, see also A. Zengin, ed., 'Death and Afterlives in the Middle East', special issue of *Comparative Studies of South Asia, Africa and the Middle East* 42, no. 1 (2022); I. Shingiray, 'An Islamicate Body: A Case Study of a Nomadic Burial from the Core Territory of the Golden Horde', *Revue des mondes musulmans et de la Méditerranée* 143 (2018), https://journals.openedition.org/remmm/10777; G. Chouin, ed., *Sillages de la peste noire en Afrique subsaharienne: une exploration critique du silence / Black Death and Its Aftermaths in Sub-Saharan Africa: A Critical Exploration of Silence*, *Afriques* 9 (2018), http://journals.openedition.org/afriques/2228; E. Aykut, 'Judicial Reforms, Sharia Law, and the Death Penalty in the Late Ottoman Empire', *Journal of the Ottoman and Turkish Studies Association* 4 (2017), 7–29; M. Ji, 'Commoditizing Tombs: Materialism in the Funerary Art of Middle Imperial China and Korea' (unpublished Ph.D. dissertation, University of Pennsylvania, 2014); E. Rebillard, 'Commemorating the Dead in North Africa: Continuity and Change from the Second to the Fifth Century CE', in *Death and Changing Rituals: Function and Meaning in Ancient Funerary Practices*, ed. J. R. Brandt, H. Ingvaldsen and M. Prusac (Oxford, 2014), pp. 269–86; M. Muravyeva, '"Till Death Us Do Part": Spousal Homicide in Early Modern Russia', *The History of the Family* 18 (2013), pp. 306–30; S. Minkin, 'History from Six-Feet Below: Death Studies and the Field of Modern Middle East History', *History Compass* 11 (2013), pp. 632–46; D. Cook, *Martyrdom in Islam* (Cambridge, 2012); K. M. Gerhart, *The Material Culture of Death in Medieval Japan* (Honolulu, 2009); T. Brook, J. Bourgon and G. Blue, *Death by a Thousand Cuts* (Cambridge, MA: 2008); R. Lee and M. Vaughan, 'Death and Dying in the History of Africa since 1800', *The Journal of African History* 49 (2008), pp. 341–59; L. Halevi, *Muhammad's Grave: Death Rites and the Making of Islamic Society* (New York, 2007); W. Diem and M. Schöller, *The Living and the Dead in Islam* (Wiesbaden, 2004); D. Howard, 'Death in Damascus: Venetians in Syria in the Mid-Fifteenth Century', *Muqarnas* 20 (2003), pp. 143–57; N. Vatin and G. Veinstein, *Le Sérail ébranlé. Essai sur les morts, dépositions et avènements des sultans ottomans (XIVe–XIXe siècle)* (Paris, 2003); N. Vatin and S. Yerasimos, *Les cimetières dans la ville: statut, choix et organisation des lieux d'inhumation dans Istanbul intra muros* (Istanbul, 2001); E. Eldem, *Death in Istanbul: Death and Its Rituals in Ottoman-Islamic Culture* (Istanbul, 2005); J.-L. Bacqué-Grammont and A. A. Tibet, ed., *Cimetières*

In keeping with these historiographical sensibilities, this volume strives to maintain a larger definition of the Middle Ages, both temporally and spatially. Just as we use the 'long Middle Ages' as an intervention to define the temporal scope of the volume, we use the Mediterranean world and its adjacent cultural zones as our spatial anchor. Being mindful of the pitfalls involved in the study of themes such as disease and death that clearly recognised no political or religious boundaries, we include a broad geographical region that stretches from Europe to the Middle East – centred on the Mediterranean – as a contact zone through which to explore the volume's themes that reveal significant convergences. As the chapters in the volume make clear, while the actual experience of death and disease was ubiquitous since people throughout western Eurasia and North Africa and around the Mediterranean basin lived in similar disease and mortality environments and were informed by a shared body of medical knowledge and practices, methods of diagnosing and explaining those experiences often diverged in different historical and local contexts. The volume's chronological and geographical spans thus highlight the reality that 'European' history cannot be understood in a vacuum.

Similarly, the myriad methods by which people tried to cope with painful experiences of disease and death, as well as their efforts toward prevention and cure, also showed surprising similarities across space and time. More specifically, the Christian, Islamic and Jewish traditions of healing addressed in this volume underscore the shared medical paradigms, notions of healthy living and attitudes toward body and illness, stemming especially though not entirely from Late Antique syntheses of Hippocratic–Galenic physiology and pathology (see Fancy's chapter 1 on the Islamicate reception of these syntheses). Clearly, religious difference alone does not guarantee an understanding of how different communities lived, became ill and died for the period under investigation. At the same time, however, there are important divergences to be noted regarding the continuity of diseases and the knowledge about them (see, e.g., Fancy's argument about the difference of medical discussions of plague in the Islamic world from those in the Latin West), new developments in medicine (e.g., Jones's chapter 8 on the rise of anatomical illustration in Europe, which was absent in the Islamic world) and the influence of law on public health (e.g., Carmichael's chapter 2 on the case of Milan). Such examples help to illustrate the diversity of experiences with disease and death across time and space.

The two historiographical sub-fields – disease and death – have long been approached and studied as inherently separate areas of research. Influenced and spurred by Ariès's work in particular,[9] death studies has developed into a thriving area of scholarship within medieval studies. The material aspects of death, dying and burial practices are topics that have long received attention from scholars, while studies in art history, literature, religion, archaeology and anthropology of the Middle Ages have shed considerable light on the portrayal of death and the myriad cultural, religious and administrative customs that

et traditions funéraires dans le monde islamique, 2 vols. (Ankara, 1996); G. Veinstein, ed., *Les Ottomans et la mort: permanences et mutations* (Leiden, 1996).

9 Ariès, *L'homme devant la mort*.

surrounded it. The Triumph of Death and the Dance of Death ('danse macabre') in artwork, the Office of the Dead in prayer books, the construction of transi tombs, 'memento mori' ('remember that you die') and other commemorative funereal monuments, the writing of testamentary wills and, of course, efforts to shorten the intermediate state after physical death spent in purgatory have all offered avenues for exploring medieval and early modern attitudes towards death. These approaches to death and disease in the long Middle Ages have been broadly informed by the anthropology of death and dying and the memorial and mourning customs that accompany human departures. As anthropologists have long reminded us, death is not simply a biological or natural process; instead, death and dying encompass moral and social obligations that are expressed culturally in mourning rituals, burial practices and commemoration. Socio-cultural historians are thus now also taking on the mantle of death to explore its medieval and early modern meanings, rituals and performances, as well as its gendered expressions.[10] The rituals surrounding the death, corpse and burial of some of the most powerful figures in the long Middle Ages – popes, kings and emperors – for example, have attracted significant attention equally from scholars of medicine, theology and politics ever since Ernst Kantorowicz's revolutionary study of the

[10] Publications in the past decade include S. Perkinson and N. Turel, ed., *Picturing Death 1200–1600* (Leiden, 2020); *World Archaeology* 52 (2020) special issue on necrogeographies; P. Booth and E. Tingle, ed., *A Companion to Death, Burial, and Remembrance in Late Medieval and Early Modern Europe, c. 1300–1700* (Leiden, 2020); T. Tomaini, ed., *Dealing with the Dead: Mortality and Community in Medieval and Early Modern Europe* (Leiden, 2018); W. J. Courtenay, *Rituals for the Dead: Religion and Community in the Medieval University of Paris* (Notre Dame, 2018); J. Hartnell, *Medieval Bodies: Life, Death and Art in the Middle Ages* (London, 2018); L. M. Becker, *Death and the Early Modern Englishwoman* (London, 2017); E. Murphy and M. Le Roy, ed., *Children, Death and Burial: Archaeological Discourses* (Oxford, 2017); J. Rollo-Koster, ed., *Death in Medieval Europe*; A. Reinis, *Reforming the Art of Dying: The* ars moriendi *in the German Reformation (1519–1528)* (London, 2016); A. Classen, ed., *Death in the Middle Ages and Early Modern Times: The Material and Spiritual Conditions of the Culture of Death* (Berlin, 2016); S. E. James, *Women's Voices in Tudor Wills, 1485–1603: Authority, Influence and Material Culture* (London, 2015); E. C. Tingle, *Dying, Death, Burial and Commemoration in Reformation Europe* (Farnham, 2015); A. Appleford, *Learning to Die in England, 1380–1540* (Philadelphia, 2015); M. Korpiola and A. Lahtinen, ed., *Cultures of Death and Dying in Medieval and Early Modern Europe* (Helsinki, 2015); T. Laqueur, *The Work of the Dead: A Cultural History of Mortal Remains* (Princeton, 2015); D. Boyer-Gardner and M. Vivas, *Déplacer les morts: voyages, funérailles, manipulations, exhumations et réinhumations de corps au Moyen Âge* (Bordeaux, 2014); Brandt, Ingvaldsen and Prusac, ed., *Death and Changing Rituals*; F. Paxton and I. Cochelin, *The Death Ritual at Cluny in the Central Middle Ages* (Turnhout, 2013); A. Kinch, *Imago Mortis: Mediating Images of Death in Late Medieval Culture* (Leiden, 2013); D. Sayer, H. Williams and H. Härke, ed., *Mortuary Practices and Social Identities in the Middle Ages: Essays in Burial Archaeology in Honour of Heinrich Härke* (Liverpool, 2013); M. D. Goggin and B. F. Tobin, ed., *Women and the Material Culture of Death* (Farnham, 2013); R. Gilchrist, *Medieval Life: Archaeology and the Life Course* (Woodbridge, 2012); C. Krötzl and K. Mustakallio, ed., *On Old Age: Approaching Death in Antiquity and the Middle Ages* (Turnhout, 2011). We primarily focus here and elsewhere in the Introduction on monograph-length works; there are significantly more journal articles that could be added.

'king's two bodies'.[11] At the other end of the spectrum, crime, martyrdom, torture and capital punishment are also receiving attention, with the body of the dead (criminal, victim or martyr) taking centre stage.[12]

These socio-cultural histories of death in the Middle Ages have demonstrated that the medieval and early modern boundaries between life and death were remarkably porous and constantly shifting according to the beliefs and social needs of particular cultures at particular times. For example, while the central importance of saints and the holy dead to medieval society has long been recognised, scholars have only recently begun to take seriously the many stories of the living in contact with the unholy and restless dead: ghosts, spirits, revenants and other types of undead that tested the meaning and supposed permanence of death.[13] The undead 'draugr' (revenant) of the Icelandic sagas has provided a particularly rich source for exploring medieval Scandinavian notions (both before and after conversion to Christianity) of how the dead continued to shape the religious customs, laws and even property boundaries of the living.[14] Other scholars have directed attention to the corpse itself of a dead person and the powers it was believed to retain or the knowledge it could deliver to the living, regardless of the persistence of an individual soul or personality. Such was the case in the popularity of 'mumia', or powdered Egyptian corpses, in both

[11] E. Kantorowicz, *The King's Two Bodies* (Berkeley, 1957). For more recent scholarship, see J. Rollo-Koster, 'Failed Ritual? Medieval Papal Funerals and the Death of Clement VI (1352)', in *Histories of Post-Mortem Contagion: Infectious Corpses and Contested Burials*, ed. C. Lynteris and N. Evans (London, 2017), pp. 27–53; A. Paravicini-Bagliani, *The Pope's Body*, trans. D. S. Peterson (Chicago, 2000) and *Il Corpo del Papa* (Turin, 1994); E. A. R. Brown, 'Royal Bodies, Effigies, Funeral Meals, and Office in Sixteenth-Century France', *Micrologus: Natura, scienze e società medievali* VII: *Il cadavere. The Corpse* (1999), 437–508.

[12] A. Gobin, *Picturing Punishment: The Spectacle and Material Afterlife of the Criminal Body in the Dutch Republic* (Toronto, 2021); A. Pinkus, *Visual Aggression: Images of Martyrdom in Late Medieval Germany* (Philadelphia, 2021); F. Sabaté, *Death Penalty in Late-Medieval Catalonia: Evidence and Significations* (London, 2019); C. Gauvard, *Condamner à mort au Moyen Âge: Pratiques de la peine capitale en France XIII–XVe siècle* (Paris, 2018); S. Tarlow and E. Battell Lowman, *Harnessing the Power of the Criminal Corpse* (Cham, 2018); J. R. Decker and M. Kirkland-Ives, ed., *Death, Torture and the Broken Body in European Art, 1300–1650* (Abingdon, 2015).

[13] To name just one key work in this vast field of the history and anthropology of medieval saints and sanctity, see A. Vauchez, *Sainthood in the Later Middle Ages* (Cambridge, 1997). Also see C. Callard, *Le temps des fantômes: spectralités de l'âge moderne (XVIe–XVIIe siècle)* (Paris, 2019); N. M. Caciola, *Afterlives: The Return of the Dead in the Middle Ages* (Ithaca, 2016); J.-C. Schmitt, *Ghosts in the Middle Ages: The Living and the Dead in Medieval Society*, trans. T. L. Fagan (Chicago, 1998).

[14] K. Kanerva, 'Rituals for the Restless Dead: The Authority of the Deceased in Medieval Iceland', in *Authorities in the Middle Ages: Influence, Legitimacy and Power in Medieval Society*, ed. S. Kangas, M. Korpiola and T. Ainonen (Berlin, 2013), pp. 205–27; T. Gunnell, 'Waking the Dead: Folk Legends Concerning Magicians and Walking Corpses in Iceland', in *News from Other Worlds: Studies in Nordic Folklore, Mythology and Culture in Honor of John Lindow*, ed. M. Kaplan and T. R. Tangherlini (Berkeley, 2012), pp. 235–66; J. D. Martin, 'Law and the (Un)Dead: Medieval Models for Understanding the Hauntings in *Eyrbyggja saga*', *Saga-Book* 29 (2005), 67–82.

European and Islamicate medicine; the development of formal autopsies in the service of criminal jurisprudence in the later Middle Ages; and the belief in cruentation, the ability of the corpse of a murder victim to bleed as if alive in the presence of the murderer.[15]

The study of death in the long Middle Ages can also be approached through the multifaceted lens of mass mortality. Scholars of disaster studies stress that premodern societies were affected by multiple natural and anthropogenic events that increased levels of mortality and, in some cases, dramatically changed social and economic structures. This approach invites new possibilities of and perspectives for studying the phenomenon of mass casualties not just as they pertained to fires, plagues and war but also earthquakes, droughts, floods, tsunamis and volcanic eruptions as well as riots, rebellions and crime, along with methods of resilience and survival.[16] Questions regarding mortality and death also intersect with urban history and the social and cultural history of cities and daily life, especially in the case of major cities of the long Middle Ages, such as London, Rome, Venice, Cairo and Istanbul.[17] So too does death linger in non-urban settings, as medical-historical, archaeological and topographical studies have shown.[18]

The study of disease has likewise long been a staple of medieval studies. Plague, as should be clear by now, has dominated the field since the first modern histories of the Black Death in the nineteenth century – largely spearheaded by the works of the early nineteenth-century German medical writer Justus Friedrich Karl Hecker. Hecker's 1832 *Der schwarze Tod im vierzehnten Jahrhundert* (The Black Death in the Fourteenth

15 W. Black, 'Animated Corpses and Bodies with Power in the Scholastic Age', in *Death in Medieval Europe: Death Scripted and Death Choreographed*, ed. J. Rollo-Koster (London, 2017), pp. 71–92; S. M. Butler, *Forensic Medicine and Death Investigation in Medieval England* (London, 2015); A. Boureau, 'La preuve par le cadavre qui saigne au XIIIe siècle, entre expérience commune et savoir scholastique', *Micrologus: Natura, scienze e società medievali* VII: *Il cadavere. The Corpse* (1999), 247–81; R. Schmitz-Esser, *The Corpse in the Middle Ages: Embalming, Cremating, and the Cultural Construction of the Dead Body*, trans. A. Classen and C. Radtke (Turnhout, 2020).

16 For a critical overview of the latest research in medieval disaster studies, see C. M. Gerrard, P. Forlin and P. J. Brown, ed., *Waiting for the End of the World? New Perspectives on Natural Disasters in Medieval Europe* (London, 2020), and especially the editors' introduction, 'Researching Natural Disasters in the Later Middle Ages', pp. 1–14. See also M. Endreß, L. Clemens and B. Rampp, ed., *Strategies, Dispositions and Resources of Social Resilience: A Dialogue Between Medieval Studies and Sociology* (Wiesbaden, 2020); J. Davies, ed., *Aspects of Violence in Renaissance Europe* (London, 2016); J. Spinks and C. Zika, ed., *Disaster, Death and the Emotions in the Shadow of the Apocalypse, 1400–1700* (London, 2016); J. Canning, H. Lehmann and J. Winter, ed., *Power, Violence and Mass Death in Pre-Modern and Modern Times* (London, 2004); J. Hanska, *Strategies of Sanity and Survival: Religious Responses to Natural Disasters in the Middle Ages* (Helsinki, 2002).

17 Recent examples include N. Varlık, 'New Methods for Governing Death in Istanbul: Early Modern Ottoman Necropolitics', *Comparative Studies of South Asia, Africa and the Middle East* 42, no. 1 (2022), 146–62; A. L. C. Emmerson, *Life and Death in the Roman Suburb* (Oxford, 2020); J. T. Walsh, *The Great Fire of Rome: Life and Death in the Ancient City* (Baltimore, 2019); J. F. Field, *London, Londoners and the Great Fire of 1666: Disaster and Recovery* (New York, 2017).

18 M. J. Dobson, *Contours of Death and Disease in Early Modern England* (Cambridge, 1997) remains a seminal study.

Century) – together with waves of cholera pandemics and the apparent re-emergence of plague – inspired a series of book chapters and monographs on the topic that continued to be produced for more than a century, as well as more specialised studies on medieval medical writing about the disease.[19] The influence of these early studies should not be underestimated: the very idea of the Black Death being black – and its heavy association with an undeveloped and sinister Middle Ages – is owed to these first histories.[20]

The darkness of early plague histories carried forward well into the twentieth century. Drawing on burial records, last wills and testaments, chronicles, letters and diaries, manorial accounts, administrative records and contemporary medical texts and literary works, scholars have sought over the past century to assess plague's purported demographic, economic, socio-cultural, political, religious and psychological impacts.[21] Among other effects, these sources have purportedly revealed abandoned settlements and depopulated towns, mass hysteria and the rise of flagellant movements, the end of feudalism, an increased cultural and artistic focus on death and decay, social unrest and violence and, ultimately, the origins of the Reformation and the Renaissance. These scholars regularly focus on claims made in contemporary narratives that highlight the culture of fear and despair that the plague wrought: the lack of enough people to bury the dead, the abandonment of families and friends, poverty and hunger, looting and violence, hostility toward and persecution of Jews, gypsies and lepers and the abrogation of moral responsibilities. While much of the historiography of the Black Death has pointed to its economic and demographic repercussions that allegedly transformed society, however, there is also a substantial body of

19 A. Coville, 'Écrits contemporains sur la peste de 1348 à 1350', in *Histoire littéraire de la France* 37 (Paris, 1938), 325–90; A. M. Campbell, *The Black Death and Men of Learning* (New York, 1931); A. C. Klebs and K. Sudhoff, *Die Ersten Gedruckten Pestschriften* (Munich, 1926); A. C. Klebs and E. Droz, *Remèdes contre la peste: facsimilés, notes et liste bibliographique des incunables sur la peste* (Paris, 1925); D. W. Singer, 'Some Plague Tractates (Fourteenth and Fifteenth Centuries)', *Proceedings of the Royal Society of Medicine* 9 (1916), 159–212; D. W. Singer, 'Survey of Medical Manuscripts in the British Isles Dating from Before the Sixteenth Century', *Proceedings of the Royal Society of Medicine* 12 (1919), 96–107; K. Sudhoff, 'Pestschriften aus den ersten 150 Jahren nach der Epidemie des "schwarzen Todes" 1348', *Archiv für Geschichte der Medizin* 2–19 (1907–27); F. A. Gasquet, *The Great Pestilence* (London, 1893); C. Creighton, *A History of Epidemics in Britain*, 2 vols. (Cambridge, 1891–94); A. Phillippe, *Histoire de la peste noire: 1346–1350 d'après des documents inédits* (Paris, 1853); J. F. C. Hecker, *Der schwarze Tod im vierzehnten Jahrhundert* (Berlin, 1832).

20 On this, see N. Varlık, 'Why Is Black Death *Black*? European Gothic Imaginaries of "Oriental" Plague', in *Plague Image and Imagination from Medieval to Modern Times*, ed. C. Lynteris (Cham, 2021), pp. 11–35.

21 The corpus of scholarship on plague, and especially on the Black Death (c. 1346–53), is immense and cannot all be listed here. For a comprehensive bibliography on the state of the field of Black Death research, see: J. Roosen and M. H. Green, 'The Mother of All Pandemics: The State of Black Death Research in the Era of COVID-19 – Bibliography', https://drive.google.com/file/d/1x0D_dwyAwp9xi9sMCW5UvpGfEVH5J2ZA/view?usp=sharing (last accessed 17 August 2021).

literature that has downplayed the impact of plague on medieval communities, seeing instead the positive changes that it may have brought about: resilience, new freedoms and opportunities for peasants being among the forefront.[22]

Since the early 2000s, there has been another seismic shift and upsurge in plague historiography, predicated on the entry into the field of scientists whose discovery and study of ancient DNA (aDNA) and better understanding of past climates and ecologies is substantially changing both what was understood about the disease and what questions are now being asked about people's experiences with it. Long-standing debates about what pathogen caused plague have now been set aside to explore new lines of enquiry.[23] How did *Y. pestis*, naturally a rodent pathogen, move across such great geographic expanses and varied topographies of Eurasia during the Middle Ages? What places did it actually reach, where no documentary records have alerted us to its presence? How and when did the various strains of the pathogen emerge and by what means did they circulate? How did these strains interact with each other and with other contemporary diseases? Does knowledge about these strains, and their longer-term presence outside Europe, invalidate the traditional delineation of three pandemics? How do factors such as climate fit into the disease narrative?[24]

The study of medieval leprosy, or more properly Hansen's disease or *mycobacterial neurodermatosis*, has also changed direction rather significantly since the 1990s. Although it is one of the least contagious of the infectious diseases, it is the one disease throughout history (and still today) that has carried a disproportionately large social stigma or negative

22 For an overview of these divergent opinions, see J. Belich, *The World the Plague Made: The Black Death and the Spread of Europe* (Princeton, 2022); J. Bolton, '"The World Upside Down": Plague as an Agent of Economic and Social Change', in *The Black Death in England*, ed. W. M. Ormrod and P. G. Lindley (Stamford, 1996), pp. 17–78 and F. M. Getz, 'Black Death and the Silver Lining: Meaning, Continuity, and Revolutionary Change in Histories of Medieval Plague', *Journal of the History of Biology* 24 (1991), 265–89.

23 For excellent summaries of both the debates and the microbiological studies that have ended them, see M. H. Green, 'Taking "Pandemic" Seriously: Making the Black Death Global', *The Medieval Globe* 1 (2014), 27–62 and L. K. Little, 'Plague Historians in Lab Coats', *Past & Present* 213 (2011), 267–90. See also Hendrik Poinar's chapter 12 in this volume.

24 For a thorough assessment and summary of palaeogenetics studies of *Yersinia pestis* and their implications for a new understanding of the history and geography of plague, see M. H. Green, 'How a Microbe Becomes a Pandemic: A New Story of the Black Death', *The Lancet Microbe* 1 (2020), e311–12; M. H. Green, 'The Four Black Deaths', *American Historical Review* 125 (2020), 1601–31; M. H. Green and L. Jones, 'The Evolution and Spread of Major Human Diseases in the Indian Ocean World', in *Disease Dispersion and Impact in the Indian Ocean World*, ed. G. Campbell and E.-M. Knoll (London, 2020), pp. 25–57 and M. H. Green, 'Putting Africa on the Black Death Map: Narratives from Genetics and History', *Afriques* 9 (2018), http://journals.openedition.org/afriques/2125. On the role of climate, see M. H. Green, 'Climate and Disease in Medieval Eurasia', in *Oxford Research Encyclopedia of Asian History* (Oxford, 2018) and B. M. S. Campbell, *The Great Transition: Climate, Disease and Society in the Late-Medieval World* (Cambridge, 2016).

connotation. It is, in some ways, one of the most meaning-laden diseases that humans have experienced. Here too, the influence of Victorian-era historiography has loomed large: negative stories and stereotypes of lepers as the medieval living dead, isolated and shunned in out-of-the-way leprosaria, were resurrected by nineteenth-century historians who decided what medieval people thought about leprosy based on their own misreading of medieval sources and architecture – and their own treatment of lepers in far-flung colonies and in the heart of the United States.[25] Research now challenges long-standing assumptions about medieval lepers and leprosy, including but not limited to whether or not they were segregated, their social status, their theological link to sin, the role and location of leprosaria, community-level persecution, medical and religious treatments and so on.[26]

While plague and leprosy have dominated medieval and early modern studies of disease, scholarship on other diseases has also increased in recent years. Malaria, cancer, epilepsy, smallpox, typhus, syphilis, parasitic infections and a host of other conditions have all received attention, as have a variety of physical and intellectual disabilities.[27] Although plague and leprosy have cast a long shadow, then, they were never alone in challenging the health of people in the past. Indeed, medieval and early modern people's attempts to keep their living spaces, and especially their cities, clean and free from disease have generated an entire sub-field of scholarship focused on what Guy Geltner has aptly called premodern 'healthscaping'.[28]

25 Marcia Gaudet, *Carville: Remembering Leprosy in America* (Jackson MI, 2004).

26 For an overview of the old history of medieval leprosy and how it has been/is being challenged, see E. Brenner, 'Recent Perspectives on Leprosy in Medieval Western Europe', *History Compass* 8 (2010), 388–406. See also E. Brenner and F.-O. Touati, ed., *Leprosy and Identity in the Middle Ages: From England to the Mediterranean* (Manchester, 2021). For the paradigm shift, see for example F.-O. Touati, *Maladie et société au Moyen Âge: La lèpre, les lépreux et les léproseries dans la province ecclésiastique de Sens jusqu'au milieu du XIVe siècle* (Brussels, 1998); L. Demaitre, *Leprosy in Pre-Modern Medicine: A Malady of the Whole Body* (Baltimore, 2007); C. Rawcliffe, *Leprosy in Medieval England* (Woodbridge, 2006). For further discussion of the historical scholarship on leprosy, see chapter 11 in this volume.

27 Among many others, see R. F. Canalis and M. Ciavolella, ed., *Disease and Disability in Medieval and Early Modern Art and Literature* (Turnhout, 2021); J. Henderson, F. Jacobs, J. K. Nelson, ed., *Representing Infirmity: Diseased Bodies in Renaissance Italy* (London, 2020); A. Foscati, *Saint Anthony's Fire from Antiquity to the Eighteenth Century* (Amsterdam, 2019); E. Connelly and S. Künzel, ed., *New Approaches to Disease, Disability and Medicine in Medieval Europe* (Oxford, 2018); C. Scarborough, *Viewing Disability in Medieval Spanish Texts* (Amsterdam, 2018); N. Varlık, ed., *Plague and Contagion in the Islamic Mediterranean* (Kalamazoo, 2017); T. P. Newfield, 'Malaria and Malaria-Like Disease in the Early Middle Ages', *Early Medieval Europe* 25 (2017), 251–300; A. Skuse, *Constructions of Cancer in Early Modern England* (Basingstoke, 2015); P. Mitchell, ed., *Sanitation, Latrines and Intestinal Parasites in Past Populations* (Aldershot, 2015); S. Scalenghe, *Disability in the Ottoman Arab World, 1500–1800* (Cambridge, 2014); K. L. Richardson, *Difference and Disability in the Medieval Islamic World: Blighted Bodies* (Edinburgh, 2012).

28 G. Geltner, *Roads to Health: Infrastructure and Urban Wellbeing in Later Medieval Italy* (Philadelphia, 2019); C. Weeda and C. Rawcliffe, ed., *Policing the Urban Environment in Premodern*

Despite the historiographical tendency to treat disease and death as separate fields of study, in reality the two experiences were conceived as a continuum for medieval and early modern people: disease and death were often part of the same narrative, whether one struggled for survival, faced the inevitable end of days or tried to understand, explain and cope with the frailties of the human body and the diseases and infirmities that wracked it. Disentangling disease from death would have been unthinkable in many instances. Leprosy's invocation of the 'living dead' and plague's so-called 'Black Death' – despite being primarily modern images imposed on medieval disease experiences – perhaps offer the most tangible links between disease and death studies. But even when approached and considered separately, historical and historiographical links abound between death and disease in medieval and early modern history. Urban mortality record keeping built upon earlier parish records but was tied, in its earliest incarnations, to epidemic outbreaks of disease. Death registers and bills of mortality enabled premodern civil governments to monitor the progress of epidemics and facilitated burial management. Post-mortem investigations of causes of death during epidemics were informed by medical diagnostic expertise and quickly integrated with emerging record-keeping practices that contributed significantly to the development of modern epidemiology. Healing practices to manage disease were, at heart, efforts to forestall death.

The field of bioarchaeology, in particular, has illuminated our understanding of disease, death and mass mortality in premodern Europe and elsewhere. Sharon DeWitte's numerous studies of the skeletal remains of medieval plague victims from the East Smithfield plague cemetery in London (which also provided the first widely convincing aDNA evidence that the Black Death was indeed plague) have challenged some of the assumptions received from traditional documentary sources, indicating, for example, that the plague did not kill everyone indiscriminately but, rather, shows patterns of selectivity according to age, gender and health.[29] DeWitte has spearheaded efforts to bring together and

---

Europe (Amsterdam, 2019); I. Fay, *Health and the City: Disease, Environment and Government in Norwich, 1200–1575* (York, 2015); C. Rawcliffe, *Urban Bodies: Communal Health in Late Medieval English Towns and Cities* (Woodbridge, 2013); M. Bradley and Kenneth Stow, ed., *Rome, Pollution and Propriety: Dirt, Disease and Hygiene in the Eternal City from Antiquity to Modernity* (Cambridge, 2012). The term healthscaping comes from G. Geltner, 'Healthscaping a Medieval City: Lucca's *Curia viarum* and the Future of Public Health History', *Urban History* 40 (2013), 395–415. On healthy living more generally and public health (especially as related to plague), see among others S. Cavallo and T. Storey, ed., *Conserving Health in Early Modern Culture: Bodies and Environments in Italy and England* (Manchester, 2017); Z. B. Tomić and V. Blažina, *Expelling the Plague: The Health Office and the Implementation of Quarantine in Dubrovnik, 1377–1533* (Montreal, 2015); S. Cavallo and T. Storey, *Healthy Living in Late Renaissance Italy* (Oxford, 2013); K. W. Bowers, *Plague and Public Health in Early Modern Seville* (Rochester NY, 2013); and J. L. S. Crawshaw, *Plague Hospitals: Public Health for the City in Early Modern Venice* (Burlington, 2012).

29 S. N. DeWitte, 'Selectivity of Black Death Mortality with Respect to Preexisting Health', *PNAS* 105 (2008), 1436–41; S. N. DeWitte, 'The Effect of Sex on Risk of Mortality During the Black Death in London, A.D. 1349–1350', *American Journal of Physical Anthropology* 139 (2009), 222–34; S. N. DeWitte, 'Age Patterns of Mortality During the Black Death in London, A.D. 1349–1350', *Journal of Archaeological Science* 37 (2010), 3394–400.

compare data from physical anthropology and economic history in the search for new or modified conclusions about the extent and impact of plague, famine and other causes of medieval mass mortality.[30] In a similar fashion, Hendrik Poinar, in his contribution to this volume (Chapter 12), reviews a decade of research (2011–21) about the blending of new palaeogenetic evidence of *Y. pestis* with historical analyses of plague. He highlights both the potential advances and pitfalls that have come from combining genetic and historical interpretations of disease and death. While much of DeWitte's work in paleopathology is based on demographic disasters in London and southern England, other scholars like Stuart Borsch remind us of the value of comparative studies in the history of death and disease by demonstrating the significantly different socio-economic outcomes of the Black Death in England and Egypt.[31]

Taken broadly, recent scholarship highlights the fact that comparative, cross-cultural and cross-chronological perspectives have much to teach us about the ways in which death and disease were conceived and addressed in the past. The chapters in this volume offer further, and at times unique, evidence that we still have much to learn.

Volume structure and chapter outlines

The chapters in this volume take advantage of several multifaceted historiographical turns that now situate the study of death and disease at the cutting edge of historical research. From the integration of previously distinct historical, archaeological and scientific sources, to a second look being given to primary sources long thought to have nothing new to offer to the history of medicine, to forays into uncharted territories and across traditional periodisations and geographies, each chapter offers original research that reaches across conventional disciplinary, sub-disciplinary and historiographical boundaries. Together, the chapters highlight some of the critical changes that have subtly been taking place in the scholarship of death and disease in recent years. As they collectively demonstrate, new historiographical interventions, together with new scientific advances, are opening the fields of death and disease to global perspectives, to a growing recognition of multi-variant cultural narratives and to greater integration of scholarly disciplines.

The volume is organised into three interrelated parts. The first part explores the ways in which death and disease were diagnosed, explained and recorded. Here, the emphasis is on the written diagnostic performance, the act of making a diagnosis (broadly defined) and of explaining the cause of disease and/or of death. Nahyan Fancy opens the volume with a pioneering chapter on the diagnosis of plague in pre-Black Death Islamicate medical texts. Contrary to the West, where discussion of plague largely ceased following the end of the First Plague Pandemic (typically dated c. 541–750 CE) and did not appear

30 S. N. DeWitte and P. Slavin, 'Between Famine and Death: England on the Eve of the Black Death – Evidence from Paleoepidemiology and Manorial Accounts', *Journal of Interdisciplinary History* 44 (2013), 37–60; S. N. DeWitte and M. Kowaleski, 'Black Death Bodies', *Fragments* 6 (2017), 1–37.

31 S. J. Borsch, *The Black Death in Egypt and England: A Comparative Study* (Austin, 2005).

in the medical canon organised in the High Middle Ages, ongoing dialogue about the disease in Arabic medical commentaries and other works suggest that Islamicate societies in western Eurasia continued to experience plague outbreaks well into the tenth century. Furthermore, after the 1240s, significantly new and detailed descriptions of the diagnostic signs of the disease strongly suggest that already by this time some Islamic physicians working in Egypt, Syria, Iraq and Iran were encountering plague outbreaks first hand or learning about them second hand. Fancy argues that these thirteenth-century commentaries corroborate recent contentions – spurred by genomic evidence and his own as well as collaborative work on outbreaks in Baghdad – that the Second Plague Pandemic may have already been in motion in the thirteenth century, rather than commencing with the European Black Death (c. 1346–53) as plague historiography has long insisted. Coinciding with or even prompted by the expansion of the Mongol Empire, these earlier outbreaks of plague described in such detail by the Islamicate writers force us to reconsider yet again what we think we know about the history of plague and about Islamicate medicine. As Fancy concludes, 'discussions of plague in the Arabic medical tradition vastly supersede those found in the Byzantine or Latin traditions in terms of their sustained efforts across three centuries to understand the disease … this led to novel observations, a refined theoretical understanding of the disease and specific treatment recommendations' that were completely absent in the West.

Ann G. Carmichael's chapter 2 on post-mortem diagnosis in late medieval Milan takes the discussion of plague in a different direction: rather than simply recording deaths and noting which persons died of plague, Carmichael's Milanese physicians and surgeons were tasked with diagnosing all causes of death. Throughout Italy plague deaths set in motion a flurry of administrative responses, but the Health Office in Milan required verifying clinical details, which were sometimes quite expansive in their step-by-step elaboration of the process of diagnosis. Thus, the cases recorded in the civic death registers provide compelling evidence of contemporary medical and epidemiological observations that we do not find in more conventional medical treatises. More important, in Carmichael's view, is that these records resemble court records in their format and language, rather than mimic typical medical case notes. Given their emphasis on testimonial and physical evidence, judgement and verdict, she argues, we should view these historical sources through a medieval juridical rather than a medical lens. The dead testified, the Health Office physicians acted rather like witnesses and prosecutors while the ducal commissioner and Health Office deputies acted as judge and jury. In sum, using a series of post-mortem records, Carmichael demonstrates the unique forensic nature of Milan's death registry over the later fifteenth century and offers an insightful and useful comparison with London's better-known *Bills of Mortality*.

In chapter 3 Nicole Archambeau uses the final book of Giovanni Villani's fourteenth-century *New Chronicle* to explore a different kind of diagnosis: explanations of epidemic illness and mortality in Europe before the Black Death. For the Florentine writer Villani, who ultimately died of plague not long after its arrival in Italy, epidemic illness and death resulted from a complex interconnection between aristocratic sin, planetary movements and warfare – especially the mercenary warfare that was increasingly typical for late medieval kingdoms and city-states. Villani did not make explicit cause-and-effect links, but Archambeau's unpacking of the chronicler's account of Louis of Hungary's invasion of the kingdom of Naples in 1347 following the assassination of his brother Andrew, purportedly at the hands of the latter's wife, Queen Johanna, clearly showcases Villani's deft weaving of pestilence and mortality into his discussion of contemporary events. This, Archambeau argues, provides 'valuable insights into contemporary views of warfare, morality, deadly natural phenomena and humans' place in the observable world' on the eve of the Black Death. Further, it locates mercenary soldiers and misbehaving aristocrats at the forefront of communities of disease- and mortality-inducing environments. During the second wave of plague in the early 1360s, contemporaries like Guy de Chauliac more directly blamed the spread of disease on mercenary soldiers; yet, as Archambeau demonstrates, this idea was already forming before plague hit the Italian shores.

Nükhet Varlık's chapter 4 on the colours of death and disease in the early modern Ottoman context rounds out the volume's first part. Varlık opens her chapter with a reflection on the disproportionate effect that COVID-19 has had on black and brown bodies – a symptom not only of socio-economic inequalities but also of the long-standing tendency of Western medicine (which includes medieval Islamicate medicine) to favour white bodies for diagnostic, prognostic and therapeutic purposes. From there, she explores the intrinsic role that colour played in the premodern cultural imagination of death and disease, and of plague in particular. As she notes, 'cultural imagination was never necessarily limited to medical definitions … [which] mostly relied on visible symptoms of diseases … Beyond medical sources … we find a rich body of testimony reflecting different experiences … [wherein] the colours that define life also define disease and death.' In Varlık's telling, colours were reflected in emotions and symbolism, in cosmologies and ways of understanding the world, as well as in the material realities that made sense of them. Yet the colours of death and disease were not universal, not even in the Ottoman Empire, where Turkic and Islamic traditions brought with them different meanings for different colours. Building on her earlier exploration of why the Black Death is black, Varlık takes us into the polychromatic world of visual, sensory, emotional and diagnostic experiences of disease and death in the Ottoman world.

The volume's second part turns to how medieval and early modern populations coped with, prevented and healed disease. Drawing again on written historical records, however, this part is more concerned with performative actions and images beyond the written text. By focusing on the musical performance that accompanied the deathbed ritual of the Franciscan liturgy for end of life, Elaine Stratton Hild's chapter 5 provides a very different vantage point from which to understand such rituals. As Stratton Hild argues, '[r]ather than accessing the rituals through their words – their intellectual content – a focus on the music invites a closer consideration of the rituals' performative aspects and, by extension, of their participants.' Taking us step by step through the five-part ritual, her attention to the role played by music – including when, how and by whom it was sung – allows us to step to the bedside as active observers. To get us there, she skilfully utilises the thirteenth-century Italian manuscript Chicago, Newberry Library, Vault Manuscript 24, which contains some of the most detailed pitch-specific music notations of this ritual, reflecting the melodic pitch for many of the ritual's deathbed chants. Importantly, as Stratton Hild remarks, the music served more than a decorative or incidental purpose; rather, it shaped the performance of the liturgy by setting the pace of the material's delivery, drawing participants into a coordinated community and shaping specific interpretations of the texts that were being sung. In short, it introduced the element of beauty into unpredictable end-of-life experiences for both the dying and those who sought to assist the dying person's soul to move onward.

In chapter 6 Jennifer Edwards takes us into the world of medieval healing saints and the constant interplay between secular and spiritual healing that was necessary for a miracle to be recognised as such. The ill typically first sought care from a secular healer, whether that be a physician, surgeon, barber, herbalist, apothecary, midwife, monastic infirmarian, astrologer or so-called wise or cunning person. It was primarily only when secular healing had failed, only in the direst cases, that people turned to saints for miraculous healing. Indeed, as Edwards notes, 'it is only when the saint demonstrates better medical talent than a secular expert that her charity is considered holy'. This does not mean, however, that hagiographies downplayed or belittled secular medicine; on the contrary, Edwards demonstrates that even when the stories emphasise the failure of secular practices to cure a petitioner – and even when they claim secular medical expertise for the saints themselves – they nevertheless express 'great respect for [secular] medical workers, since it is only when the best possible secular care has failed that the saint's cure [can be] deemed remarkable'. In other words, the secular medical care previously received by the petitioner must have been of a high standard and the health practitioner of excellent repute for the saint's miraculous cure to be accepted. Edwards utilises the detailed descriptions of secular medical practices found in hagiographies (saints' lives) to discuss both their treatment of medical experts and the differential attention and roles accorded to males and females, whether secular healers or saintly ones.

Jenni Kuuliala's chapter 7 continues the theme of miraculous healing, but from the perspective of petitioners who were so ill or disabled that they sought death rather than to be cured (or death if they could not be cured). Drawing from canonisation inquests (the process and documents for officially recognising a person as a saint with the Roman Church) recorded between the thirteenth and fifteenth centuries in France and Italy, Kuuliala explores not only medieval notions of curability and incurability but also the types of conditions – medical and social – that caused the diseased and disabled to wish for death, and the narrative performance of those wishes as they played out during the inquests. As she demonstrates, canonisation inquests were highly structured: 'witnesses were not allowed to recite their memories freely, but were, rather, interrogated' by papal commissioners who typically followed a set script comprised of ready-made questions.

Their responses were recorded not necessarily verbatim but, again, through the lens of the inquest's formulaic requirements and language. The inquests were also sites of the performance of lived religion, wherein the participants acted out the appropriate emotions, sentiments and reactions that were important aspects of the veneration of saints. The death wishes themselves played an important role in the canonisation testimonies: the severity of the patient's condition, coupled with the futile attempts of secular medicine to heal them and the utter despair felt by the patient, helped to prove the miraculous nature of the saint's cure.

In chapter 8 Lori Jones turns our attention back to secular healing by addressing a unique set of therapeutic diagrams found in a small number of fifteenth- and sixteenth-century plague treatises that, in effect, repurposed generalised phlebotomy instructions and wound man imagery specifically for the treatment of plague. Phlebotomy played a large role in plague prevention and cure, and many treatises included detailed written instructions on which veins to bleed, when and for what duration. Yet diagrams of any kind are exceptionally rare in these texts, as are images of plague patients in other types of medical writings. For a disease that was typically diagnosed by visual notice of its most ubiquitous signs and symptoms, especially the bubo, and for which phlebotomy therapy was based on anatomical knowledge, this absence is somewhat surprising from a modern perspective in which disease and therapy is best imagined and even understood visually, rather than just textually. Yet these few illustrations, which have been identified thus far in German and English manuscripts as well as printed texts from Basel, Venice and Lyon, offer some insight into the performance of fifteenth-century plague therapy. Visual, didactic and closely attuned to their accompanying texts – at least in the earliest incarnations – such diagrams offer a novel representation of plague not for diagnostic or descriptive purposes but for active and practical treatment.

In chapter 9 Andrew Berns also examines the contents of a plague treatise, not for its images but instead for its 'traditional advice common in Galenic medicine [that] sits comfortably aside … a rich blend of kabbalistic doctrines, appeals to non-physical worlds and psalm recitations'. Abraham Yagel's *Moshi'ah Ḥosim*, a Hebrew plague treatise published in Venice in 1587, starkly challenges old historiographical assumptions of a clear dichotomy between medical and spiritual healing. For Yagel, medical and spiritual text could be one and the same. Throughout the treatise, he explores his belief in a triadic universe consisting of three interconnected realms: natural, astral and divine; the causes of plague could appear in any or all of these realms, as could the signs by which the disease is known and methods to prevent and cure it. While Christian and Muslim treatises of the era often also invoked active spiritual practice and performance to forestall or cure plague, what specifically sets Yagel's treatise apart is that he approaches his discussion of plague from the perspective of Hebrew literature and that he utilises the Torah as medicine. According to Yagel, reciting Psalm 38 aloud functioned to deter plague by strengthening one's immunity to infection. By interpreting, glossing and performing the psalm in this way, Yagel effectively medicalises a spiritual text and treats liturgy as prophylaxis.

Nichola Harris rounds out the second part in chapter 10, by drawing upon methodologies related to the history of ideas and the history of the book to explore the evolution of medieval and early modern lapidary treatments for paediatric and obstetric diseases. Utilising a variety of written and iconographic sources, she uses the practice of lapidary medicine as a lens through which to view both the evolution of medical theories, demonstrating a millennia-long continuity in Western pharmacology, and the ways in which ideas change as intellectual traditions merge and interact. Harris also challenges traditional categorisations applied to amuletic uses of mineral pharmaceuticals, arguing that ligatures and suspensions were simply one of many orthodox methodologies for employing the healing virtues found in natural objects. Focusing, in particular, on the use of red coral for the treatment of illnesses and ailments related to birth, infancy and early childhood, Harris takes us through the evolution of medical thinking from ancient pharmacopoeias to early modern popular advice manuals. Along the way, she points to significant textual innovations that brought about new interpretations of established uses for red coral that, in turn, led to a vast expansion of the healing properties ascribed to it. The study concludes with evidence demonstrating the wide availability of Mediterranean coral in seventeenth-century London apothecary shops and considerations of audience and authorship within the medical marketplace of early modern England.

The third and final part of the volume highlights the scientific study, analysis and interpretation of premodern diseases. Some material trappings of death and disease available to historical analysis exist on the scale of microbes, rather than on that of human culture. Harnessed in large parts by the efforts of Monica Green,[32] the new genetics paradigm has provided further opportunities for historians to envision global connections via patterns in the spread of infectious disease. This part of the volume thus examines the contributions that modern science, considered alongside contemporary primary sources, brings to a new understanding of death and disease in the medieval and early modern eras. In chapter 11 Fabian Crespo explores the relationship and interactions between leprosy and other diseases. In a truly interdisciplinary study, Crespo incorporates biological, archaeological and historical evidence to determine how, or whether, medieval Europeans developed some measure of immunity to leprosy by means of co-infection with the disease of tuberculosis, caused by a related species of *Mycobacterium*. Inspired by Ann Carmichael's revolutionary study of the interrelationship between plague and other contemporary, infectious diseases in early modern Florence,[33] Crespo applies a similar 'syndemic approach' to medieval disease in which he studies the bio-social implications of leprosy and tuberculosis within a single population. Crespo's tentative conclusions, defined primarily by the field of immunology, should nonetheless shape any future historical and cultural interpretations of the rise and apparent disappearance of leprosy and other diseases in later medieval Europe.

[32] See, for example, Green, 'Putting Africa on the Black Death Map'; Green, 'How a Microbe Becomes a Pandemic'; Green, 'The Four Black Deaths'; and Green and Jones, 'The Evolution and Spread of Major Human Diseases'.

[33] A. G. Carmichael, *Plague and the Poor in Renaissance Florence* (Cambridge, 1986).

In chapter 12 Hendrik Poinar's elucidation of the evolution and current state of palaeogenetic research, the opportunities that it offers to the historical study of past disease and death – and the challenges faced when interpreting aDNA evidence – closes out the volume. As Poinar argues, '[i]n much the same way that a single historical document or object can offer only a snapshot of a particular moment or place in time and cannot nor should not readily be extrapolated, an aDNA sequence without proper context derived from additional historical, biochemical, archaeological and other evidence likewise remains anecdotal.' In today's world, technological and scientific advances appear with dizzying regularity and offer new information about premodern diseases and mortality. The resulting reinterpretations of the past can highlight inconsistencies in existing data or historical narratives, conclude long-standing debates or verify long-held assumptions. In this light, Poinar's chapter serves simultaneously as a follow-up to Lester Little's 2011 review article about the microbiological discovery of *Y. pestis*,[34] as an exciting springboard to what is possible in future studies of death and disease in the past and as a cautionary tale of how science can be misused when its limitations are not adequately recognised.

Cross-cutting themes

While the volume is organised as noted above, several critical themes also cut across the chapters in different parts of the book, tying them together in multiple ways. Sister Eufemia's death from plague takes us into the heart of a gendered space – the nuns' convent – and thus witnesses an oft-repeated anthropological observation: that it is women and other feminised agents of health who provided the day-to-day physical and spiritual caregiving for the sick and dying. While a male physician may have attended to Eufemia, and a male confessor likely provided her with the viaticum, it was her sisters who accompanied her at the bedside for the complete duration of her illness. Historians of the long Middle Ages have worked to include such feminised bedside forms of care, including the maintenance of the six non-naturals, and the provision of other kinds of healthcare by women on the broader map of health and healing practices. In doing so, they have recentred histories of premodern health and healing by calling attention to the critical role of the daily maintenance of the non-natural environment, a burden that most often fell on women. The presence of women as caregivers extended beyond their roles in maintaining healthy daily regimens, however; it also included providing regulatory and palliative forms of sick care and caring for the dead. It was women, and very often semi-religious women such as beguines, who prepared corpses for burial, watched over them during the night while chanting the psalms and escorting them to burial. Women also played a greater role in the broader provision of healthcare than has long been assumed.[35]

34 Little, 'Plague Historians in Lab Coats'.

35 Among many others, see S. Ritchey, *Acts of Care: Recovering Women in Late Medieval Health* (New York, 2021); M. E. Boyle and S. E. Owens, ed., *Health and Healing in the Early Modern Iberian World: A Gendered Perspective* (Toronto, 2021); S. Ritchey and S. Strocchia, ed., *Gender,*

Analysis of gender in relation to disease and death threads through several of the chapters in this volume. Edwards's (chapter 6) discussion of healing saints and their miraculous cures shows us that not all such saints were created equally. Instead, there is a significant gender difference in how male and female saints were represented in terms of their abilities and their relationship with secular healing, especially in the popular thirteenth-century *Golden Legend* written by Jacobus de Voragine. While hagiographers obviously celebrated female saints' thaumaturgic healing power, they largely focused on the more mundane healing interventions – bathing, feeding, bandaging wounds or broken limbs, applying ointment – that these women offered as charity to the sick and the poor. Where female saints are described as having demonstrated a miraculous healing, even a resurrection, their efforts tend not to have been discussed in terms of what a secular healer might have done. Their male counterparts, however, purportedly offered healing that was patently superior to the medical abilities of secular healers; indeed, they often acted as physicians themselves or intervened early enough to allow the patient to avoid unnecessary, and often painful, secular treatment. As Edwards observes, this discrepancy can be linked to 'institutionalising trends that, by the thirteenth century, placed greater emphasis on the university training that limited and marginalised women's roles in the professional medical fields' as well, perhaps, to the fact that the number of male saints vastly outnumbered their female counterparts. It might also explain why, among those saints credited with working healing miracles, many holy women seem to have been able to perform such miracles only after their own deaths.

In Harris's chapter 10, gender appears not in the guise of a healer but, rather, as the target of healing therapies. Because of its ancient sympathetic connection with blood and bleeding, the medical uses of red coral became increasingly gendered in medieval and early modern pharmacology. Long associated with bleeding and the protection of children within the Hippocratic and Galenic traditions, Salernitan and mendicant texts merged and expanded these properties in the twelfth and thirteenth centuries to identify coral as a

---

Health, and Healing, 1250–1550 (Amsterdam, 2020); L. Astbury and E. Leong, 'Medical Knowledge and Practice', in *The Routledge History of Women in Early Modern Europe*, ed. A. L. Capern (Abingdon, 2019), pp. 181–98; S. T. Strocchia, *Forgotten Healers: Women and the Pursuit of Health in Late Renaissance Italy* (Cambridge MA, 2019); C. Caballero-Navas, 'Virtuous and Wise: Apprehending Female Medical Practice from Hebrew Texts on Women's Healthcare', *Social History of Medicine* 32 (2019), 691–711; E. Leong, *Recipes and Everyday Knowledge* (Chicago, 2018); C. Sautter, 'Women, Dance, Death, and Lament in Medieval Spain and the Mediterranean: Jewish, Christian, and Muslim Examples', in *Death in Medieval Europe*, ed. Rollo-Koster, pp. 107–27; S. Ritchey, 'Affective Medicine: Later Medieval Healing Communities and the Feminization of Health Care Practices in the Thirteenth-Century Low Countries', *Journal of Medieval Religious Cultures* 40 (2014), 113–43; M. Shefer-Mossensohn, 'A Sick Sultana in the Ottoman Imperial Palace: Male Doctors, Female Healers and Female Patients in the Early Modern Period', *Hawwa* 9 (2011), 281–312; M. H. Green, 'Gendering the History of Women's Healthcare', *Gender & History* 20 (2008), 487–518; M. Cabré, 'Women or Healers? Household Practices and the Categories of Health Care in Late Medieval Iberia', *Bulletin of the History of Medicine* 82 (2008), 18–51.

multipurpose therapeutic that would work to not only staunch postpartum and menstrual bleeding but also prevent complications for the labouring mother and child. The obstetric and gynaecological use of red coral continued to evolve in the early modern era, becoming widely endorsed by midwives and in printed manuals of popular healing for the prevention of miscarriage, hysteria, puerperal eclampsic convulsions and menstrual bleeding. During this period, the use of red coral also extended to remedying barrenness in women and the treatment of various types of venereal disease – again primarily in women. With the exception of a few texts purportedly authored by women, the pharmaceutical history of coral, however, was written by male physicians, friars, herbalists, apothecaries and lapidaries.

In chapter 3 Archambeau notes that, for Giovanni Villani, the most common cause of pestilence and mortality was warfare. The last book of his *New Chronicle* recounts the mercenary warfare that wrought devastation on Italy in the years and months leading up to the Black Death. Unlike previous episodes, however, this was mercenary warfare that had a specifically gendered origin, pointing to later medieval expectations of wives in the context of disease and death: the betrayal and murder of Andrew of Hungary by his wife, Queen Johanna of Naples, and her subsequent marriage to his rival. For Villani, Johanna's lack of grief over her husband's death validated rumours that she had played a role in – and possibly even instigated – the assassination. Johanna's immoral acts and egregious sins turned many of her lords against her and the pope had cartloads of her supporters killed. While various members of the wider Angevin royal family were accused of complicity, it is Johanna – the queen – who receives the bulk of Villani's scorn and whose behaviour he most vehemently excoriates.

Sister Eufemia's story also enables us to explore the role of emotions as they pertain to disease and death. Although we have no records to tell us about how Eufemia experienced her rapid decline or how her sisters at Santa Maria Maddalena dealt with the emotional blow of her illness and passing, the burgeoning field of the history of emotions offers us a window into their long-ago world. Of course, the melancholic temperament, influenced by the dominance of black bile within an individual, was an integral aspect of the humoral system. Melancholy itself, caused by an excess of black bile, was a 'diagnosable' condition with particular mental and physical symptoms. Nichola Harris, in particular, highlights in her chapter 10 the use of coral in treating conditions stemming from excess black bile.

Emotions, or passions, have long been recognised as one of the Galenic non-naturals whose balance was a necessary component of health, and many regimens of health provided advice on how to create and maintain a positive state of mind. Fear of plague was considered to be such a risk factor of infection that numerous plague tracts included a discussion of the topic. Fear of the deliberate spread of plague poison led to violent reprisals against suspected perpetrators. More than that, though, recent research is demonstrating the central role that emotions played in everyday life, health and death in the long Middle

Ages, how they were understood and the many ways in which they were expressed and managed.[36]

The history of emotions is evident in the chapters by Stratton Hild, Kuuliala, Varlık, Carmichael and Berns. For Stratton Hild in chapter 5, liturgical ritual acts as a way to manage emotions associated with dying and death. Focusing on the music of the deathbed liturgy rather than on its words 'invites a closer consideration of the rituals' performative aspects and, by extension, the rituals' participants ... Far from being an incidental component, or a neutral mechanism for conveying texts, music shaped the liturgy' and embodied the emotional act of mourning and sending the deceased person's soul into the next world. Deathbed rituals were by their very nature emotional: for the dying persons themselves, for their mourning families and friends and for those brought in to conduct the last rites and to assist 'the final agony (when the "soul is struggling to exit")'. Performing the sung litany engaged all those gathered at the bedside together in a responsorial fashion, enabling them to channel their emotions to a singular purpose and to be drawn into the 'detailed, vibrant images of the soul's successful passage' that the prayers invoked. The dying person's and his/her family's anxieties about death were likewise incorporated into the ritual, eased by the melodic performance of Psalms 117 and 118 and by the aural images of the soul's safe passage that these melodies roused. As Stratton Hild notes, 'The deliberate, disciplined use of time might well have added an element of calm and reassurance for both the attending community and the dying person. At the moment of highest anxiety, the ritual prescribes texts depicting a loving, powerful God, conveyed with beautiful sound'.

In Kuuliala's case (chapter 7), unpacking expressions of grief and desperation at the core of the death wishes recorded in canonisation inquests likewise recasts them as part of an emotional ritual and devotional practice. Testimony related to the damaging emotional impact of severe illness or disability, to the anxious hope for a cure and to the outpouring of joy and gratitude at its deliverance lay at the very heart of miracle narratives. By their nature, Kuuliala argues, 'miracle narratives are therefore emotional scripts'. Yet, while emotions generally take centre stage in these narratives, Kuuliala digs deeper into the questions of whose emotions were important, which emotions were appropriate and how and by whom these emotions were recorded to reveal the ways in which juridical and theological requirements guided the entire emotional process for all involved. These scripts served not only to 'make' the miracle, but, by being made publicly available in collections of miracles and saints' lives, they also 'guided people in their emotional practices and in the ways they later reported their [own miraculous] experiences'.

[36] Among others, see B. H. Rosenwein and R. Cristiani, *What is the History of Emotions?* (Cambridge, 2018); N. Cohen-Hanegbi, *Caring for the Living Soul: Emotions, Medicine and Penance in the Late Medieval Mediterranean* (Leiden, 2017); S. Broomhall, ed., *Early Modern Emotions: An Introduction* (Abingdon, 2016); D. Boquet and P. Nagy, *Sensible Moyen Âge: Une histoire des émotions dans l'Occident médiéval* (Paris, 2015); J. Plamper, *The History of Emotions: An Introduction* (Oxford, 2015); R. F. McNamara and U. McIlvenna, 'Medieval and Early Modern Emotional Responses to Death and Dying', *Parergon* 31 (2014), 1–10; E. Carrera, *Emotions and Health, 1200–1700* (Leiden, 2013).

Varlık's chapter 4 takes us into the cultural imagination of colour in the long Middle Ages and the emotional responses that different colours elicited. From social standing to medical diagnosis and prognosis, colours 'were invoked and recorded to *colour* imagination. They allowed those experiencing disease and death to engage in their own kind of personal and cultural diagnosis'. From the bright colours typically associated with life, to the dark colours typically associated with death, each colour evoked a culturally specific and symbolic emotional response: joy, love and hope; fear, dread and anguish. As Varlık points out, even the nineteenth-century Gothic imaginary of plague, which brought us the now ubiquitous term 'Black Death', was predicated on an emotional view of the Middle Ages as dark, dangerous and deadly. Yet we cannot assume that emotional landscapes of colour were (or are) universal: each culture had its own colour correspondences, and in multicultural societies like the Ottoman Empire the same colour could elicit different emotional responses depending on the context.

While Carmichael's chapter 2 may less obviously evoke the history of emotions, here too we can see emotions in play. The dispassionate nature of the often-cursory records of cause of death belied both household anxieties about the implications of a plague diagnosis and the physicians' struggles and sense of burden to make the 'right' diagnosis. Treating patients experiencing significant pain or who were 'restless and in terror of death' could never have been an easy mental exercise, nor could have exposing oneself to the corruption of plague. 'Existential fear' during recurrent outbreaks was real, even among the recording physicians and surgeons who did not openly express their feelings about what they witnessed. Yet hints remain: their notations about the family and neighbours' fear, their remarks about patients being in terror of death and their defensive comments about their own diligence and carefulness in making a judgement. Even when not articulated explicitly, emotions underscored Milan's *Books of the Dead.*

So too do emotions permeate Abraham Yagel's plague treatise, as Berns's chapter 9 notes. Yagel likely wrote his work in the wake of a deadly outbreak in Venice in 1575–77 that may have taken the lives of up to a third of the city's population. Death – and the dying – was everywhere, and few would have been spared the sights, smells or sounds of plague. In a medical tract published just one year before Yagel's, a physician had recommended 'exercising the mind by singing psalms and listening to theological stories [because these] would delight and invigorate the soul and spirits, which in turn would help the body to better resist infirmity'. For Yagel, the recitation of scripture also had salubrious effects and his exegesis of Psalm 38 provides emotional elaborations on the meaning of simple phrases: 'I groan' becomes the 'moaning of my heart' due to the 'agony of my sickness', a fluttering heart means being surrounded by grief and overcome with weakness. Yagel's investing of the sacred text with contemporary meaning and his imbuing of it with medical significance was more than just an intellectual exercise; it was an emotional one that was meant to heal both bodies and minds.

Recent forays into material culture and the archaeology of death and disease have emphasised how material objects mediate memories of the dead and give cultural meaning to death and disease through materialisations.[37] Artefacts like monuments, clothes and photographs influence memory because they are relational constructs produced through a mutual constitution of material objects and human beings. During the long Middle Ages, only the elite enjoyed the privilege of leaving behind some material presence by which to be remembered after they died. While monuments, works of art and artefacts were limited to a very small minority, the majority of the population would have left, at best, a grave with a tombstone. Eufemia's grave likely had a tombstone, bearing her name and the singular identifier of her order – Humiliati. Even though her death was one suspected of plague, she may still have been buried in the monastery's graveyard, in a somewhat orderly fashion. Within weeks, plague would have spread to the city, taking hundreds of lives every day. In such extraordinary circumstances of extremely high mortality, other people's bodies were buried irregularly, sometimes multiple bodies buried in one grave, other times, though very rarely, thrown into large pits. In retrospect, Eufemia was fortunate to have escaped that dreaded fate of sheer erasure from collective memory.

In effect, most cultures of the long global Middle Ages maintained rituals to ensure the remembrance of the dead. The materiality of funerary cultures and practices reflects the social conventions that both united and separated the world of the living from that of the dead, preserving firm boundaries and yet leaving them porous to allow only regulated types of interaction to assuage the spiritual and emotional needs of the living. As Karen Gerhart has observed in medieval Japanese death rituals, the material trappings of death memorialisation are designed for the community of the living. The funeral choreography of colour, smell, sound and sight served to separate the living from the dead, containing and enclosing dead bodies even while designing them in ways that facilitate communication with the deceased or to improve the situation of the deceased in the afterlife.[38] If it were not for the suspicion of plague, Eufemia's body would have received a proper funeral in which her body would have been carefully prepared for burial. And even though it would have had to be a quick burial, it is not entirely implausible that the sisters washed her body despite the fear of contagion. They must have faced a dilemma about whether to wash Eufemia's body or not. This decision may even have created a little drama in the monastery. Did the sisters wash Eufemia's body anyway because they saw no buboes, which would be the only definite sign of plague for them, even though the city doctors hedged their bets and called it plague without that sign? Or did they give in to the fear of corpse contagion? We may never know. What we do know is that sometimes religious devotion overrode health concerns, as was documented to be the case in some Muslim records of this period. Washing the body of the deceased, even of those suspected of or showing clear signs of plague, was common in the Ottoman Empire.[39]

37 E. Hallam and J. Hockey, *Death, Memory, and Material Culture* (Abingdon, 2020).

38 K. Gerhart, *The Material Culture of Death in Medieval Japan* (Honolulu, 2009).

39 As discussed in Varlık, *Plague and Empire*, pp. 264–71.

Chapters in the volume engage with the materiality of death and disease in unique ways. Some chapters examine the materiality of texts, by carefully tracing their provenance and circulation or their reception and impact. For example, Stratton Hild's chapter 5 traces the life story of the Newberry MS 24, as it examines the manuscript and its many lives. In doing so, the chapter goes beyond the materiality of the manuscript as a text; it engages with the materiality of the music that accompanied deathbed rituals of the Franciscan liturgy for the end of life. In other words, the chapter uses the materiality of the music to connect us to a deathbed scene in the thirteenth century. Fancy's detective work in tracing references to plague in late medieval Islamic medical commentaries offers another way of engaging with the materiality of texts. His chapter 1 presents a very close reading of Arabic medical texts of the thirteenth century to find traces of plague, a disease that was long believed to be absent at that time. Careful reading of the sources, however, suggests otherwise; the chapter demonstrates the presence of the disease through its traces in the text and hence presents a very strong case that texts can offer a lens to the materiality of history with what they reveal or what they hide.

Other chapters in the volume tackle the materiality of disease and death in a different way. Carmichael's chapter 2 offers a very close reading of sources to detect disease and death as experienced by their past actors. To that end, it goes to great lengths to find where plague buboes were located on a victim's body and hence demonstrates that a careful examination of the sources can reveal even the most intimate individual experiences. Other chapters in the volume go altogether beyond texts and dig deeper into the materialities of disease and death through novel ways. In chapter 8 Jones's work on the diagrams that accompany plague tracts shows us that visual instruction and learning extended far beyond the text: pictures, perhaps, offered greater clarity. Poinar's chapter 12 takes us as close as possible to the bones and cells of plague victims that carry the traces of ancient pathogens' signatures. Exploring the story of the bones and genomes of past victims of infectious diseases affords us a better knowledge of their experiences of disease and death – a spectacular opportunity for historians to incorporate into their toolkits. Similarly, Harris's chapter 10 traces the long healing history of coral in its materiality, allowing us to connect to the disease experience of women and children in the past and their hopes for healing. Tracing red coral across time and space reveals its pervasive presence, over millennia, in the lives of women who searched for relief during labour, as well as for infants and children.

As different chapters in the volume find creative ways to deal with the materiality of texts, music, stories, architecture, art, artefacts, bones, genomes and gemstones, they enrich the study of past disease and death. They each do this, not only with the acumen of exemplary scholarship, but also with the historical sensibilities to connect to past lives through shared universal experiences of disease and death.

Eufemia's life was spent straddling worlds and crossing boundaries. She was in regular contact with the world of the poor and the needy, while also living a secluded life. She straddled the religious and secular spheres of urban life, at least in her visits to give alms but also possibly while seeking treatment. Certainly she did when her body came into contact (even post-mortem) with secular health authorities. She likely never imagined that her dead, and perhaps naked, body would be inspected by men that she did not know. By centring cultural and biological approaches to death and disease, the chapters in this volume also reveal continuities and contact across multiple cultures, languages and faith traditions in the long Middle Ages. An increasing attention among scholars to disease environments has slowly shifted the geographic imaginary from regions of seeming cultural isolation to broad zones of contact and exchange across the Mediterranean and into the Indian Ocean. Travellers along these commercial circuits carried with them health knowledge and practices, along with concrete forms of 'materia medica' (medical material) and, quite often, pathogenic microbes.[40] Knowledge and experience of disease and death then spread beyond these zones of contact through book exchange that was further accelerated with the processes of print and vernacularisation.[41]

Zones of contact and exchange in various guises – and sometimes the lack thereof – appear in the chapters by Fancy, Jones, Harris, Varlık, Crespo and Poinar. In chapter 1 Fancy traces the textual conventions of writing about the clinical aspects of plague across Byzantine Greek, Syriac and Arabic traditions, including descriptions found in chronicles, medical commentaries and other works. In doing so, he carefully dissects both the continuities that run through them – highlighting where information has been passed on or gleaned through shared knowledge practices – and the singularly unique interpolations that suggest first-hand knowledge of plague after the 1240s. Remarkable in all of this is

40 Campbell and Knoll, ed., *Disease Dispersion*; M. Marsden, *Beyond the Silk Roads* (Cambridge, 2021), especially pp. 77–81; R. Yoeli-Tlalim, *ReOrienting Histories of Medicine: Encounters along the Silk Roads* (London, 2021); E. Lambourn, *Abraham's Luggage: A Social Life of Things in the Medieval Indian Ocean World* (Cambridge, 2018), especially pp. 219–39; Campbell, *Great Transition*; N. Varlık, *Plague and Empire in the Early Modern Mediterranean World* (Cambridge, 2015); I. McCleery, 'From the Edge of Europe to Global Empire: Portuguese Medicine Abroad (Thirteenth to Sixteenth Centuries)', in *Travels and Mobilities in the Middle Ages: From the Atlantic to the Black Sea*, ed. M. O'Doherty and F. Schmieder (Turnhout, 2015), pp. 55–90; M. Abattouy, 'The Arabic–Latin Intercultural Transmission of Scientific Knowledge in Pre-Modern Europe: Historical Context and Case Studies', in *The Role of the Arab-Islamic World in the Rise of the West* (London, 2012), pp. 167–219. Relevant here, too, is the large literature on the so-called 'Columbian Exchange', the movement of flora, fauna and microbes between Africa, Europe and the Americas during European exploration and colonialism and the transatlantic slave trade.

41 On the spread of knowledge and practice related to death and disease through books, see also O. Merisalo, M. Kuha and S. Niiranen, ed., *Transmission of Knowledge in the Late Middle Ages and the Renaissance* (Turnhout, 2019), especially the four chapters on medical knowledge; E. Leong and A. Rankin, 'Introduction: Secrets and Knowledge', in *Secrets and Knowledge in Medicine and Science, 1500–1800*, ed. E. Leong and A. Rankin (Aldershot, 2011), pp. 1–20; F. Günergun and D. Raina, ed., *Science Between Europe and Asia: Historical Studies on the Transmission, Adoption and Adaptation of Knowledge* (London, 2010), especially the four chapters on medicine and medical practices; M. Nicoud, *Les régimes de santé: naissance et diffusion d'une écriture médicale, XIIIe–XVe siècle* (Rome, 2007). For the mobility of books and the ideas contained within them more generally, see also S. Shep, 'Books in Global Perspectives', in *The Cambridge Companion to the History of the Book*, ed. L. Howsam (Cambridge, 2015), pp. 53–70.

that although medieval Islamicate and Latin European medical knowledge and practice was predicated on the same corpus, and although the European tradition owed much to the translation of Arabic texts, the sustained discussion of plague that Fancy traces in the Arabic texts is entirely absent in the Latin tradition.

In chapter 10 Harris's work on the use of coral for paediatric and childbirth-related diseases and conditions likewise shows both the transmission of medical knowledge across the centuries and the creation and integration of new knowledge as cultures came into contact with each other. Perhaps the most obvious example of this is the medieval reinterpretation of classical lapidary medicine through a Christian lens and the subsequent blending of this perspective with the ideas found in Byzantine and Arabic texts. The later emergence and dissemination of the new theories and techniques of chemical medicine advocated by Paracelsus and his followers then further expanded again the paediatric applications of coral that carried forward into the early modern era.

Jones's chapter 8, by contrast, shows the emergence of strikingly similar anatomical diagrams in fifteenth-century plague texts produced in southern Germany and northern England, with no known connection between the illustrators and/or scribes in the two locations. Even the plague treatises to which the respective diagrams are attached are different: the earlier German diagram followed a plague treatise by Jakob Engelins von Ulm, an early fifteenth-century physician or surgeon at the Viennese Habsburg court of Duke Albrecht IV of Austria, while the slightly later English diagram was embedded in a versified version of the treatise attributed to John of Burgundy, a mid-fourteenth-century physician from Liège. In this case, although any specific zones of contact and exchange remain to be identified, the small number of surviving diagrams of a similar nature, and their complete absence from other cultures and geographies before the age of print, point to the likelihood that such zones did exist in this case.

Varlık's discussion in chapter 4 of the colours of disease and death emphasises that fact that the symbolic meaning of colours is not universal. Each of the major ancient medical cultures had its own 'systematic body of correspondences, in which colours were thought to correspond to certain key properties for health' – but which colour aligned with which element or which temperament, and thus with what health status, differed across them. In a multicultural society like the early modern Ottoman Empire that emerged from more than one distinct lineage – in this case Turkic and Islamic – the same colours could also serve distinctly different purposes, depending on the context. As Varlık notes, 'Ottoman colour cosmologies represent a hybridity of influences' that, in turn, reflect 'overlaps, interactions and exchanges' that played out in how colour words were used, or not, to describe diseases.

For its part, Crespo's chapter 11 on syndemics – including possible 'cross immunity between the biologically related pathogens responsible for leprosy and tuberculosis' – provides an important perspective on zones of contact not only at the societal level or at the microbiological level, but at the bio-social level. As Crespo explains, 'an individual's capacity to mount a proper immunological response against leprosy' inherently brought together all of the environmental and social factors that influenced his or her life. It was not just (unfortunately) coming into sustained contact with the leprosy bacillus that mattered; just as important were living conditions, diet and, perhaps surprisingly, local social attitudes towards leprosy. These multivariate factors were heterogeneous across the long Middle Ages – and indeed across the geographies covered by the volume – and, as a result, so too was the prevalence and persistence of Hansen's disease.

In chapter 12, in exploring the opportunities and challenges offered to the study of disease and death by palaeogenetics research on aDNA, Poinar offers us a window into a different kind of contact zone: multidisciplinary collaborations that cross what have traditionally been completely separate disciplinary fields. As Poinar rightly notes, scientists have long drawn from historical studies to contextualise their findings, and humanist scholars have increasingly been drawn to rapidly evolving microbiological findings. Yet, without a clear understanding of what can – and more importantly cannot – be known or understood from either discipline, without a proper awareness of the all-important context, simply utilising findings without a clear comprehension of what they mean can easily lead one astray.

Finally, the diversity of experiences regarding disease and death, as universal as they may have been, still requires paying special attention to the inequalities (resulting from differences in class, race, gender, age, etc.) that persisted across time and space. People of different socio-economic levels did not have the same living standards and life expectations and, as such, lived and died differently. As much as deadly pandemics of the past like the Black Death are often regarded as the 'Great Equalizer', historical scholarship suggests otherwise. The chapters in this volume take stock of these inequalities at many levels. They collectively remind us that our historical actors were not equal in the face of disease and death. As we read in some chapters, these differences sometimes resulted from differences in class (e.g., Archambeau's chapter 3 reveals the stark contrast between the living standards of the aristocratic elite and the mercenary soldiers in late medieval Italy), gender (e.g., Harris's chapter 10 puts the perils of childbirth under spotlight), race (e.g., Varlık's chapter 4 reflects on the implications of disease diagnosis by coloured markers on white skin) and age (e.g., Carmichael's chapter 2 draws attention to disease and death among children in the Milanese registers).

Other chapters take a historiographical stand to intervene in past injustices. They address the inequalities that result from the differences in the availability of, or access to, sources as they try to restore the epistemic inequity where it is due. Chapters in this volume help to make some of the voices of the past more accessible (e.g., Kuuliala's chapter 7 helps us to hear the death wishes of those nearing death; Edwards's chapter 6 highlights the experiences of those who were in search of a cure; Crespo's chapter 11 underscores the experiences of stigmatised 'lepers'). Some chapters bring to light sources that have received little attention (e.g., Berns's chapter 9 on Abraham Yagel's little-known plague treatise) or offer a fresh reading of them (e.g., Archambeau's reading of Giovanni Villani's chronicle in chapter 3). Other chapters enrich the written sources by underlining the value of music, visualisation and colour (e.g., Stratton Hild's, Jones's and Varlık's chapters 5, 8 and 4, respectively) that accompany them. When written sources are not available, it is possible to close the gap in knowledge by using genomic materials (e.g., Poinar's chapter 12).

In our quest to explore experiences of death and disease in the long Middle Ages, nothing drives the point home better than stories like Eufemia's. Her story matters: as we follow it, we see the ills of long-ago societies through the lens of her sick and then dead body. A voice long lost to us, Eufemia guides us to future research – meanwhile gently reminding us that along with the joys of scholarship, the study of disease and death also comes with its own baggage of human suffering and pain.

PART I

Diagnosing, Explaining and Recording

1

Knowing the Signs of Disease: Plague in the Arabic Medical Commentaries between the First and Second Pandemics

NAHYAN FANCY[1]

Introduction

The new religion of Islam emerged during the course of the First Plague Pandemic. Also referred to as the Justinianic Plague after the Byzantine Emperor Justinian (r. 527–65), in whose reign the plague pandemic is traditionally assumed to have begun (541), the origins of this significant disease episode are being studied anew.[2] Historians, chief amongst them Lawrence Conrad, have examined the impact of this first pandemic on the burgeoning Islamic polity in Western Asia and North Africa, as well as on Islamic religious thought over the subsequent centuries.[3] Although plague was discussed often in literary works throughout the Abbasid period (750–1258), scholars have generally

1 I would like to thank Jasmeet Kaur, Lori Jones, Emilie Savage-Smith, Justin Stearns and Nükhet Varlık for their helpful comments and suggestions, including recommendations for further reading. This chapter would not have been possible at all without Monica Green's published works and our conversations about the implications of new phylogenetics and bioarchaeology work for historians; she also generously read and commented upon multiple drafts of this paper.

2 Recent phylogenetic work on *Yersinia pestis* (the bacterium that causes plague) suggests that the First Pandemic may have begun in Central Asia three centuries earlier; see M. Keller et al., 'Ancient *Yersinia pestis* Genomes from Across Western Europe Reveal Early Diversification during the First Pandemic (541–750)', *PNAS* 116 (2019), 12363–72. The study's implications for historians are laid out in M. H. Green, 'When Numbers Don't Count: Changing Perspectives on the Justinianic Plague', *Eidolon* 18 November 2019, https://eidolon.pub/when-numbers-dont-count-56a2b3c3d07, last accessed 9 June 2020.

3 See L. I. Conrad, 'The Plague in the Early Medieval Near East' (unpublished Ph.D. dissertation, Princeton University, 1981); L. I. Conrad, '*Ṭāʿūn* and *Wabāʾ*: Conceptions of Plague and Pestilence in Early Islam', *Journal of the Economic and Social History of the Orient* 25 (1982), 268–307; L. I. Conrad, ''Umar at Sargh: The Evolution of an Umayyad Tradition on Flight from the Plague', in *Story-Telling in the Framework of Non-Fictional Arabic Literature*, ed. S. Leder (Wiesbaden, 1998), pp. 488–528; and J. van Ess, *Der Fehltritt des Gelehrten: Die 'Pest von Emmaus' und ihre theologischen Nachspiele* (Heidelberg, 2001).

concurred with Conrad's judgement that the end of the First Pandemic coincided with the Abbasid dynasty's rise in 750.[4]

Historians also have generally believed that the Second Pandemic, whose first wave is known as the Black Death, began in the 1330s in Central Asia, arrived in Eastern Mediterranean societies in the late 1340s and lasted until the eighteenth century in Western Europe (and the nineteenth century in Islamic Mediterranean societies).[5] However, as Monica Green has argued, recent genomic studies of the plague bacillus *Yersinia pestis* using archaeological DNA samples (primarily from Europe, but also Kyrgyzstan and Russia) have allowed historians to revisit historical literary sources and to expand both the geography and chronology of past plague pandemics.[6]

This chapter builds upon Green's invitation to revisit our historical sources in light of the new genomic evidence, much as Ann Carmichael and Robert Hymes have done for Italian and Chinese sources, respectively.[7] I focus here on Arabic medical works from the ninth to the thirteenth centuries, particularly the medical commentary corpus. Sustained, at times detailed, discussions of plague in the commentaries and other medical works suggest the distinct possibility that Islamic societies in Western Eurasia continued to witness plague outbreaks well into the tenth century. Yet their derivative writing suggests that physicians from Egypt, Syria, Iraq and Iran did not have much direct experience with the disease. Medical commentaries composed after the 1240s, however, demonstrate significant changes in how plague was characterised, suggesting that by this era some Islamic physicians working in these regions were encountering or learning about plague outbreaks during their lifetimes. These commentaries corroborate Green's argument that the Second Pandemic may have begun already in the thirteenth century, coinciding with the expansion of the Mongol Empire into East, Central and Western Asia in the middle of the century.[8]

4 See, for example, L. Little, 'Review Article: Plague Historians in Lab Coats', *Past and Present* 213 (2011), 267–90 (pp. 270–1). Conrad did note the possibility of isolated plague outbreaks in the tenth century, but considered the pandemic over in 750; 'Plague in the Early Medieval Near East', p. 311.

5 Little, 'Plague Historians', p. 271; M. Dols, *The Black Death in the Middle East* (Princeton, 1977); and N. Varlık, ed., *Plague and Contagion in the Islamic Mediterranean* (Kalamazoo, 2017).

6 M. H. Green, 'Editor's Introduction to *Pandemic Disease in the Medieval World: Rethinking the Black Death*', *The Medieval Globe* 1 (2014), 9–26; M. H. Green, 'Putting Africa on the Black Death Map: Narratives from Genetics and History', *Afriques: Débats, méthodes et terrains d'histoire* 9 (2018), https://journals.openedition.org/afriques/2125, last accessed 27 September 2019; and M. H. Green, 'Four Black Deaths', *American Historical Review* 125 (2020), 1601–31.

7 A. G. Carmichael, 'Plague Persistence in Western Europe: A Hypothesis', *The Medieval Globe* 1 (2014), 157–91; R. Hymes, 'Epilogue: A Hypothesis on the East Asian Beginnings of the *Yersinia Pestis* Polytomy', *The Medieval Globe* 1 (2014), 285–308.

8 Green, 'Four Black Deaths'.

Arabic medical works before 1240

The Arab Muslim encounter with plague in Syria (c. 638) during the conquests is well documented in religious and literary sources and gave rise to robust theological debates about contagion, God's decree, martyrdom, etc. The pandemic had been ravaging Syria, Egypt and Iraq for the preceding century and it is likely that many of Muhammad's followers – merchants who traded with communities in these regions – were familiar with the disease.[9] Arabic literary sources record many plague outbreaks over the next hundred years across Iraq, the Levant and Egypt, claiming that outbreaks ceased with the rise of the Abbasid dynasty in 750.[10]

The death and destruction wrought by plague on the nascent Muslim community left its mark on the Islamic religious tradition, the subject of numerous studies since the 1970s.[11] The First Pandemic's impact on the Arabic medical tradition has received less attention. Dols and Conrad examined how the Arabic medical authors used Hippocratic humoral and miasmatic theories to understand the cause of the disease. However, given their limited access to sources, especially commentaries on the Hippocratic *Aphorisms*, they could not uncover the pandemic's lasting impact on the Arabic medical tradition – an impact that supersedes what is found in the Byzantine Greek or Latin traditions.[12]

Greek and Syriac sources chronicle numerous plague outbreaks throughout Egypt, the Levant and Anatolia between 541 and 750.[13] However, the extant Greek or Syriac medical texts from this period (and beyond) have little to say about plague. Instead, Greek

9 The fact that there are traditions ascribed to Muhammad concerning plague (*ṭāʿūn*), such as whether or not to flee or enter plague-ridden areas, suggests that the Prophet and some of his companions were familiar with the disease prior to the Muslim army's encounter with it in Syria in 638. It is worth noting that the absence of plague from Mecca and Medina became a dogmatic theological position in the period between the First and Second Pandemic; see Conrad, '*Ṭāʿūn* and *Wabāʾ*', pp. 285–6.

10 Conrad, '*Ṭāʿūn* and *Wabāʾ*', p. 288; Conrad, 'Plague in the Early Medieval Near East', p. 311; and Little, 'Plague Historians', pp. 270–1.

11 Conrad, ''Umar at Sargh'; Conrad, '*Ṭāʿūn* and *wabāʾ*'; van Ess, *Der Fehltritt des Gelehrten*; Dols, *Black Death*; and J. Stearns, *Infectious Ideas: Contagion in Premodern Islamic and Christian Thought in the Western Mediterranean* (Baltimore, 2011). Also, see M. Shefer-Mossensohn, 'A Historiography of Epidemics in the Islamic Mediterranean', in *Plague and Contagion*, ed. Varlık, pp. 3–26.

12 For the Latin tradition, see L. Jones, *Patterns of Plague: Changing Ideas about Plague in England and France, 1348–1750* (Montreal, 2022). As this chapter was in its final stages of production, two new studies were published with which I have not been able to engage fully in this chapter. The first is on the genre of Arabic plague treatises: M. Arıcı (trans. F. Akyıldız), 'Silent Sources of the History of Epidemics in the Islamic World: Literature on *Ṭāʿūn*/Plague Treatises', *Nazariyat* 7 (2021), 99–158. The second is a follow-up study on Greek medical responses to plague: J. Mulhall, 'Confronting Pandemic in Late Antiquity: The Medical Response to the Justinianic Plague', *Journal of Late Antiquity* 14 (2021), 498–528.

13 See M. Morony, '"For Whom does the Writer Write?": The First Bubonic Plague Pandemic According to Syriac Sources', in *Plague and the End of Antiquity: The Pandemic of 541–750*, ed. L. Little (Cambridge, 2007), pp. 59–86; and D. Stathakopoulos, 'Crime and Punishment: The

authors, such as Aetius of Amida (sixth century) or Paul of Aegina (seventh century), take an encyclopaedic approach wherein they copied 'a section on this disease by Rufus of Ephesus (late first century), as Oribasius (fourth century) had done in his turn'.[14] Rufus did not encounter plague himself but recorded its presence in North Africa and Syria on the authority of earlier Greek writers. In the oft-cited passage, Rufus differentiated between common swellings ('bubōnes') that can arise with or without fevers and those that are pestilential ('loimōdeis'). The latter are swellings that are 'large, hard and not suppurating' and accompanied by sharp fever and terrible pain, sometimes causing delirium. The swellings are said to occur behind the knee, in the groin and in the bend of the arms, which largely matches modern clinical diagnoses of plague. We also know that the onset of disease is quite sudden and is often accompanied by other non-specific symptoms such as chills, headaches, palpitations, vomiting and dryness and swellings in the tongue and face.[15]

The fact that Paul and Aetios included Rufus's distinction between the two kinds of swellings ('bubōnes') in their works is significant. These works were compiled during the First Pandemic, when literary authors such as Procopius (d. 570) were using 'bubōnes' unrestrictedly to refer to plague swellings.[16] Their citation of Rufus might have been a way to educate their audiences about the difference between a regular swelling and a plague bubo. It is also worth emphasising that Paul and Aetios did not mistakenly claim that 'boubōn' in the Hippocratic corpus referred to plague buboes – a mistake that many modern historians have made and one that is found in the Syriac translation of the Hippocratic corpus.

Plague in translations of Hippocrates and Galen (eighth/ninth centuries)

The Hippocratic *Aphorisms* IV.55 states 'fevers following "boubōn" are all bad, except for those that last one day [i.e. ephemeral fevers]'. The same aphorism also appears verbatim in *Epidemics II*.[17] Yet 'boubōn' in the Hippocratic corpus had a broad semantic range.

Plague in the Byzantine Empire, 541–749', in *Plague and the End of Antiquity*, ed. Little, pp. 99–118.

14 Stathakopoulos, 'Crime and Punishment', pp. 110–11.

15 J. Mulhall, 'Plague Before Pandemics: The Greek Medical Evidence for Bubonic Plague before the Sixth Century', *Bulletin of the History of Medicine* 93 (2019), 151–79 (pp. 165–7). The translation of Rufus's text is taken from Mulhall's article. For a modern clinical understanding of the disease, see V. Nikiforov et al., 'Plague: Clinics, Diagnosis and Treatment', in *Yersinia Pestis: Retrospective and Perspective*, ed. R. Yang and A. Anisimov (Utrecht, 2016), pp. 293–312. Swellings behind the knee are uncommon: M. H. Green, 'Taking "Pandemic" Seriously: Making the Black Death Global', *The Medieval Globe* 1 (2014), 27–62 (p. 41). Mulhall incorrectly states on the authority of Manfred Ullmann that this Rufus passage 'has not been identified in Arabic sources' (p. 165, n. 52). Lutfallah Gari has identified it in the plague tract of al-Masīḥī and it is also found in the work of al-Rāzī (see below).

16 Mulhall, 'Plague before Pandemics', p. 160.

17 Mulhall, 'Plague before Pandemics', p. 161; and G. C. Kühn, *Galeni opera omnia*, 20 vols. (Leipzig, 1821–33), XVII, 733–4. The translation is taken from Mulhall. The same statement appears

Anatomically, it referred to 'the groin or, occasionally, the groin lymph gland' or an 'area under the abdomen and between the thighs'. Pathologically, the word was more vague and referred to some kind of glandular swelling but was never associated with a specific disease or condition and certainly not with plague.[18] The Syriac translator of this aphorism (eighth or early ninth century), however, assigned the specific term 'sharʿūṭā' to 'boubōn', a term that was used by ninth- and tenth-century Syriac writers to refer specifically to a plague bubo.[19] By translating 'boubōn' as 'sharʿūṭā', the Syriac translator captured the interpretation of a medical community that had chosen to read plague back into the Hippocratic corpus, however incorrectly. Thanks to Ḥunayn ibn Isḥāq (d. 873) and the translator of the *Alexandrian Summary* of *A Method of Medicine to Glaucon*, this interpretation then was carried into the emerging Arabic medical tradition, where it gave rise to a rich tradition of plague discussions in the *Aphorisms* commentaries.[20]

Ḥunayn, famous for translating much of the Galenic corpus into Arabic, was an Iraqi Nestorian physician. He studied under a leading Syriac physician and acted as 'a broker of knowledge between' the Syriac medical community and the 'Arab Muslim political ascendancy'.[21] Although Ḥunayn claims in his *Risāla* (Epistle) that he had corrected an earlier Syriac translation of the *Aphorisms*, he did not produce the extant Syriac version (preserved in a bilingual, parallel Syriac–Arabic manuscript).[22] Ḥunayn translated *Aphorism* IV.55 into Arabic thus: 'Every fever that accompanies a swelling of the soft flesh that is in the groin or other [members] like it is bad, except the one that lasts for a day ('kull ḥummā takūn maʿa waram al-laḥm al-rakhw alladhī fī al-ḥālibayn wa-ghayrihi mimmā ashbahahu fa-hiya radīʾa illā an takūn ḥummā yawm')'.[23] Ḥunayn chose not to translate

in the *Epidemics II*; Galen, *Commentary on Hippocrates' Epidemics Book II, Parts 1–VI*, Arabic ed. and trans. U. Vagelpohl with S. Swain, 2 vols. (Berlin, 2016), I, 476–7.

18 Mulhall, 'Plague before Pandemics', pp. 160–1.

19 Earlier writers, such as John of Ephesus (d. 578/9) and the author of the *Chronicle of Zūqnīn*, both of whom lived during the First Pandemic, use the more generic *mawtānā* (epidemic) or *mawtānā rabbā* (the great epidemic, or plague) to refer to various plague outbreaks. *The Chronicle of Zūqnīn* exists in an autograph manuscript copy from 776; see Morony, 'First Bubonic Plague Pandemic', pp. 60–1; and *The Chronicle of Zūqnīn, Parts III and IV: A.D. 488–775*, trans. A. Harrak (Toronto, 1999), pp. 12–17.

20 I am extrapolating from Robert Wisnovsky's excellent study, *Avicenna's Metaphysics in Context* (Ithaca, 2003), in which he shows the central role played by the neo-Platonic interpretations of Aristotelian texts within Hellenistic philosophical communities on the Arabic translations of Aristotle's works.

21 G. Cooper, 'Ḥunayn ibn Isḥāq and the Creation of an Arabic Galen', in *Brill's Companion to the Reception of Galen*, ed. P. Bouras-Vallianatos and B. Zipser (Leiden, 2019), pp. 179–95 (p. 180).

22 T. Mimura, 'A Reconsideration of the Authorship of the Syriac Hippocratic *Aphorisms*: The Creation of the Syro-Arabic Bilingual Manuscript of the *Aphorisms* in the Tradition of Ḥunayn ibn Isḥāq's Arabic Translation', *Oriens* 45 (2017), 80–104. Taro Mimura graciously helped me with the Syriac version of the *Aphorisms*.

23 Galen, *Commentary on the Hippocratic Aphorisms, Book IV*, Arabic ed. P. E. Pormann et al. (Manchester, 2017), p. 68, https://doi.org/10.3927/51931732, last accessed 10 September, 2019.

'boubōn' as 'ṭāʿūn', the Arabic term for plague bubo equivalent to the Syriac 'sharʿūṭā', even though contemporary literary and religious scholars were using the term to document plague outbreaks of the preceding centuries.[24] Nonetheless, the long gloss for 'boubōn' in Arabic ('swelling of the soft flesh that is in the groin or other [members] like it') captures the original sense of the term, while leaving the door ajar for the aphorism to be linked to plague buboes.

Ḥunayn's translation of Galen's commentary on this aphorism further encouraged his readers to read plague into the Hippocratic aphorism. In the Greek, Galen's text does not gloss the term 'boubōn'. It only clarifies the difference between a 'boubōn' that occurs due to a visible cause and one that does not.[25] Ḥunayn, though, translated the first occurrence of 'boubōn' in Galen's commentary as 'a swelling of the soft flesh like that in the groin ('al-urbiyyatayn')' and the second occurrence of the term as 'swellings that occur in this flesh ('al-awrām allatī taḥdath fī hādhā al-laḥm')'.[26] The *Aphorisms* and Galen's commentary were mainstays of medical education in Islamic societies well into the fourteenth century.[27] Ḥunayn's translation choices kept the disease's memory alive within the Islamic medical community, especially since another key work for early Islamic medical education, the Arabic version of the *Alexandrian Summaries* (*Jawāmi al-Iskandarāniyyīn*), connected *Aphorisms* IV.55 (and Galen's commentary on it) to plague even more explicitly.[28]

Plague buboes are discussed in the *Summary of Glaucon* (*Jawāmiʿ Ighlūqan*) – the Alexandrian summary of the Galenic work, *A Method of Medicine to Glaucon*.[29] The original discussions of swellings (including glandular swellings), whether in the Greek texts of Galen's larger, *On the Method of Medicine*, or the shorter, *A Method of Medicine to Glaucon*, do not refer to swellings in the specific regions of the groin, armpits and behind the ears,

---

Ḥunayn's translation of this aphorism in *Epidemics II* is identical; see Galen, *Commentary on Hippocrates' Epidemics*, I, 476–7.

24 Conrad had mistakenly assumed that the Hippocratic *Aphorism* unequivocally refers to plague buboes and then had faulted (incorrectly) Ḥunayn for not using *ṭāʿūn* in his translation of the aphorism; '*Ṭāʿūn* and *Wabāʾ*', pp. 292–3.

25 Kühn, *Galeni opera*, XVII.2, 733–4. I would like to thank James Wells for helping me with the Greek text.

26 Galen, *Commentary on the Aphorisms*, p. 68.

27 P. E. Pormann and N. P. Joosse, 'Commentaries on the Hippocratic *Aphorisms* in the Arabic Tradition: The Example of Melancholy', in *Epidemics in Context: Greek Commentaries on Hippocrates in the Arabic Tradition*, ed. P. E. Pormann (Berlin, 2012), pp. 211–49 (p. 211).

28 See A. Z. Iskandar, 'An Attempted Reconstruction of the Late Alexandrian Medical Curriculum', *Medical History* 20 (1976), 235–58; P. E. Pormann and E. Savage-Smith, *Medieval Islamic Medicine* (Washington D.C, 2007), pp. 12–15; P. E. Pormann, 'Medical Education in Late Antiquity from Alexandria to Montpellier', in *Hippocrates and Medical Education: Selected Papers Presented at the XIIth International Hippocrates Colloquium, Universiteit Leiden, 24–26 August 2005*, ed. M. Horstmanshoff (Leiden, 2010), pp. 419–41; and I. Garofalo, 'Galen's Legacy in Alexandrian Texts Written in Greek, Latin, and Arabic', in *Brill's Companion*, ed. Bouras-Vallianatos and Zipser, pp. 62–85.

29 I would like to thank Cristina Álvarez-Millán for directing me to this work.

nor do they mention plague.[30] The *Summary of Glaucon*, on the other hand, supplements Galen's brief reference to the different indications of pulse, face and urine in ephemeral fevers caused by buboes ('boubōnes') as follows.[31]

> The swelling that is known in Greek as 'boubōn', meaning 'ṭāʿūn', is a swelling that occurs in the soft flesh. The soft flesh in which this swelling appears can either be in the groin, or in the armpits, or in the neck, or behind the ears. The one in the groin receives, in most cases, wastes from the liver and so the swelling that occurs in it becomes an intense[32] swelling which is the plague bubo. The one in the armpits receives, in most cases, wastes of the heart and for that reason the swelling that occurs in it is extremely hot and it is the harmful, bad plague bubo. The one in the neck and behind the ears receives wastes from the brain and for that reason the swelling that occurs in it, in most cases, is cold.[33]
>
> ('al-waram al-musammā bi-l-yūnāniyya būbon tafsīrahu al-ṭāʿūn huwa waram yaḥdath fī al-laḥm al-rakhw wa-l-laḥm al-rakhw yuḥdath fīhi hādhā al-waram immā fī al-ḥālibayn wa-immā fī al-ibṭayn wa-immā fī al-ʿunuq wa-khalf al-udhunayn wa-mā huwa fī al-ḥālibayn fa-shaʾnuhu an yaqbal fī akthar al-ḥālāt faḍl al-kabid wa-lidhālik ṣāra al-waram al-ḥādith fīhi waraman ḥā[dd]an wa-huwa al-ṭāʿūn wa-mā huwa fī al-ibṭayn fa-shaʾnuhu an yaqbal fī akthar al-amr faḍl al-qalb wa-lidhālik ṣāra al-waram alladhī yaḥdath fīhi ashaddu ḥarāra wa-huwa al-ṭāʿūn al-khabīth al-radīʾ wa-mā huwa fī al-ʿunuq wa-khalf al-udhunayn fa-shaʾnuhu an yaqbal faḍl al-dimāgh wa-lidhālik ṣāra al-waram alladhī yaḥdath fī akthar al-ḥālāt bāridan').

30 In *On the Method of Medicine*, Galen says: 'I think I should remind you also of what has been demonstrated often – that the superfluities thrust out from the stronger parts on account of amount or quality pass down to the weaker [parts] and, because of this, the glands also receive the flux, especially those that are by nature looser in texture'. This is why glands in the groin and armpit swell due to wounds in a foot or hand, respectively, whereas glands in the neck or behind the ears swell from wounds 'in the head or neck'. 'They call glands swollen in this way "buboes" (*boubōnes*)'; Galen, *On the Method of Medicine*, ed. and trans. I. Johnston and G. H. R. Horsley, Loeb ed., 3 vols. (Cambridge MA, 2011), III, 327–9 (ed. Kühn, X, 880).

31 Galen, *On the Constitution of the Art of Medicine, The Art of Medicine and A Method of Medicine to Glaucon*, ed. and trans. I. Johnston, Loeb ed. (Cambridge MA, 2016), p. 357 (ed. Kühn, XI, 14): 'In the ephemeral fever due to buboes, the pulse becomes very large, rapid and frequent … In fevers such as these, … the patients generally become red and more swollen in the face, and the urine is whitish'.

32 There is at least one letter missing. Based on al-Rāzī's notes in the *Ḥāwī* (see below), I have inserted the missing letter *d* to make it 'ḥāddan' (intense).

33 *Jawāmiʿ al-Iskandrāniyyīn: Alexandrian Summaries of Eight Medical Treatises by Galen*, London, British Library: Oriental Manuscripts, Add. MS 23407, fols. 85a–b, https://www.qdl.qa/en/archive/81055/vdc_100022522872.0x000001, last accessed 15 June 2020. Arıcı uses the following edition: Ḥunayn ibn Isḥāq, *Kitāb Jālīnūs ilā Ighlūqan fī-l-taʾattī lī shifāʾ al-amrāḍ*, Muḥammad S. Salīm (Cairo, 1982). The editor, however, has incorrectly classified the work as Ḥunayn's translation of Galen's original *Method of Medicine to Glaucon*. Both of these claims are incorrect (see below).

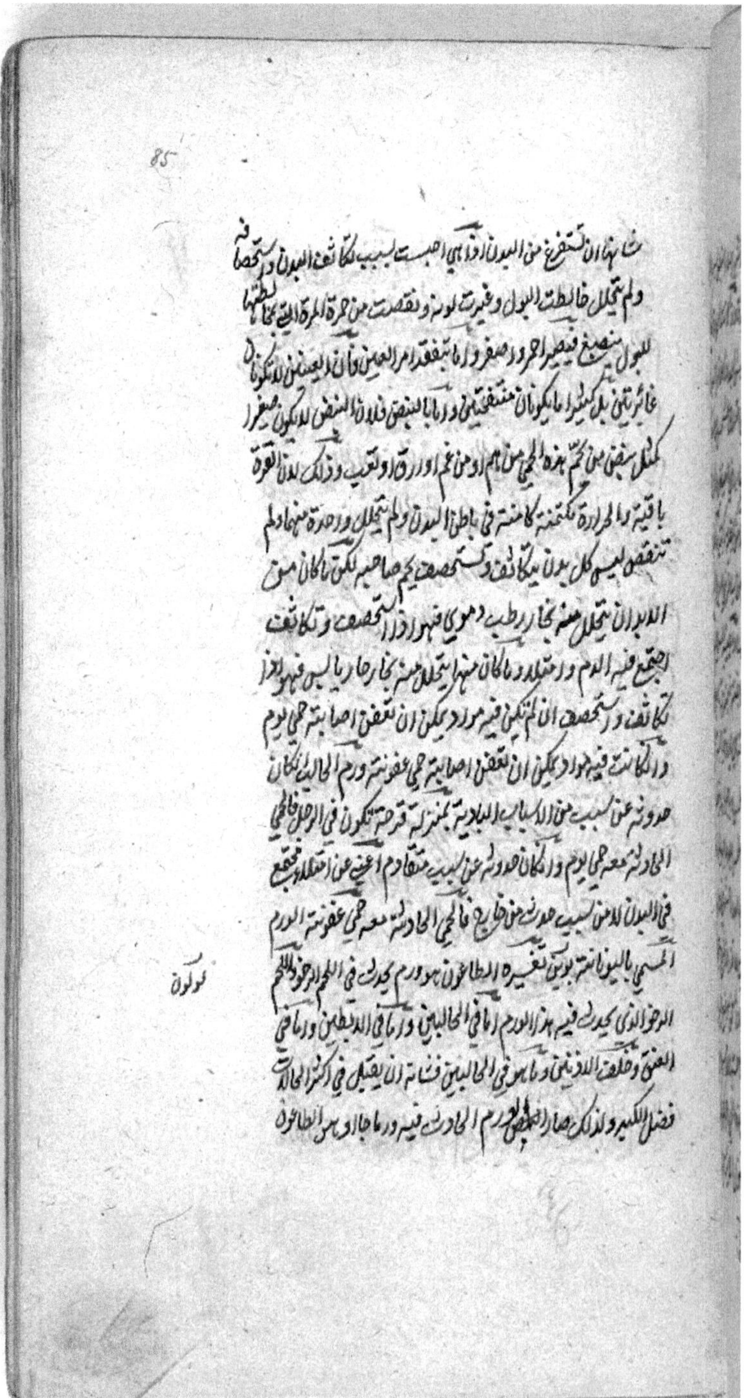

Fig. 1.1. Passage on plague from the *Summary of Glaucon* text. The bottom of the folio states clearly that the Greek term *boubon* is rendered *ta'un*. London, British Library, Oriental Manuscripts, Add. MS 23407, fol. 85a, available under a Public Domain Mark.

This long excerpt from the *Summary of Glaucon* confirms much of what Peter Pormann and Ivan Garofalo have stated about the Alexandrian summaries, generally, and *To Glaucon*, specifically.[34] The pedagogical method of classifying by divisions and subdivisions ('diairesis') is apparent in the excerpt, as the swellings in the soft flesh are subdivided into classes and treated separately. The excerpt also shows that *Summary of Glaucon* deviates significantly from Galen's Greek text, suggesting that it is, strictly speaking, not a summary but, rather, a commentary.[35]

Both the accurate identification of plague buboes and the application of Galenic principles to understand their cause are missing in other extant Alexandrian commentaries on this text.[36] For example, plague buboes are not mentioned in the corresponding passage of the abridgment of *A Method of Medicine to Glaucon* by the Alexandrian, Yaḥyā al-Naḥwī (John the Grammarian).[37] Stephanus of Alexandria's (fl. late sixth century) commentary on Galen's work also does not mention plague swellings in these specific sites, nor does it suggest that the chief organs send their wastes to these locations.[38] The *Summary of Glaucon*'s detailed and explicit discussion of plague buboes suggests that its milieu was different from that of John and Stephanus, or perhaps that the extant *Summary* was composed at a

34 P. E. Pormann, 'The *Alexandrian Summary* (*Jawāmi*ʿ) of Galen's *On the Sects for Beginners*: Commentary or Abridgment', *Bulletin of the Institute of Classical Studies* 83 (2004), 11–33; Pormann, 'Medical Education'; and Garofalo, 'Galen's Legacy'.

35 Bos and Langermann have argued that it is best to see these summaries as not only teaching texts but also as works that bring 'Galen up-to-date'; G. Bos and Y. T. Langermann, *The Alexandrian Summaries of Galen's* On Critical Days*: Editions and Translations of the Two Versions of the* Jawāmiʿ*, with an Introduction and Notes* (Leiden, 2014), p. 1.

36 Savage-Smith has reviewed the fragility of the evidence that even connects the summaries to an Alexandrian context; E. Savage-Smith, 'Galen's Lost Ophthalmology and the *Summaria Alexandrinorum*', in *The Unknown Galen*, ed. V. Nutton (London, 2002), pp. 121–38.

37 *Kitāb Ikthiṣār al-sittat ʿashr li-Jālīnūs, talkhīṣ Yaḥyā al-Naḥwī*, London, British Library: Oriental Manuscripts, MS Arundel Or. 17, fol. 14b, https://www.qdl.qa/en/archive/81055/vdc_100000041053.0x000001, last accessed 15 June 2020. There is much debate over whether this is John Philoponus (d. 574), or John of Alexandria (fl. 600–42); see Pormann, '*Alexandrian Summary*', pp. 21–2.

38 K. Dickson, *Stephanus the Philosopher and Physician: Commentary on Galen's Therapeutics to Glaucon* (Leiden, 1998), pp. 47, 75 (ed. Kühn, XI, 6, 14). Stephanus here refers more generally to glands receiving excess humours since the former are weaker parts of the body where these humours can then putrefy and cause swellings. A similar discussion is found in Stephanus's *Commentary on the Aphorisms*; however, there he singles out the three traditional sites of plague buboes as receiving the wastes from the chief organs in buboes that are pestilential. Nonetheless, he then adds that they are neither 'dangerous' nor 'deadly' but, rather, treatable even if they are 'bad'. This does not match up with how plague buboes were understood in the Arabic *Summary to Glaucon* or in the subsequent Arabic commentary tradition on the *Aphorisms*; L. Westerink (ed. and trans.), *Stephani Atheniensis In Hippocratis Aphorismos commentaria* (Berlin, 1992), pp. 345, 347. Mulhall has recently argued that Stephanus in his *Commentary on Aphorisms* was describing his experience with the first plague pandemic; Mulhall, 'Confronting Pandemic in Late Antiquity', pp. 513–17.

later date, possibly even originally in Syriac rather than Greek.[39] It is also noteworthy that the Arabic text of the *Summary of Glaucon* translates 'boubōn' as 'ṭāʿūn', unlike Ḥunayn's translations.[40]

The supplementary discussion of plague in the *Summary of Glaucon* ends by applying Galen's commentary on *Aphorisms* IV.55 to plague swellings, i.e. that the fever accompanied by swellings is bad when it is due to hidden causes. The Alexandrian summary states that if the swelling of the soft flesh is what causes the fever, then that fever is not bad since it is an ephemeral fever. However, if the swelling accompanies the fever 'but is not its cause then the fever is bad and harmful ('wa-laysa huwa sababuhā fa-l-ḥummā radiyya wa-khabītha')', since it indicates that the fever is due to a corruption in the chief organs ('al-aʿḍāʾ al-jalīla'). The *Summary of Glaucon* thus explicitly connects *Aphorisms* IV.55, Galen's commentary on it and his discussion on swellings in *A Method of Medicine to Glaucon* to plague buboes, based on the medical community's (Greek, Syriac and/or Arabic) direct experience with the disease during the First Pandemic. The Arabic commentaries on the *Aphorisms* drew upon this passage from the *Summary of Glaucon* while commenting on IV.55, even though Ḥunayn's Arabic text does not use the word 'ṭāʿūn'.

Commentaries on the Aphorisms (eleventh to thirteenth centuries)

Of the seven extant, pre-1240 Arabic commentaries on the *Aphorisms*, only four include and discuss *Aphorisms* IV.55.[41] Maimonides's (d. 1204) commentary does not connect the aphorism to plague at all. He merely reiterates Galen's claim that swellings accompanied

39 Garofalo has argued that the *Summary of Glaucon* was translated directly from the Greek since it is very close to Stephanus's commentary; see I. Garofalo, 'La traduzione araba dei compendi alessandrini delle opere del canone di Galeno: Il compendio dell'*Ad Glauconem*', *Medicina nei secoli* 6 (1994), 329–48 (p. 333). However, as I have shown, in the discussion on buboes it overlaps slightly with Stephanus's *Commentary on the Aphorisms* (not on *Therapeutics to Glaucon*), but is also substantially different.

40 Although the Arabic translation of the *Alexandrian Summaries* has often been attributed to Ḥunayn, Garofalo and Pormann have questioned this attribution; I. Garofalo, 'La traduzione araba del *De Sectis* e il sommario degli alessandrini', *Galenos* 1 (2007), 191–210 (p. 206); Garofalo, 'Galen's Legacy', p. 66; and Pormann, *Alexandrian Summaries*, p. 18. Ḥunayn's Arabic translation of Galen's *On Method of Medicine to Glaucon* also does not render *boubōn* as *ṭāʿūn* but, rather, as 'the glandular swelling that is in the groin or armpit'; *Kitāb Jālīnūs ilā Ighlūqan fī shifāʾ al-amrāḍ* in Galen, *Majmūʿa fī al-ṭibb*, Princeton, Princeton University: Islamic Manuscripts, MS Garrett no. 1G, fols. 283b, 287a, https://catalog.princeton.edu/catalog/4808744, last accessed 15 June 2020.

41 Pormann and his team have edited all extant Arabic commentaries on the *Aphorisms*. They are all listed here: http://hummedia.manchester.ac.uk/schools/salc/subjects/clah/projects/arabiccommentaries/List-of-Scholarly-Editions.pdf, last accessed 8 June 2020. Al-Nīlī's (d. 1029), Ibn Riḍwān's (d. 1067) and Ibn al-Minfākh's (d. 1258) extant, edited commentaries do not contain this aphorism.

by non-ephemeral fevers are dangerous since they are due to swellings in internal organs.[42] The other three commentators all connect the aphorism directly to plague swellings.

Ibn Abī Ṣādiq al-Nīsābūrī (d. after 1067), a Persian physician whose commentary survives in over forty manuscripts,[43] explained that when a non-ephemeral fever is caused by a swelling of the soft flesh, such 'a swelling is bad because such members receive harmful materials ('fa-l-waram radī' li-anna al-mawād al-khabītha')' from the chief organs. He further added that 'many swellings of [the soft glandular] flesh belong to the genus of plague buboes, whose fevers are extremely bad ('fa-inna akthar awrām hādhihi al-luḥum hiya min jins al-ṭawāʿīn wa-ḥummayātuhā radīʾa jiddan')'. He also classified the swellings from safest to most dangerous, claiming that those in the jaws ('al-laḥyayn') are the safest ('aslamhā'), since they receive wastes from the brain, while 'most of the swellings that arise in the armpits are dangerous as they are from wastes of the heart ('wa-aktharuhā khaṭaran mā yakūn fī al-ibṭayn li-annahā min fuḍulāt al-qalb')'. The swellings in the groin fall 'in between the two ('mutawassiṭ baynahumā')' in terms of danger since they receive waste from the liver.[44] The commentary clearly relies on the *Summary of Glaucon* and unmistakably refers to plague ('ṭawāʿīn', sing. 'ṭāʿūn') and its specific symptoms, i.e. glandular swellings and dangerous fever. The Persian physician al-Sinjārī (fl. twelfth c.) did not use the term 'ṭāʿūn' specifically, but his commentary is heavily indebted to Ibn Abī Ṣādiq, as it also refers to swellings in the jaws, rather than the neck or behind the ears.[45]

ʿAbd al-Laṭīf al-Baghdādī (d. 1231), a physician-philosopher who spent much of his time in Syria and Egypt, also used 'ṭāʿūn' in his commentary on *Aphorisms* IV.55. However, the rest of his text is distinct from Ibn Abī Ṣādiq's work and even (partly) from the *Summary of Glaucon*. His commentary first states that non-ephemeral fevers caused by swellings can be of different types. Some follow the course of fevers that result from abscesses classified as phlegmone ('al-khurājāt al-falghamūniyya'), i.e., bloody abscesses. Plague buboes are not classified as such in the *Summary of Glaucon*. He then adds, in cases when 'the swellings of the soft flesh are not due to any apparent cause, but rather are

42 Maimonides, *Commentary on the Hippocratic Aphorisms*, ed. P. E. Pormann et al. (Manchester, 2017), Aphorism 55, pp. 76–7, https://doi.org/10.3927/53356462, last accessed 1 September 2019; and Galen, *Commentary on the Aphorisms*, p. 68.

43 Pormann and Joosse, 'Commentaries on the Hippocratic *Aphorisms*', pp. 222–3. Ibn Abī Ṣādiq's commentary also represents a marked transition away from Galen's textual authority; see K. Karimullah, 'Transformation of Galen's Textual Legacy from Classical to Post-Classical Islamic Medicine: Commentaries on the Hippocratic *Aphorisms*', *Intellectual History of the Islamicate World* 5 (2017), 311–58; and R. M. Batten, 'The Arabic Commentaries on the Hippocratic *Aphorisms*: Arabic Learned Medical Discourse on Women's Bodies (9th–15th cent.)' (unpublished Ph.D. dissertation, University of Manchester, 2018).

44 Ibn Abī Ṣāḍiq, *Commentary on the Hippocratic Aphorisms, Book Four*, ed. P. E. Pormann et al. (Manchester, 2017), Aphorism 54, pp. 53–4, https://doi.org/10.3927/51932186, last accessed 1 September 2019.

45 al-Sinjārī, *Commentary on the Hippocratic Aphorisms, Book Four*, ed. Pormann et al., Aphorism 55, pp. 36–7, http://doi.org/10.3927/52132455, last accessed 1 September 2019.

accompanied by hot[46] swellings ('wa-qad yakūn hādhā al-waram fī al-laḥm al-rakhw lā ʿan sabab ẓāhir bal maʿa awrām ḥārra')', such swellings are plague bubo-like ('ṭāʿūniyya'), harmful ('khabītha') 'and the fever in such cases is bad ('wa-l-ḥummā fīhā radīʾa')'.[47]

In short, three pre-1200 commentaries on the *Aphorisms*, including Ibn Abī Ṣādiq's widely disseminated work, connected *Aphorisms* IV.55 to plague and two commentators, like the *Summary of Glaucon*, linked each of the three primary bubo sites to wastes expelled from the three chief organs. Yet, the commentaries also contain some additional information, such as classifying the varying dangers of the buboes and how they are related to other swellings and abscesses. From where did they get their supplemental information? For that, we need to turn to the medical encyclopaedias of the tenth century.

Plague in tenth- and early eleventh-century medical compendia

Plague appears in the medical compendia of Abū Bakr al-Rāzī (d. c. 925), ʿAlī ibn ʿAbbās al-Majūsī (d. c. 994) and Ibn Sīnā (d. 1037). Some physicians even composed special tracts on the disease, the most famous of which are the plague treatises of Qusṭā ibn Lūqā (d. 912) and Abū Sahl al-Masīḥī (d. 1010).[48] Although much material was recycled over the century, one still finds new things highlighted in Ibn Sīnā's later work. One should also give these writers credit for applying Greek humoral and miasma theories to plague, since, outside of the *Summary of Glaucon* and brief remarks from physicians like Rufus, Greek sources had little to say about the disease itself. The sustained Arabic medical discussions of plague in the tenth century medical works suggest that outbreaks continued to occur in Islamic societies after 750. Syriac and Arabic literary sources refer to many epidemics/pestilences ('mawtānā/wabāʾ') during the early Abbasid period and Arabic sources also record a plague outbreak ('ṭāʿūn') in 913–14 in Baghdad itself![49]

Conrad has already provided a brief overview of the plague discussions in the medical encyclopaedias. My goal here is to explain how plague was described and characterised by tenth-century physicians and to recognise the depth of their engagements, in order to be in a better position to judge the novel elements found in the post-1240 texts. In his encyclopaedia, *al-Ḥāwī fī al-ṭibb* (The Comprehensive Book on Medicine), al-Rāzī discusses plague ('ṭāʿūn') in three different sections, only two of which Conrad knew. The first is in a long section (eighty-eight pages in its modern edition) on abscesses and swellings. Here,

46 The edition has 'ḥādda' but it should be 'ḥārra' as found in one of the manuscripts, since that matches Galen's own discussion in his commentary.

47 ʿAbd al-Laṭīf al-Baghdādī, *Commentary on the Hippocratic Aphorisms, Book Four*, ed. Pormann et al., Aphorism 165, pp. 43–4, https://doi.org/10.3927/51689018, last accessed 1 September 2019.

48 For more pre-1240 medical works that discuss plague, see Dols, *Black Death*, p. 28, n. 52; and now Arıcı, 'Silent Sources', pp. 110–17.

49 Conrad, 'Plague in the Early Medieval Near East', pp. 307–10. The later writer, Ibn Abī Hajala (d. 1375), lists numerous outbreaks of plague in Iraq, Iran and even in Egypt over the course of the tenth and eleventh centuries; Ibn Abī Hajala, *Dafʿ al-niqma fī ṣalāh ʿalā nabī al-raḥma*, Madrid, Escorial Library, MS 1772, fols. 64a–69b.

al-Rāzī cites the *Summary of Glaucon* to characterise the plague bubo as 'a swelling that occurs in the soft flesh'. The swellings behind the ear, in the armpits and in the groin are due to wastes expelled from the three chief organs: brain, heart and liver, respectively. He describes the swellings behind the ear as 'cold and non-pulsing ('bārid sākin')', while the swellings in the armpit are characterised as 'harmful, hot ('khabīth ḥārr')' and those in the groin as less intense.[50]

Al-Rāzī's work also contains a section dealing with smallpox ('al-judarī'), measles ('al-ḥaṣba') and plagues ('al-ṭawāʿīn'). Most of the section is devoted to smallpox and measles. He discusses plague very briefly, citing an Alexandrian physician and presbyter, Ahrun (fl. seventh c.).[51] Here, a plague bubo is characterised as 'a warm swelling that occurs in the groin and armpit and kills within four to five days ('waram ḥārr yaʿruḍ fī al-urbiyyāt wa-l-ibṭ wa-yaqtul fī arbaʿa aw fī khamsa'. The black and green swellings are deemed the worst, almost always resulting in death, the red and white are deemed the safest, while the yellow swellings are deemed to be in the middle. Al-Rāzī also states (on the authority of Ahrun) that nothing is more beneficial in treating plague than bleeding, so long as the patient can bear it, after which one should apply coats of Armenian bole.[52] We thus see some additional information to what is found in the *Summary of Glaucon*. The speed and the greater danger associated with buboes of the armpits and groin (as Ibn Abī Ṣādiq and al-Sinjārī will later note) is much more explicit in this passage from Ahrun than in the *Summary*. Other new material includes the classification of the colour of the buboes and how to treat patients afflicted with plague.

Finally, al-Rāzī refers to symptoms that accompany plague in his section on endemic diseases and pestilences ('wabāʾ') and how one should modify one's dietary regime according to the changing seasons. The passage is from Paul on the authority of Rufus.[53] It states that 'delirium accompanies the pestilential plague ('yaʿruḍ maʿa al-ṭāʿūn al-wabāʾī ikhtilāṭ al-ʿaql')', along with a host of other symptoms including cold extremities, abdominal

50 Abū Bakr al-Rāzī, *al-Ḥāwī fī al-ṭibb*, ed. M. M. Ismail, XXIII books in 8 vols. (Beirut, 2000), XII, 77. The edited text has 'ḥādd'.

51 Little is known about this physician, although his work was translated into Arabic and quite popular in the early period. There is also a debate about whether he flourished in the sixth or seventh century; see M. Ullmann, *Die Medizin im Islam* (Leiden, 1970), pp. 87–9 and A. Dietrich, *Encyclopaedia of Islam*, 2nd ed., ed. P. Bearman et al. (Leiden, 1960–2007), s.v. 'Ahrun'.

52 al-Rāzī, *al-Ḥāwī fī al-ṭibb*, XVII, 4–5. The Arabic text here is not as straightforward, which led Dols to mistakenly claim 'Ahrun describes the spitting of blood' (*Black Death*, p. 30). The text states, 'wa-idhā iḥtamal al-ʿalīl irsāl al-dam fa-lā shayʾ fī ʿilāj al-ṭāʿūn ablagh minhu'. My thanks to Kevin Blankinship for confirming my reading.

53 The quote follows one attributed to both Paul and Oribasius. However, given that the quotation leaves out Rufus's discussion of the sites of the plague buboes, this quote must have been taken from Paul, since Paul also left out that part of Rufus's passage; see Rebecca Flemming, 'Pandemics in the Ancient Mediterranean World: Essay Version 2', *Isis Cumulative Bibliography*, Special Issue on Pandemics, ed. S. P. Weldon and N. Sankaran, May 2021, p. 6, https://isiscb.org/special-issue-on-pandemics/essay.html?essayID=13.

pain and distension, nosebleeds, a hot and painful chest, a black tongue, thirst and a loss of appetite, amongst other bad things.[54] Rufus's description of the buboes themselves is missing in this citation and many of the symptoms are not specific to plague; however, the reference to a pestilential plague, as opposed to just plague, along with the highlighting of delirium, suggests that al-Rāzī is liberally quoting from the Rufus passage but mixing it with other symptoms of pestilential diseases (Greek 'loimos', Arabic 'wabāʾ'), such as those described by Galen for the Antonine plague.[55]

Al-Rāzī's quotation continues by recommending what one should do as the temperament starts to change during a bout of pestilential plague, which is to counter the excessive moisture by purging, bloodletting and exercise, and counter the excessive warmth by cooling treatments.[56] He then quotes a recipe for a medicine made from aloe, myrrh and saffron which 'Rufus claimed he had not seen anyone drink this medicine who then died during a pestilence ('fa-zaʿama rūfus annahu lam yar aḥadan shariba hādhā al-dawāʾ fa-māta fī al-wabāʾ')'.[57] This same recipe is quoted earlier, towards the end of a discussion by al-Rāzī on what to do to protect oneself from a 'wabāʾ', especially its putrid heat. In one such case, al-Rāzī cites a long passage from al-Yahūdī on what to do at the time of a 'wabāʾ'. Al-Yahūdī suggests staying away from moist foods, amongst other things, and to consume many sour and astringent things, like oxymel, Armenian bole with water and vinegar, pomegranates, plums, gourd, Indian pea, etc. He also recommends sprinkling vinegar and asafetida in the house. He ends by saying, 'This even protects one from plague ('fa-in hādhā amān min al-ṭāʿūn')'.[58]

In his seminal article, Conrad had shown that in the early Islamic period, 'wabāʾ' was understood to be 'a pestilential corruption of the natural environment', while 'ṭāʿūn' referred to 'a well-known disease'. However, the relationship between the two is not entirely clear. Al-Yahūdī (Māsarjawayh) clearly differentiated between the two, since he emphasised that

54 al-Rāzī, *al-Ḥāwī fī al-ṭibb*, XV, 215–16.

55 Rebecca Flemming, 'Galen and the Plague', in *Galen's Treatise* Περὶ Ἀλυπίας *(De Indolentia) in Context: A Tale of Resilience*, ed. C. Petit (Leiden, 2019), pp. 219–44 (p. 229).

56 The treatments provided by al-Rāzī differ from those found in Paul of Aegina's work, suggesting that he is incorporating other sources or mixing his own recommendations based on his theoretical conception of the disease; see Mulhall, 'Confronting Pandemic in Late Antiquity', pp. 518–19.

57 al-Rāzī, *al-Ḥāwī fī al-ṭibb*, XV, 216. Al-Rāzī also quotes a treatment for 'mawtān' (plague?) mentioned by Rufus in *On Regimen*, which too suggests cooling the body and avoiding activities that would heat it, such as over-exerting oneself.

58 al-Rāzī, *al-Ḥāwī fī al-ṭibb*, XV, 208, 210–11. According to Ibn Abī Uṣaybiʿa's thirteenth-century biographical dictionary, al-Yahūdī is the Jewish physician of Basra, Māsarjawayh (fl. 715). He translated the medical compendium ('kunnāsh') of Ahrun from Syriac into Arabic and compiled his own medical compendium in addition to works on diet and on the eye; E. Savage-Smith, S. Swain and G. J. van Gelder, ed., *A Literary History of Medicine* (Leiden, 2020), passage 8.19, https://dh.brill.com/scholarlyeditions/library/urn:cts:arabicLit:0668IbnAbiUsaibia, last accessed 16 July 2020.

his suggestions for 'wabā'' help with plague too. It seems as though al-Yahūdī had direct experience treating plague patients. Al-Rāzī too kept 'wabā'' and 'ṭāʿūn' distinct for the most part, since he does not emphasise fevers in the case of 'ṭāʿūn', unlike 'wabā''.[59] Yet, there is a sense in his work that the corruption that is part of a 'wabā'' causes fevers and similar corruption causes plague.[60] This connection between the two was strengthened by later encyclopaedic writers who defined 'wabā'' as any disease caused by a corruption that impacts many people in one region and 'ṭāʿūn' as a specific kind of lethal 'wabā''.

In summary, although al-Rāzī includes plague in his encyclopaedia, he does so only on the authority of other, earlier physicians. He devotes very little space to the disease when compared to smallpox and measles, even though plague had ravaged the larger Islamic Mediterranean for more than two centuries and even devastated the jewel of the Islamic world, Baghdad, during his own lifetime. All of this suggests that, despite his vast clinical experience in Rayy and Baghdad, including in 'bīmāristāns' (hospitals), al-Rāzī did not have personal experience with the disease and so merely copied the little he found in other medical works. By contrast, his detailed discussion of smallpox and measles suggests personal experience with those diseases.

Unlike al-Rāzī, al-Majūsī and Ibn Sīnā devoted much more space to plague, adding material that built upon the theoretical understanding of swellings found in the *Summary of Glaucon*. In the *Royal Book*, al-Majūsī discusses plague in sections on fevers and epidemic diseases ('al-amrāḍ al-wabʾiyya'), thus connecting 'ṭāʿūn' more specifically with 'wabā'' than al-Rāzī had done.[61] While categorising various types of swellings that can accompany fevers, al-Majūsī states that when a blood-based, hot swelling occurs in 'the soft flesh such as under the armpits, the groin, or in the eye, or behind the ear, and it takes place quickly, it is called the plague bubo and abscess ('fī al-laḥm al-rakhw alladhī taḥta al-ibṭayn wa-l-urbiyyatayn aw fī al-ʿayn aw khalf al-ādhān wa-tawallud fīhi al-mudda bi-surʿa qīla

59 Also see his *al-Kitāb al-Manṣūrī fī al-ṭibb*, Washington DC, Library of Congress, MS Manṣūrī Collection SM 55, https://www.wdl.org/en/item/4276/, last accessed 28 May 2020, fols. 47b–8b, 163a–5a.

60 That a *wabāʾ* causes fevers is found in the Alexandrian summary of Galen's *On the Differences of Fevers*, a text that al-Rāzī cites just before quoting the aforementioned passage from Paul on the pestilential plague; *[Jāwāmiʿ] Kitāb Jālīnūs fī aṣnāf al-hummayāt* in Galen, *Majmūʿa fī al-ṭibb*, fol. 71b. The text also goes on to add that some regions are prone to corruption because of vapours from swampy lands or water that mixes with the air, thus corrupting it, or because their dead never disintegrate. The latter is deemed the reason for the prevalence of *wabāʾ* in Ethiopia (fol. 72a). Galen's original text (citing Thucydides) claims that Ethiopia was the source of the Athenian plague for this same reason (ed. Kühn, VII, 289–90). I thank Glen Cooper for identifying that passage in Galen's original work.

61 Al-Majūsī's encyclopaedia was a response to and a critique of al-Rāzī's *al-Ḥāwī*; see E. Savage-Smith, 'Medicine', in *Encyclopedia of the History of Arabic Science*, 3 vols., ed. R. Rashed with R. Morelon (London, 1996), III, 903–62 (pp. 917, 919).

lahu al-ṭāʿūn wa-l-khurāj')'.[62] He also deems the blood-based swelling that changes into a bilious one (or vice versa) and one into which pus flows as plague buboes. He concurs with al-Rāzī's interpretation of the *Summary of Glaucon* that the buboes in the armpits are the worst and most harmful 'since these glands receive wastes from the heart, and they are the hottest ('li-anna hādhihi al-ghudad taqbal fuḍūl al-qalb wa-hiya ashaddu ḥarāra')'.[63]

In his section on epidemic diseases, al-Majūsī explains that when a 'wabāʾ' arises due to something entering the body from the outside, it is due to either: (a) changes in the temperament of the air; or (b) changes in the substance of the air ('jawhar al-hawāʾ'). The latter 'generates bad, lethal diseases in people like plagues, harmful, deadly fevers, smallpox and the like ('fa-yaḥdath fī al-nās amrāḍan radīʾatan qattālatan bi-manzilat al-ṭawāʿīn wa-l-ḥummayāt al-khabītha al-muhlika wa-l-judarī wa-ghayra dhālik')'. No epidemic disease, however, affects every person. Even an epidemic arising from a change in the substance of the air affects only those people whose bodies' natural constitution inclines towards that corruption or is unable to counteract it. Consequently, in line with humoral theory, he recommends that precautions be taken to prevent the disease using the principle of opposites. Since this corruption of the substance of air happens 'most often due to excessive heat and moisture ('fī akthar al-amr min ifrāṭ al-ḥarāra wa-l-ruṭūba')', the primary preventative measures are bloodletting, the use of purgatives, the use of cooling and drying regimens, etc. He then provides many specific suggestions, well known to scholars of plague, such as using fragrances for changing the air (sandalwood, camphor), vinegar, drinks (pomegranate juice, sumac water), consuming sour things (apples, quinces, Armenian bole), etc.[64] All these recommendations are rooted in Galenic–Hippocratic theory and many are based on Galen's own recommendations for treating swellings and epidemic/pestilential fevers generally.[65] However, only a few (e.g. bloodletting and Armenian bole) were explicitly recommended for treating plague by earlier Greek physicians, such as Ahrun and Rufus.[66]

In his *Canon of Medicine*, Ibn Sīnā concurs with much of what is found in al-Majūsī's work.[67] He too discusses plague ('ṭāʿūn') in sections devoted to swellings and epidemic fevers. In *Canon* I.2.1 (book one, part two, lesson one), Ibn Sīnā uses the example of

62 The classification scheme of swellings is heavily indebted, but not identical, to what is found in Galen's works; *On Method of Medicine*, pp. 319–29 (ed. Kühn, X, 874–81) and *To Glaucon*, pp. 447–57 (ed. Kühn, XI, 71–7).

63 al-Majūsī, *Kitāb Kāmil al-ṣināʿa al-ṭibbiyya: al-maʿrūf bi-l-Malakī*, Yale University, Cushing Medical Library, MS Arabic 4, fol. 169b, http://www.wdl.org/en/item/9716/, last accessed 1 June 2020.

64 al-Majūsī, *Kāmil al-ṣināʿa*, MS Arabic 4, fols. 267a–b. Compare with Dols, *Black Death*, pp. 98–109.

65 Dols, *Black Death*, p. 102.

66 The exception here is al-Yahūdī, who listed many of these suggestions to treat 'wabāʾ' but then added that they can also protect one from 'ṭāʿūn'.

67 While Ibn Sīnā does not cite his sources, his introductory discussion has been read as a veiled critique of al-Majūsī; see Savage-Smith, 'Medicine', p. 922.

swellings to explain the nature of compound diseases. Like al-Majūsī, he categorises the various types of swellings, but then departs slightly by claiming that an abscess is when both blood and yellow bile are found together in a swelling. Only when 'this abscess occurs in the soft flesh, such as the armpits, behind the ears, and the groin, and it is of a corrupt kind, it is called a plague bubo ('wa-idhā waqaʿa al-khurāj fī al-luḥūm al-rakhw wa-l-maghābin wa-khalf al-udhnayn wa-l-urbiyya wa-kāna min jins fāsid summā ṭāʿūnan')', and these he claims he will discuss later.[68]

Ibn Sīnā discusses plague specifically in a chapter within the first 'maqāla' (article) of part three of book four (*Canon* IV.3.1), amid a larger discussion of hot swellings and pustules. However, he also makes scattered remarks about plague buboes across book four. For example, following the dominant interpretation of *Aphorisms* IV.55, Ibn Sīnā discusses plague swellings in his section on ephemeral fevers (*Canon* IV.1.1). Like al-Sinjārī's *Commentary*, Ibn Sīnā does not mention plague buboes specifically, but reworks the passage from the *Summary of Glaucon* to claim that fevers accompanied by swellings due to hidden causes include abscesses that form in the soft, glandular flesh, 'such as those that occur in the groin out of the wastes of the liver, and the armpit out of the wastes of the heart, and behind the ear out of the wastes of the brain ('mathal allatī taqaʿ fī al-urbiyya ʿan fuḍūl al-kabid wa-l-ibṭ ʿan fuḍūl al-qalb wa-taḥta al-udhun ʿan fuḍūl al-dimāgh')'. If these swellings are merely due to the warmth of the wastes, then the resulting fever could still be ephemeral, but if the warmth is accompanied by corruption, then it is not. Ibn Sīnā states that Hippocrates called the latter kind 'harmful ('khabītha')'.[69] We thus see that the Arabic commentators on *Aphorisms* IV.55 were relying on a theoretical understanding of plague swellings found in the *Summary of Glaucon* that was also accepted by al-Rāzī, al-Majūsī and Ibn Sīnā.

Like al-Majūsī, Ibn Sīnā connected plague directly to epidemic diseases. In his introductory discussion of swellings (*Canon* IV.3.1), Ibn Sīnā classifies the various kinds of swellings just as al-Majūsī (and Galen) had. He then adds, 'When the matter in a hot swelling is abundant and the swelling becomes very large, then [the swelling] is one of the lethal plague swellings ('wa-idhā katharat māddat al-waram al-ḥārr wa-ʿaẓuma al-waram jiddan fa-huwa min jumlat al-awrām al-ṭāʿūniyya al-qattāla')'. Such lethal plague swellings prevail 'in the year of an epidemic ('fī sanat al-wabāʾ')'.[70] Although Ibn Sīnā does not single out plague ('ṭāʿūn') in his general discussion of epidemic fevers (*Canon* IV.1.2), the explicit connection he makes between plagues and epidemics implies that many of the symptoms, causes and treatments he described for epidemics may apply to plague too. For example, in addressing al-Majūsī's assertion that lethal epidemics such as plague are caused by a corruption in the substance ('jawhar') of air, Ibn Sīnā explains that, like water, air is only corrupted when it is mixed with bad vapours and never in its simple, elemental

68 Ibn Sīnā, *al-Qānūn fī al-ṭibb*, 3 vols., ed. M. A. al-Dinnawi, (Beirut, 1999), I, 107–8.

69 Ibid., III, 20–1.

70 Ibid., III, 153–4.

state.[71] As a philosopher, Ibn Sīnā used terms such as essence or substance ('jawhar') very carefully and any corruption caused by mixing with vapours, no matter how bad, could not technically be a corruption of the essence of the simple element, air. In an earlier passage from book one, Ibn Sīnā similarly explains that the phrase 'corruption in the substance of air' does not imply a corruption of the simple element air, but, rather, of the ambient air that is a mixture of elements.[72]

Ibn Sīnā explained that air could be corrupted in many ways. Once corrupted, air ruins the spirit in the heart, which is then distributed throughout the body through arteries. This corruption can generate symptoms such as heavy breathing, shortness of breath, thirst, loss of appetite, delirium ('ikhtilāṭ al-ʿaql'), cough, tiredness, etc. Many of these symptoms are found amongst plague patients, but Ibn Sīnā's list is not restricted to plague.[73] He also listed numerous earthly and cosmic signs that portend the coming of an epidemic. One such earthly sign is the sight of rats and other ground-burrowing animals fleeing to the surface. Since rodents are now known to be hosts of *Y. pestis* and the vectors (fleas) that transmit the disease to humans, Dols had highlighted this passage for its novelty, as it is not found in Galen's works.[74] Notably, however, Ibn Sīnā maintained that fleeing rats signified epidemics ('wabāʾ') generally speaking, not plague ('ṭāʿūn') specifically. As far as I know, no Arabic commentary on the *Aphorisms*, the *Canon* or the *Epitome* ever connected rats specifically to plague. For treatment and prevention, Ibn Sīnā recommended bloodletting, evacuations, purging, cooling fragrances, vinegar and sour foods and juices. In short, almost all the recommendations for treatment and prevention associated with 'wabāʾ' in the works of al-Rāzī and al-Majūsī are found in the *Canon* and, hence, in plague tracts from the 1350s onwards.[75]

Ibn Sīnā begins his section on plague buboes in the *Canon* by reconstructing a terminological history of 'ṭāʿūn'. He states that the ancients characterised a swelling in glandular flesh (sensitive or not) with a term translated into Arabic as 'ṭāʿūn'. The word was then used to characterise a potentially lethal, hot swelling in these areas. Ibn Sīnā explains that lethal swellings arise because their matter is transformed into a poisonous substance that corrupts members. And, if such a swelling leaks blood and/or pus, it harms the heart and initiates vomiting, palpitation and fainting. If these symptoms intensify, the patient dies. He then clarifies that this last type of swelling is what the ancients called 'qūmāṭa' – a

71 Ibid., III, 87.

72 Ibid., I, 125. Medical and religious works on plague from the 1350s onwards regularly claimed that plague is caused by a corruption in the 'essence of air', where the latter phrase is understood, following Ibn Sīnā, to mean the corruption of the ambient air and not the simple element; Dols, *Black Death*, pp. 87–90.

73 Ibn Sīnā, *al-Qānūn fī al-ṭibb*, III, 87–9.

74 Ibid., III, p. 89. Dols suggested the possibility that Ibn Sīnā had either learned of this phenomenon from 'earlier Arabic medical commentaries …, from non-medical writers' or perhaps his own observations; *Black Death*, p. 89.

75 Ibn Sīnā, *al-Qānūn fī al-ṭibb*, III, 89–90; and Dols, *Black Death*, pp. 98–109.

lethal swelling that often occurs in weak members, the most dangerous being those 'in the armpits and behind the ears, due to their proximity to the members that are the most chief ('fī al-ābāṭ wa-khalf al-udhun li-qurbihā min al-aʿḍāʾ allatī hiya ashaddu riyāsa')'.[76] Ibn Sīnā thus changed a mainstay of the *Summary of Glaucon* and earlier commentaries, which suggested that the swelling behind the ears (or in the jaws) is less lethal than the swelling in the groin. It is unclear whether Ibn Sīnā made the change based on his own experience or on his theoretical understanding of the chief organs and their roles in the body. He also stated that the safest ('aslam') bubo is red in colour, the next safest green, while buboes that tend towards black almost always kill. This same colour classification is present in Ahrun's work cited by al-Rāzī.[77]

Ibn Sīnā's suggested treatments for plague are similar to those proposed for other epidemics, such as bloodletting and evacuations to remove corrupted humours and various foods, juices and fragrances to strengthen the heart, such as lemon, pomegranate juice, roses and water lilies. More specifically, he recommends using specific bandages and dressings for treating the buboes and their poison. In linking specific bandages to the buboes' stage of development, Ibn Sīnā moved beyond al-Majūsī and other earlier authors, although he may have deduced his specific treatment recommendations theoretically, since he referred his readers to an earlier discussion on bandaging abscesses ('khurāj').[78]

al-Masīḥī's treatise on epidemics

One final text from the tenth/eleventh century is worth considering here, a treatise devoted to epidemics and how to protect oneself from them. The treatise has been characterised as a plague treatise, although the text actually deals with epidemics more generally.[79] Entitled *Risāla fī taḥqīq amr al-wabāʾ wa-l-iḥtirāz minhu wa-iṣlāḥihi idhā waqaʿa* (Treatise on the investigation of the state of the epidemic, protecting [oneself] from it and treating it when it strikes), it was the work of Ibn Sīnā's teacher, Abū Sahl al-Masīḥī (d. 1010).[80]

Much of al-Masīḥī's text provides an overview of the standard Hippocratic/Galenic theory of diseases based on *Airs, Waters and Places*. It defines a non-lethal epidemic ('wabāʾ') as follows: 'a disease that [affects] most bodies in a single region due to the

76 Ibn Sīnā, *a-Qānūn fī al-ṭibb*, III, 164–5. Conrad dismissed Ibn Sīnā's history of the term *ṭāʿūn* and its Greek equivalents, stating that 'Ibn Sīnā is at this point very much misinformed'; '*Ṭāʿūn* and *Wabāʾ*', p. 295. However, Conrad's dismissal is premised on the notion that the 'term ṭāʿūn does not figure significantly in the Arabic translations of the Greek medical corpus', which I have just shown is not correct.

77 Ibn Sīnā, *al-Qānūn fī al-ṭibb*, III, 164–5.

78 Ibid., III, 165; cf. Dols, *Black Death*, pp. 105–9.

79 Dols, p. 28, n. 52.

80 G. Karmi, 'A Mediaeval Compendium of Arabic Medicine: Abū Sahl al-Masīḥī's "Book of Hundred"', *Journal for the History of Arabic Science* 2 (1978), 270–90 (p. 272); and L. Gari (Qārī), '*Risāla fī taḥqīq amr al-wabāʾ wa-l-iḥtirāz minhu wa-iṣlāḥihi idhā waqaʿa* taʾlīf Abī Sahl al-Masīḥī', *Journal for the History of Arabic Sciences* 13 (2005), 5–56.

corruption of the air ('huwa al-maraḍ al-ʿāmm li-akthar al-abdān fī buqʿa wāḥida min jiha fasād al-hawāʾ)'.[81] By contrast, a lethal epidemic is caused by corruption of the air such that it has the rank of poison and this generates a 'mawtān'. The text characterises three distinct causes for epidemics: excessive heat and moisture, excessive dryness and 'the air changing to a strange quality, or mixing with a vapour possessing a strange quality that is inappropriate for the human body such that it has the rank of poison. A "mawtān" is most often caused by this ('yataghayyar al-hawāʾ ilā kayfiyya gharība aw yukhāliṭuhu bukhār gharīb al-kayfiyya ghayra munāsib li-l-badan al-insānī ḥattā yakūn bi-manzilat al-samm wa-min hādhā yakun al-mawtān akthar')'.[82] 'Mawtānā' was the word used to describe plague outbreaks in pre-ninth-century Syriac chronicles. Some Arabic plague tracts also used the term 'mawtān' to refer to plague outbreaks.[83] It is possible that al-Masīḥī was describing plague ('mawtān') as an epidemic caused by air that had acquired a poison-like quality; this would align with al-Majūsī and Ibn Sīnā's contemporary understanding of plague ('ṭāʿūn').

Al-Masīḥī devoted part of his text to describing the various signs and symptoms of epidemic diseases, as the ancients had confirmed. According to al-Masīḥī, Galen had maintained that patients suffering from epidemic diseases suffer from bilious swellings in the mouth, a hot chest, abundant urine (thick or thin, cloudy or with dregs of black bile), excessive thirst, a desire for cold water and hot, burning eyes.[84] Al-Masīḥī, then, like al-Rāzī, quoted the Rufus passage from Oribasius stating that 'delirium accompanies a pestilential plague ('yaʿruḍ maʿa al-ṭāʿūn al-wabāʾī ikthilāṭ al-ʿaql')'.[85] But, like al-Rāzī, al-Masīḥī did not refer to any swellings in the glandular regions, even though the original text of Oribasius describes the swellings in detail.[86] Later, when al-Masīḥī turned to his 'experience ('jarrabtu')' to describe symptoms of 'wabāʾ', he described pustules – but not in the glandular flesh – and omitted delusions.[87] It seems highly unlikely, then, that al-Masīḥī had any direct experience with plague.

Summary of the pre-1240 texts

Comparing the compendia and al-Masīḥī's plague tract as a whole to the earlier *Summary of Glaucon* and the later *Aphorisms* commentaries reveals many similarities, but also some noteworthy differences. First, both al-Mājūsī and Ibn Sīnā devoted considerable time to understanding the causes of plague and recommending preventative measures and treatments, unlike the *Aphorisms* commentators, who briefly described and classified the various plague swellings but offered no recommendations. Second, the encyclopaedists explained

81 Gari, '*Risāla fī taḥqīq*', p. 21.
82 Ibid., p. 27.
83 Dols, *Black Death*, pp. 316–17.
84 Gari, '*Risāla*', p. 37.
85 Ibid.
86 The Greek text and translation can be found in Mulhall, 'Plague before Pandemics', p. 166.
87 Gari, '*Risāla*', p. 39.

the causes of plague in far more detail than did the *Aphorisms* commentaries. Third, unlike for other glandular swellings, al-Majūsī (but not Ibn Sīnā) claimed that plague buboes erupt quickly, an observation that is absent in the *Summary of Glaucon* and the *Aphorisms* commentaries but that accords well with our modern clinical understanding of the disease. These differences reveal that for al-Majūsī and Ibn Sīnā plague was a real concern, perhaps because the disease was still ravaging some communities in Iraq and Iran into the early tenth century. Moreover, al-Majūsī and Ibn Sīnā's theoretical conceptualisation of plague as a lethal, epidemic disease ('wabāʾ') caused by a corruption in the substance of air moves beyond what is found in the *Summary of Glaucon* and earlier Greek, Syriac and Arabic works. In terms of treatment recommendations too, the encyclopaedists added to the early medical communities' enshrined experience of plague.

Despite their clear interest in and awareness of the disease, however, none of the encyclopaedists succinctly brought together the various symptoms and conditions of a plague patient. For example, Ibn Sīnā reconstructed a linguistic history for plague swellings, interspersing it with descriptions of symptoms and how they arise, rather than providing a quick description of the symptoms that a physician could use to identify the disease. Moreover, from his work, one learns that: (a) plague involves a hot, corrupt swelling/abscess made of blood and yellow bile that occurs in the soft flesh, especially armpits, groin and behind the ears and prevails in times of epidemics; (b) the swellings in the armpits and ears are the most lethal; (c) the swellings can cause vomiting, palpitation and fainting; and (d) the red-coloured bubo is the safest, followed by the green, while the black is almost always fatal. Ibn Sīnā did not say much about the intensity of pain or fever, though that may be inferred. He talked about neither the quick eruption of the swellings nor the speed with which an afflicted person dies. This suggests that even if the communal memory of plague was fresher in their time, al-Rāzī, al-Masīḥī and Ibn Sīnā (and possibly even al-Majūsī) had no direct personal experience with the disease, unlike with smallpox.[88] The commentators from the mid-thirteenth century onwards, by contrast, articulated the symptoms of plague much more precisely and concisely, suggesting that these authors had more hands-on knowledge of the disease.

Post-1240 Arabic medical writings

Palaeogenetic and phylogenetic evidence suggest that four lineages of *Yersinia pestis* could have emerged in the thirteenth century. Arabic and Persian literary sources from that period claim that an epidemic disease ('wabāʾ') accompanied the destruction of Baghdad and other cities during the second Mongol invasion of the Middle East in the late 1250s, spreading all the way to Syria (and possibly Egypt). The medical commentaries of that era, as I shall show, support Green's claims that the strain of *Yersinia pestis* that might have given rise to the Second Pandemic in Western Eurasia was brought by Mongols from the

88 For example, compare Ibn Sīnā's discussions of these diseases; *al-Qānūn fī al-ṭibb*, III, 90–2 (smallpox) and 164–5 (plague).

Tian Shan mountains and seeded in Iran and its surrounding regions during the second half of the thirteenth century.[89]

The earliest of the thirteenth-century works that adds new information about plague is Ibn al-Nafīs's (d. 1288) *Commentary on the Canon* – the first lemmatic commentary on all five books of Ibn Sīnā's *Canon*. Book one of the *Commentary* was completed at the latest by 1242, somewhere in Syria or Egypt.[90] While commenting on two separate passages of the *Canon* – the exact passages in which Ibn Sīnā discusses plague in books one and four – Ibn al-Nafīs refers to his friend, Shams al-Dīn al-Makkī, witnessing plague in Ethiopia. At least two subsequent scholars, whose works were widely read in the fourteenth and fifteenth centuries, included this account of plague in Ethiopia in their works.[91] Ibn al-Nafīs never mentions encountering plague himself, nor does he suggest that plague had broken out in Syria and Egypt at this time.

While commenting on *Canon* I.2.1, Ibn al-Nafīs explains some of the technical terms, such as abscesses, and their relationship to swellings. He also clarifies that moist, soft flesh is by nature more susceptible to being corrupted by the hot and moist matter that causes plague. He further cites *Aphorisms* IV.55, i.e. non-ephemeral fevers accompanied by a swelling in certain areas are bad, to emphasise the danger that plague buboes pose. This represents the continuing use of this particular *Aphorism* for plague discussions. At this point, Ibn al-Nafīs recounts his friend's experience in Ḥabasha (Ethiopia), a passage worth quoting in full.[92]

> A friend of mine had traveled to the region of the Ethiopians, and upon returning to ʿAqal[93] related to me that many of its people die due to plague. They call it there

[89] Green, 'Four Black Deaths'. Also see, N. Fancy and M. H. Green, 'Plague and the Fall of Baghdad', *Medical History* 65 (2021), 157–77.

[90] For the dating of his work and biography, see N. Fancy, *Science and Religion in Mamluk Egypt: Ibn al-Nafīs, Pulmonary Transit and Bodily Resurrection* (New York, 2013). The UCLA manuscript (Biomedical Library, MS Ar. 80) of his *Commentary on the Anatomy*, which was appended to the commentary on book 1 of the *Canon*, was copied in 1242; E. Savage-Smith, 'Attitudes Toward Dissection in Medieval Islam', *Journal of the History of Medicine and Allied Sciences* 50 (1995), 67–110 (p. 99). All copies of Ibn al-Nafīs's commentary on book 1 that I have accessed post-date the fourteenth century.

[91] Dols, *Black Death*, p. 15.

[92] For most of Ibn al-Nafīs's contemporaries and predecessors, 'ḥabasha' signified the coastal region of the Horn of Africa and not the Ethiopian highlands; however, as I show below, Ibn al-Nafīs actually meant Ethiopia when he used the term 'ḥabasha'.

[93] I am not certain of this transcription. ʿAqal is a coastal region in the Qatar peninsula; J. G. Lorimer, *Gazetteer of the Persian Gulf, ʿOmān and Central Arabia, Volume II: Geographical and Statistical* (Calcutta, 1908), part 1, pp. 88–9. There is also an ʿAqal in modern south-western Saudi Arabia. Ḥaql was a port in the Gulf of Aqaba, close to which the Mamluk Sultan Baybars (r. 1260–77) had built a lodge ('khān') to serve Ḥajj pilgrims; S. S. 'Abd al-Malik, 'The *Khans* of the Egyptian Hajj Route in the Mamluk and Ottoman Periods', in *The Hajj: Collected Essays*, ed. V. Porter and L. Saif (London, 2013), pp. 52–64.

'jaghala'/'jufla'.[94] It occurs most often in the glandular flesh. Most of the deadly ones do not attain the size of a walnut when they are accompanied by extreme pain, excessive distress, and vomiting of various colours. The sound one from amongst them is that which is very small in size from which a piece like dead flesh emerges when slit. In such a case, one recovers quickly. He [i.e., Shams al-Din] said: when it enters a region, it spreads amongst its people. Whenever one person in a house is afflicted by it, it spreads to all its residents. He said: when it strikes, the people of that region see an army that descends amidst drum beats with swordsmen, spearmen, banners and the rest. Whosoever sees that army deems that if one of them were to throw at him an arrow, or a spear or the like, then the plague bubo would occur on the location where that [spear, etc.] struck. Those struck thus hear the discourse of [the soldiers] and see their movements. I say: it is not unlikely that in its first instance, the disease corrupts the imagination such that one sees that. Perhaps it was originally named from the root word [for piercing] a 'ṭāʿūn' for that reason.[95]

(ṣadīq lī sāfara ilā arḍ al-ḥabasha fa-rajaʿa ilā ʿAqal ḥakā an akthar mawt ahlihā bi-l-ṭāʿūn wa-hum yusammūnahu hunāk jaghala wa-taḥdath aktharahu fī al-luḥūm al-rakhwa wa-ghālib al-qātil minhu lā yablugh qadr al-jawza wa-yaʿruḍ maʿahu alam shadīd wa-karb mufriṭ wa-qayʾ mukhtalif al-alwān wa-l-salīm minhu wa-huwa qalīl jiddan bi-ʿiẓam wa-idhā buṭṭa ukhrijat minhu qiṭʿa ka-annahā laḥm mayyit wa-bariʾa bi-surʿa qāla wa-idhā dakhala bi-balda ʿamma ahlahā wa-ayy bayt aṣāba wāḥidan fīhi ʿamma ahlahu wa-ʿindamā yaḥdath yushāhid ahl dhālik al-balad ʿaskaran qad nazala bi-hum bi-ṭubūl wa-l-suyūf wa-l-ḥirāb wa-l-bayāriq wa-ghayrihā wa-man yushāhid dhālik al-ʿaskar raʾa qad rashaqahu aḥaduhum bi-sahm aw bi-ḥarba aw ghayra dhālik fa-yaḥdath al-ṭāʿūn fī al-mawḍiʿ alladhī aṣābahu bi-tilka wa-in dhālik alladhī uṣība yasmaʿu kalāmahum wa-yushāhid ḥarakātahum aqūl lā yabʿud an yakūn dhālik al-maraḍ yalzam awwal ḥudūthihi fasād fī al-khayāl ḥattā yushāhid dhālik wa-laʿalla mabdāʾan tasmiyya fī al-aṣl ṭāʿūnan innamā kāna ka-dhālik.)

94 Dols transcribed the word as *jaghala*, since that is how it appears in plague treatises that cite Ibn al-Nafīs's account (*Black Death*, p. 15). Selassie was unable to find a corresponding word to 'jaghala' in Ethiopic languages. The closest he found was 'hglah', which is described as a famine that occurred in the Muslim sultanate of Shewa in 1272/3. Y. G. Selassie, 'Plague as Possible Factor for the Decline and Collapse of the Aksumite Empire: A New Interpretation', *Ityopis* 1 (2011), 36–61 (p. 50). Unfortunately, this event occurred thirty years after Ibn al-Nafīs composed his commentary, so it cannot be the event described by him. The word in Fazıl Ahmed Paşa's manuscript resembles more 'jufla' (or 'ḥufla' or 'khufla'), as does the quoted passage in the Ayasofya manuscript of Quṭb al-Dīn al-Shīrāzī's commentary (see below).

95 Ibn al-Nafīs, *Sharḥ al-Qānūn*, Istanbul, Süleymaniye Library, MS Ayasofya 3648, fol. 141b; Istanbul, Süleymaniye Library, MS Fazıl Ahmed Paşa 969, fol. 48b; and London, Wellcome Library, MS Arabic 51, fol. 67a. http://wellcomelibrary.org/item/b20294979#?c=0&m=0&s=0&cv=3&z=-0.6572%2C-0.0788%2C2.3144%2C1.5751, last accessed 11 September 2019.

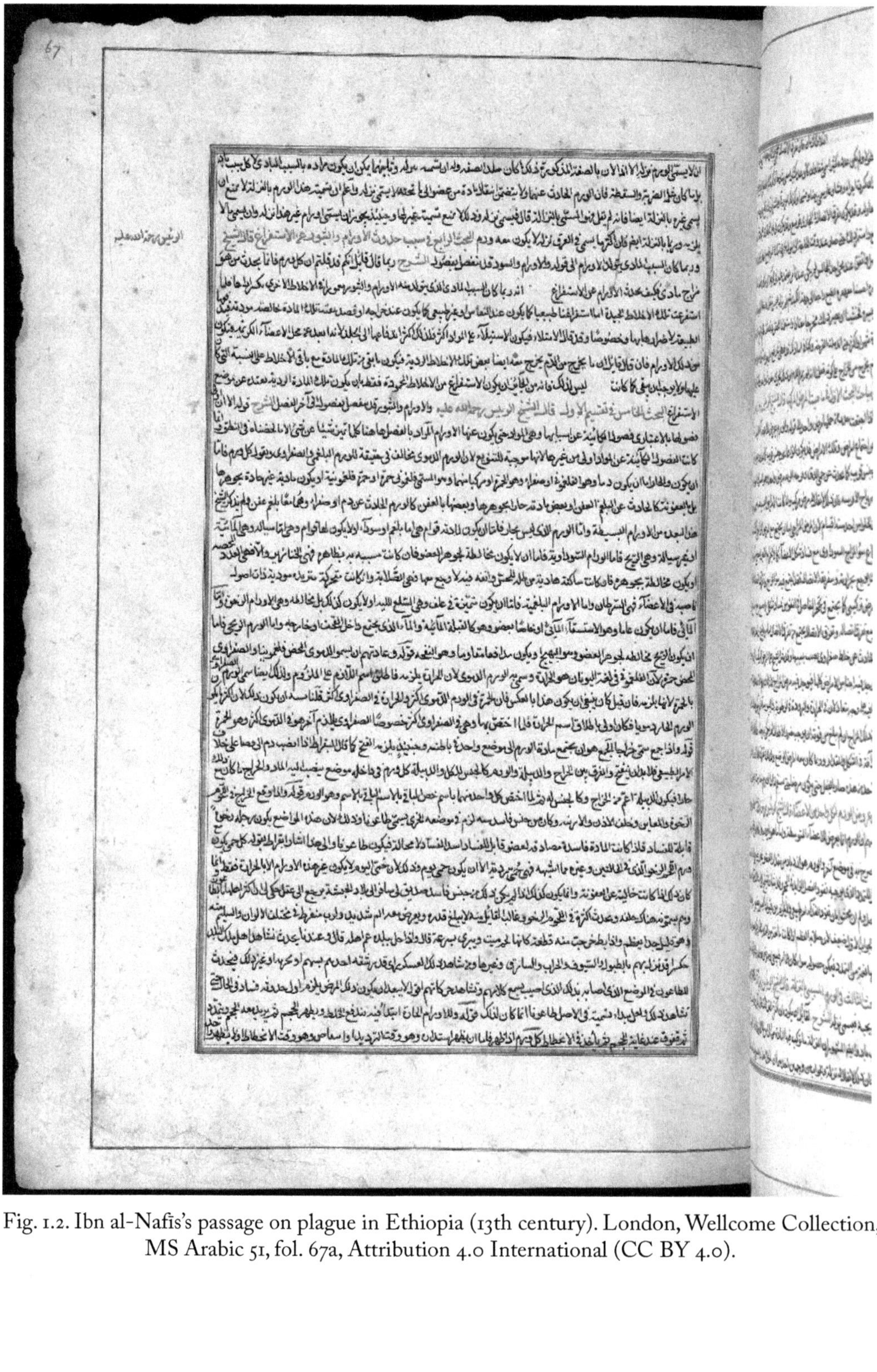

Fig. 1.2. Ibn al-Nafīs's passage on plague in Ethiopia (13th century). London, Wellcome Collection, MS Arabic 51, fol. 67a, Attribution 4.0 International (CC BY 4.0).

Given the earlier Arabic medical tradition on plague, this description is truly remarkable. It confirms that Ibn al-Nafīs's friend encountered the disease in the Ethiopian highlands.[96] Extreme pain and vomiting are associated with plague, as are delirium, fever and buboes. The delirium is very clearly described in the words of Shams al-Dīn. The imagery of the army marching downhill accompanied by drum beats and banners is not uniquely Ethiopian; it is, however, significantly different from descriptions of plague delusions found in other works, such as those of Procopius or Ibn Ḥajar al-ʿAsqalānī (d. 1449).[97] Ibn al-Nafīs directly equated these visions with a corruption of the imagination, even going so far as to suggest that plague was probably called 'ṭāʿūn' in Arabic due to these visions of piercing.[98] It is worth highlighting that the disease was not new in Ethiopia: it already had a name in an Ethiopic language, suggesting a long-standing experience with plague.

That Ibn al-Nafīs's friend visited inner Ethiopia and not just the coastal regions of the Horn of Africa is confirmed by a later passage in book one of his *Commentary on the Canon*. In a passage on the effects of habitats (*Canon* I.2.2), Ibn Sīnā had claimed that the land of Ḥabasha (the Horn of Africa for him) is extremely hot, which is why its people are dark and age quickly. Ibn al-Nafīs, on the authority of Shams al-Dīn and some 'ḥabashī' male servants, corrected Ibn Sīnā by pointing out that Ḥabasha (inland Ethiopia for Ibn al-Nafīs) is much more temperate and akin to Damascus. It is also very fertile and filled with trees.[99] This correction of Ibn Sīnā's assertions and description of inland Ethiopia lends further credibility to Shams al-Dīn's report on plague.

Ibn al-Nafīs mentioned Shams al-Dīn's account again while commenting on *Canon* IV.3.1. In this passage too, Ibn al-Nafīs suggests that 'these swellings are called buboes ('ammā tasmiyya hādhihi al-awrām bi-l-ṭawāʿīn')' due to the fact that the manner in which

96 Marie-Laure Derat has only been able to find references to plague outbreaks in the Horn of Africa that occurred later in the thirteenth century, e.g. in the Muslim sultanate of Šawā (modern day Somalia) in 1262 and 1274–75 CE. 'Du lexique aux talismans: occurrences de la peste dans la Corne de l'Afrique au XIIIe et XVe siècle', *Afriques: débats, méthodes et terrains d'histoire* 9 (2018), https://journals.openedition.org/afriques/2090, last accessed 27 September 2019. In the absence of archaeological samples of *Yersinia pestis* from Ethiopia and the Horn of Africa we cannot be certain, but it is possible that the plague outbreaks that Shams al-Dīn witnessed in Ethiopia were due to a First Pandemic lineage of the bacterium.

97 Procopius, *History of the Wars*, trans. H. B. Dewing, Loeb Classical Library, 6 vols. (New York, 1914), I, 455; Ibn Ḥajar al-ʿAsqalānī, *Badhl al-māʿūn fī faḍl al-ṭāʿūn*, ed. A. Q. al-Kātib (Riyadh, n.d.), pp. 102–22.

98 The connection between piercing by lances and plague is captured in a famous, non-canonical Prophetic tradition and in Arabic lexicographical works; see Conrad, '*Ṭāʿūn* and *Wabāʾ*', p. 292. This tradition plays a key role in Ibn Ḥajar's claim that plague is caused by the jinn; see Dols, *Black Death*, pp. 115–17.

99 Ibn al-Nafīs, *Sharḥ al-Qānūn*, MS Arabic 51, fols. 78a–b; MS Ayasofya 3648, fols. 162b–3a; and MS Fazıl Ahmed Paşa 969, fol. 64b. Also see my 'Verification and Utility: Authorial and Exegetical Practices in the Commentaries on the *Canon of Medicine* of Fakhr al-Dīn al-Rāzī (d. 1210) and Ibn al-Nafīs (d. 1288)', *Journal of the History of Medicine and Allied Sciences* 75 (2020), 361–82 (pp. 377–8).

'their matter penetrates the affected member ('māddatuhā tanfudh ilā al-ʿuḍw alladhī yuʿriḍ lahu')' is quite like 'something that pierces, like a lance, and the like ('nufūdh mā yaṭʿan bihi wa-huwa al-rumḥ wa-naḥwahu')'.[100] He then repeats his friend's story about the delusional visions of infected Ethiopians, noting that the disease is prevalent in the region and called 'jaghala'/'jufla'. Not much is added to the earlier description, but Ibn al-Nafīs mentions that his friend was a jurist who stayed in Ethiopia for some time and is more commonly known as Ibn ʿAsū.[101] He also clarifies that the afflicted mistakenly deem the delusions to be real.

The remaining commentary on this section glosses Ibn Sīnā's text. For example, Ibn al-Nafīs explains that buboes occur in soft, glandular flesh because these regions are by nature the most susceptible to corruption. He deems the location behind the ears to be the primary site of such corruption due to its proximity to the moist brain.[102] In terms of treatment, Ibn al-Nafīs objects to Ibn Sīnā's recommendation to use cooling and compressing treatments on the buboes, considering this treatment to be 'a grave mistake ('fa-huwa ʿindī min al-ghalaṭ al-ʿaẓīm')'.[103] He explains that since a bubonic swelling's matter is so corrupt, it would be 'extremely dangerous ('ghāʾila shadīda')' if any of it were to return to 'the body's interior depth ('ʿamq al-badan')', particularly since the sites for plague buboes receive materials from the respective chief organs.[104] Ibn al-Nafīs never claimed to have encountered plague, so either his recommendation was based on his theoretical understanding of the disease or, perhaps, Shams al-Dīn informed him about suppurating buboes and how they can improve the health of a patient.[105] Recall that in the first passage Shams al-Dīn stated that an object like dead flesh emerging from an opened bubo often signalled a quick recovery.

Unlike his *Canon* commentary, Ibn al-Nafīs's commentary on *Aphorisms* IV.55 is brief. Ibn al-Nafīs explains that non-ephemeral fevers accompanied by swellings in the soft glandular flesh are bad, corrupt fevers, since this type of flesh is excessively moist and thus susceptible to corruption.[106] If the corruption is excessive, then the swelling turns into a plague bubo ('ṭāʿūn') 'which is lethal ('wa-huwa qattāl')'.[107] Ibn al-Nafīs's commentary on this aphorism is different from earlier commentators, although like his predecessors his focus in this work was to briefly explain how buboes form and why they are bad, not

[100] Ibn al-Nafīs, *Sharḥ al-Qānūn*, Istanbul, Süleymaniye Library, MS Şehid Ali Paşa 2051, fol. 691a.

[101] The name is slightly erased in the Şehid Ali Paşa manuscript but is more clearly visible in the Wellcome manuscript: MS Arabic 51, fol. 528a.

[102] Ibn al-Nafīs, *Sharḥ al-Qānūn*, MS Şehid Ali Paşa 2051, fol. 691a.

[103] Ibid., fol. 691a; and Ibn Sīnā, *al-Qānūn fī al-ṭibb*, III, 165.

[104] Ibn al-Nafīs, *Sharḥ al-Qānūn*, MS Şehid Ali Paşa 2051, fol. 691a.

[105] Modern clinical experience suggests that if buboes suppurate, the patient's health improves dramatically, though it may not always lead to recovery, since the risk of secondary infection is high in such cases; Nikiforov et al., 'Plague', p. 299.

[106] Ibn al-Nafīs, *Sharḥ Fuṣūl Abuqrāṭ*, ed. Y. Zaydan (Cairo, 1991), p. 319.

[107] Ibid., p. 320.

treating them. In both the *Aphorisms* commentary and the *Canon* commentary, however, we detect a distinct shift away from the material found in the *Summary of Glaucon*.

Ibn al-Nafīs's contemporary, Ibn al-Quff al-Karakī (1232–86), a Christian physician-surgeon from Syria and modern-day Jordan, also composed well-known commentaries on the *Aphorisms* and the *Canon*. Although I have not been able to examine his passage on plague swellings found in book one of the *Canon*, his commentary on *Aphorisms* IV.55, completed in 1282, moves beyond what is found in the earlier commentaries.[108]

Ibn al-Quff divided his comments on this aphorism into three investigations ('mabāḥith').[109] In the first, he briefly explained that both ephemeral and non-ephemeral fevers are linked because the swellings that occur in the soft flesh can result in a corrupt fever or an ephemeral fever. The corrupt fever occurs if the swelling causes corrupt vapours to rise to the heart.[110] In the second investigation, he addressed the specific sites of these swellings, namely the soft, glandular flesh of the groin, etc. Ibn al-Quff suggested that these areas accept matter easily due to 'their weakness ('li-sakhāfatihā'), their instability of form ('takhalkhulihā')' and their inability to expel this matter because of 'their weak expulsive faculty ('li-ḍuʿf dāfiʿatihā')'. As a result, the matter collects and becomes corrupted, causing corrupt vapours to rise from them and generate intense corrupt fevers. The three specific locations that he noted – the groin, armpits and behind the ears – likewise act as 'recipients for [the wastes of] the chief organs ('maghāyaḍ li-l-aʿḍāʾ al-raʾīsa')'. Thus, when these sites are harmed, the harm proceeds to the chief organs. The matter that flows from the swellings in these sites is especially harmful because the collected matter 'changes into a poisonous kind ('tastaḥīl ʿalā kayfiyya sammiyya')' and much of the poisonous matter 'becomes a plague bubo ('yaṣīr ṭāʿūnan')'.[111]

Whereas the first two investigations are largely similar to what is found in the *Aphorisms* commentary tradition going back to the *Summary of Glaucon*, the third investigation includes some genuinely novel aspects. Here, Ibn al-Quff first explains that the word buboes was used in the past to refer to all swellings that occurred in 'the three recipients ('al-maghāyaḍ al-thalātha')', namely the groin, armpits and behind the ears. Then, people restricted ('thumma khaṣṣaṣū') the word to mean 'a cold or hot swelling that occurs under the armpits and is changed into a poisonous kind ('bi-l-waram al-bārid aw al-ḥārr al-ḥāṣil taḥta al-ibṭayn al-mustaḥīl ilā kayfiyya sammiyya')'.[112] This passage is reminiscent of the passage in Ibn Sīnā's *Canon* (IV.3.1) that recounts the terminological history of the Arabic

108 Pormann and Joosse, 'Commentaries on the Hippocratic *Aphorisms*', p. 236, n. 167.

109 For more on Ibn al-Quff's exegetical style and its reliance on Fakhr al-Dīn al-Rāzī's method of 'taḥqīq' (verification), see K. Karimullah, 'The Emergence of Verification (*Taḥqīq*) in Islamic Medicine: The Exegetical Legacy of Fakhr al-Dīn al-Rāzī's (d. 1210) Commentary on Avicenna's (d. 1037) *Canon of Medicine*', *Oriens* 47 (2019), 1–113.

110 Ibn al-Quff, *Commentary on the Hippocratic Aphorisms, Book Four*, ed. Pormann et al., pp. 85–6, http://doi.org/10.3927/52132103, last accessed 11 September 2019.

111 Ibid., p. 86.

112 Ibid.

term and its Greek counterparts. The discussion in the *Aphorisms* commentary, however, deviates from the *Canon* significantly, since Ibn al-Quff had no interest in correlating the Arabic term to its possible Greek predecessors. Moreover, he stated that the term had come to signify a 'cold or hot' swelling located specifically in 'the armpits' (the *Canon* does not confine its location as such).[113] Ibn al-Quff then added more information about the disease at the conclusion of this investigation:

> From amongst the characteristics of the [bubo] are a bad odour, black colour around the swelling, fainting on some occasions, and cold sweat. All this (happens) when the poisonous vapours reach the heart from it ('min ʿalāmatihi ridāʾat al-rāʾiḥa wa-sawād lawn mā ḥawla al-waram wa-ḥuṣūl ghashy fī baʿḍ al-awqāt wa-ʿaraq bārid kull hādhā la-mā yaṣil minhu ilā al-qalb min al-abkhira al-sammiyya').[114]

These clinical descriptions are very precise. They are not brought together as concisely in either the earlier *Aphorisms* commentaries or the encyclopaedias. There is thus a distinct possibility that Ibn al-Quff either had direct experience with the disease or knew someone who had, since no physician, including Ibn al-Nafīs, whose friend had witnessed plague, mentioned the odour of the buboes or chills/cold sweat.[115] We know that Ibn al-Quff's teacher's patron, the Ayyubid ruler of Karak, al-Malik al-Nāṣir Dāwūd, died of plague in 1258 in Syria.[116]

The works of Quṭb al-Dīn al-Shīrāzī (d. 1311) increase the possibility that Ibn al-Quff was aware of plague outbreaks that had taken place across Syria and Iraq during his lifetime.

[113] Ibn al-Quff provides a similar terminological history of the term for plague in his earlier encyclopaedic work on surgery; *Kitāb al-ʿumda fī ṣināʿat al-jirāḥa*, London, British Library, Oriental Manuscripts, MS 23409, fol. 41b, https://www.qdl.qa/en/archive/81055/vdc_100022565463.0x000001, last accessed 1 June 2020. Here too, Ibn al-Quff restricts the swelling to the armpits: 'This word [i.e. 'ṭāʿūn'/'ṭawāʿīn'] was first applied in the Greek language to every swelling that occurs in the glandular flesh, such as behind the ears, in the armpits and in the groin, regardless of whether (the swelling) is cold or hot. Then it was restricted after that and applied to hot swellings that obtain in the aforementioned places. Then it was restricted and applied to only those that occur under the armpits. Then only to a blood-based swelling that has been transformed into a bad, poisonous quality'. He follows up this passage with two possible ways in which such plague buboes are generated, either by the poisonous matter slowly drifting into these regions or being expelled there. This part is not from the *Canon*. The rest of the discussion is either identical to or builds upon what is found in the *Canon* passage on plague, e.g. 'plague mostly occurs during an epidemic year and in corrupt regions'; 'the safest [bubo] is that whose colour inclines to red'; and 'the worst is that whose colour inclines to black'.

[114] Ibn al-Quff, *Commentary on the Aphorisms*, p. 86.

[115] Ibn Sīnā included fainting along with palpitations as plague symptoms. Ibn al-Quff's claim that fainting and chills occur when the vapours reach the heart from the swelling echoes Ibn Sīnā's own theoretical assessment of why fainting occurs; see *al-Qānūn fī al-ṭibb*, III, 164. Al-Rāzī had mentioned the different colours of buboes while quoting Ahrun, but he did not refer to smells or chills.

[116] Fancy and Green, 'Plague and the Fall of Baghdad', pp. 163, 167.

Not only did al-Shīrāzī serve under the Mongols and their vassals in the second half of the thirteenth century in Iran and Eastern Anatolia, he also composed a commentary on book one of the *Canon* and possibly penned a *History of the Mongols* (*Akhbār-i Moghūlān*).[117] Both of these texts were produced after al-Shīrāzī returned to Tabriz from his travels in Syria and Egypt in 1282. As Green has recently shown, the numerous incidences of 'wabā'' (epidemic) mentioned by al-Shīrāzī (and other chroniclers) during the Mongol army's advance through Western Iran on their way to Baghdad in the 1250s were in all likelihood plague outbreaks.[118] We also know now that plague broke out in Syria three months after the Mongol destruction of Baghdad in 1258.[119]

In his commentary on the first book of the *Canon* (completed 1307), entitled *al-Tuḥfa al-Saʿdiyya* (The Gift to Saʿd, the vizier of the Mongol Ilkhanid ruler Öljeytü), al-Shīrāzī describes the causes and symptoms of plague ('ṭāʿūn') quite clearly. While commenting on *Canon* I.2.1, he elaborates on the various types of swellings, much of which is copied verbatim (often without citation) from Ibn al-Nafīs's *Commentary on the Canon*, which he obtained during his visit to Egypt in 1282.[120] After explaining the difference between abscesses and swellings, al-Shīrāzī states, echoing Ibn al-Quff, that when the abscess is generated from poisonous matter whose poison is carried to the heart through the arteries, this can 'cause palpitations and fainting, and in most cases is fatal, and <u>is known as plague</u> ('fa-yaḥdath al-khifqān wa-l-ghashī wa-huwa fī akthar al-amr qattāl <u>sammā ṭāʿūnan</u>')'.[121] The symptoms of the disease are thus described as succinctly as we find in Ibn al-Quff's commentary on the *Aphorisms*, though the style is similar to the *Canon*, since these comments appear in the midst of his *Canon* commentary. Al-Shīrāzī then shifts to explaining why soft, glandular flesh is prone to corruption by quoting (again) from Ibn al-Nafīs's *Commentary on the Canon*. He ends this discussion by citing *Aphorisms* IV.55 to claim that not all such swellings are bad.[122]

At this point, al-Shīrāzī follows in the footsteps of Ibn Sīnā and Ibn al-Quff and provides a terminological history of 'ṭāʿūn'. Al-Shīrāzī's passage is heavily indebted to Ibn al-Quff's work, but with a crucial difference at the end (underlined text mirrors

[117] G. Lane, *The Mongols in Iran: Quṭb al-Dīn al-Shīrāzī's Akhbār-i Moghūlān* (London, 2018), pp. 9–11. The treatise's authorship is disputed. Some claim it was composed by Quṭb al-Dīn al-Shīrāzī himself, while others reject that possibility. What we can definitively say though is that al-Shīrāzī found this text important enough to copy in his own hand during the same period in which he was composing his *Canon* commentary. I thank Monica Green for bringing this text to my attention.

[118] Green, 'Four Black Deaths'; Lane, *Mongols in Iran*, pp. 52–5.

[119] Fancy and Green, 'Plague and the Fall of Baghdad'.

[120] Quṭb al-Dīn al-Shīrāzī, *al-Tuḥfa al-Saʿdiyya*, Istanbul, Süleymaniye Library, MS Ayasofya 3649–56, 3651, fol. 186a; and Ibn al-Nafīs, *Sharḥ al-Qānūn*, MS Fazıl Ahmed Paşa 969, fol. 48b.

[121] al-Shīrāzī, *al-Tuḥfa*, MS Ayasofya 3651, fol. 186a; and Ibn Sīnā, *al-Qānūn fī al-ṭibb*, I, 108. The underlined phrase is part of the original *Canon* text being commented upon.

[122] al-Shīrāzī, *al-Tuḥfa*, MS Ayasofya 3651, fols. 186a–b; and Ibn al-Nafīs, *Sharḥ al-Qānūn*, MS Fazıl Ahmed Paşa 969, fol. 48b.

what is found in Ibn Sīnā's *Canon* IV.3.1; italicised text mirrors what is found in Ibn al-Quff's works):

> *Know that the word ṭāʿūn was applied by the Greeks to every swelling that occurs in the aforementioned glandular flesh. Then after that it was applied to the hot swelling that occurs in the aforementioned locations. Then after that it was applied to the hot swelling that has turned into something poisonous and occurs under the armpits specifically.* This [latter] is what is common[ly known] in our time – this is amongst physicians – as the plague.
>
> (wa-iʿlam anna lafẓ al-ṭāʿūn kānat tuṭlaq ʿinda al-yūnān ʿalā kull waram yaḥdath fī al-luḥūm al-ghadadiyya al-madhkūra thumma baʿd dhālik uṭliqat ʿalā al-waram al-ḥārr al-ḥāṣil fī al-mawāḍiʿ al-madhkūra thumma uṭliqat ʿalā al-waram al-ḥārr al-mustaḥīl ilā kayfiyya sammiyya al-ḥāditha taḥta al-ibṭayn khāṣṣatan wa-hādhā huwa al-mashhūr fī zamāninā hādhā bayn al-aṭibbāʾ bi-l-ṭāʿūn.)[123]

Like Ibn al-Quff, al-Shīrāzī did not list any Greek terms and preferred to use the verb from the root *ṭ-l-q* rather than the more generic 'qīla' (it was said) that Ibn Sīnā used. Likewise, al-Shīrāzī stated that the term applied only to swellings of the insensitive glandular flesh of the armpits, groin, etc. and not of sensitive flesh like that of the breasts and tongue, as Ibn Sīnā had maintained. Most importantly, al-Shīrāzī restricted the use of the term plague bubo to a hot, poisonous swelling that arises specifically in the armpits. This restriction to the armpits is a peculiar feature of the commentaries composed after the Fall of Baghdad and is also found in the commentary of Muwaffaq al-Dīn al-Sāmirī (d. 1282), a Syrian physician and commentator on the *Canon* who also taught Ibn al-Quff.[124] These subtle changes across the medical tradition lend further support to Green's claim that plague was indeed brought to western Eurasia by the Mongols (unwittingly) during the thirteenth century.

Conclusion

The discussions of plague in the Arabic medical tradition vastly supersede those found in the Byzantine or Latin traditions in terms of their sustained efforts across three centuries to understand the disease, which led to novel observations, a refined theoretical understanding of the disease and specific treatment recommendations. This despite the fact that a key text for the Arabic tradition, the one that enshrined the Mediterranean medical community's experience with the First Pandemic, was the *Alexandrian Summary* of Galen's *A Method of Medicine to Glaucon*. The *Summary of Glaucon* has always been presumed to have been composed in Greek, though the original is no longer extant. The Arabic version of this text provided key observations of the disease, explaining them using Galenic

[123] al-Shīrāzī, *al-Tuḥfa*, MS Ayasofya 3651, fol. 186b; Ibn Sīnā, *al-Qānūn fī al-ṭibb*, III, 164; Ibn al-Quff, *Kitāb al-ʿumda*, fol. 41b; and Ibn al-Quff, *Commentary on the Aphorisms*, p. 86.

[124] Fancy and Green, 'Plague and the Fall of Baghdad', p. 167.

medical theory and *Aphorisms* IV.55. The Arabic commentaries on the *Aphorisms* and the various medical encyclopaedias of the tenth and eleventh centuries engaged with plague by building upon this foundational knowledge, sometimes by drawing upon other medical authorities (such as Rufus and Ahrun, whose testimony captured ancient and late antique experiences with plague) and at times elaborating further its causes and suggesting new treatments. None of these Arabic works from the tenth through the twelfth centuries, however, cites direct experience with the disease. On the other hand, the shift in how the disease is described and understood in the works of Ibn al-Quff and al-Shīrāzī strongly suggests that people in Syria and the surrounding regions were experiencing plague outbreak(s) during the second half of the thirteenth century.

Let me conclude by providing two more pieces of evidence to support this latter claim. First, al-Shīrāzī concluded his discussion of plague by quoting Ibn al-Nafīs's passage on plague in Ethiopia.[125] He thus highlighted the fact that plague patients experience delirium and reported on other specific symptoms, such as the size of the bubo and what happens when one cuts it. As Dols noted, this description of plague in Ethiopia was also cited by Ibn Abī Ḥajala (d. 1375), who composed three treatises on the disease nearly a century later and soon died of plague.[126] Al-Shīrāzī's decision to end his discussion of plague by quoting explicitly from Ibn al-Nafīs's account may have been driven by a similar desire to accurately describe a disease his contemporaries/immediate predecessors were experiencing/had experienced.

Second, another contemporary of Ibn al-Nafīs and Ibn al-Quff, the Syrian religious scholar and traditionalist al-Nawawī (d. 1277), provided perhaps the most succinct and clear description of the disease in the midst of his large commentary on the 'sound ('ṣaḥīḥ')' Prophetic traditions of Muslim ibn al-Ḥajjāj (d. 875). Muslim's collection of traditions is preceded by a long introduction wherein he discusses the unreliability of various transmitters. In that introduction, Muslim assesses the veracity of a specific transmitter by first determining his dates using the onset of the Plague of the Torrent ('al-jārif'). In the commentary, al-Nawawī seizes this opportunity to add a lengthy excursus on the history of plague in Islamic societies. But before he presents the history, he describes the disease thus:

> As for the plague, it is a well-known kind of pestilence involving pustules and extremely painful swellings, the eruption of which is accompanied by a fiery inflammation. The surrounding area blackens, and darkens or reddens into a dingy purple; and with this there also occurs palpitation of the heartbeat and nausea.[127]

[125] al-Shīrāzī, *al-Tuḥfa*, MS Ayasofya 3651, fol. 186b; and Ibn al-Nafīs, *Sharḥ al-Qānūn*, MS Fazıl Ahmed Paşa 969, fol. 48b.

[126] Dols, *Black Death*, p. 15.

[127] L. I. Conrad, 'Arabic Plague Chronologies: Social and Historical Factors in the Formation of a Literary Genre', *Studia Islamica* 54 (1981), 51–93 (p. 66) and al-Nawawī, *Ṣaḥīḥ Muslim bi-sharḥ al-Nawawī*, 2 vols. (Cairo, 1929–30), I, 105. Translation as found in Conrad.

This succinct and accurate description of plague is not found in any of the pre-1240 medical works. Al-Nawawī's own account dates from the latter part of his life, since commentaries on canonical 'ḥadīth' texts (reports on the Prophet Muhammad's sayings and actions) were generally composed during one's later years.[128] The earliest extant manuscript (possibly an autograph) was completed months before al-Nawawī died in 1277.[129] Al-Nawawī's description is not identical to that found in post-1240 medical works, yet accords with the succinct, new characterisations of plague found in the contemporary works of Ibn al-Nafīs, al-Sāmirī and Ibn al-Quff.[130] These new depictions of plague should encourage us to shift the chronological and geographical focus of the Second Pandemic to Western and Central Asia during the thirteenth century.

[128] J. Blecher, '*Ḥadīth* Commentary in the Presence of Students, Patrons, and Rivals: Ibn Ḥajar and *Ṣaḥīḥ al-Bukhārī* in Mamluk Cairo', *Oriens* 41 (2013), 261–87 (p. 265).

[129] Conrad, 'Arabic Plague Chronologies', p. 66, n. 3.

[130] See also Fancy and Green, 'Plague and the Fall of Baghdad', pp. 167–9.

2

The Legal Foundations of Post-Mortem Diagnosis in Later Medieval Milan

ANN G. CARMICHAEL[1]

Introduction

Two lengthy death reports made to Milan's Health Office ('Magistrato alla Sanità') in 1479 illustrate the questions and problems that concern me in this chapter. In both cases, the Health Office needed to decide whether a particular individual had died of plague. The clinical and physical details provided in these reports are striking, steeped in detailed medical and epidemiological observations. Even though the content of these civic death registers is compelling, the record format and the language of the court suggest that these reports would be better situated in a juridical, rather than medical, context.

The first report, submitted on 5 May 1479, concerned Venturino, a sixteen-year-old servant or retainer ('famulus') of Lord Azzone Visconti.[2] Visually assessing the boy's body post mortem, the primary physician for the Sanità established a cause of death. Giovanni Catelano judged – 'Iudicio Cat[elani]' – that Venturino's cadaver was cachectic (or, emaciated, 'cachechiam') in appearance.[3] It was also covered by very black and corrupted 'measles' ('morbilis valde denigrates') on both sides of the 'anterior' (ventral, 'anterius parte corporis') aspect of his body, visible on the abdomen, arms, chest, hands and on the digits 'all the way to the nails' ('digitos usque ad ungues'). Catelano then added: 'he died before the third day of his supposed relapse' ('extinctus citra tertiam sui fallacis lapsus'), not accepting that the death was caused by mistaken diagnosis: 'nor was it likely that [his demise] was caused by the earlier fever' ('nec verisimile a decipiente et ipsa febre exeuntum fuisse'). At some point, discussion about the duration of the young man's actual cause of death must have occurred.

Although this particular record entry does not reveal office procedures, contemporary legislative evidence shows that community physicians and surgeons were required to

1 I am especially grateful to Guy Geltner and to Joanna Vitiello for their very helpful comments and suggestions, as well as to the two editors of the volume for their encouragement and patience at all stages of my work.

2 Archivio di Stato Milano, Atti di Governo, Popolazione, Parte Antica, *Registri dei Morti di Milano*. Hereafter specific death reports will be cited as ASMi, *Pop. p.a.*, c. [box or cartella], then day and year.

3 ASMi, *Pop. p.a.*, c. 75, 5 May 1479.

report to an 'anziano' (parish or neighbourhood prior) all persons who were in their care for more than three days. An earlier initial notification to the Health Office could have established the onset of Venturino's illness independently.[4] If Venturino's fever were the recurrence of an earlier illness, rather than a sudden departure from prior good health, plague as the cause of death could be doubted. Catelano's report instead asserted that the team had already established the timing of the onset of Venturino's most recent illness. It is possible that members of the household, anxious to prevent quarantine or even removal of the family and servants to an isolation area outside the city, may have offered an alternative explanation, the persistent fever.

Weighing the evidence – the judges here would have included the ducal commissioner and the judicial and medical deputies appointed to the Office – the Sanità came to its verdict: Venturino died on the third day of his illness, making this a plague death. Their final decision was made in a one-word sentence: 'they accused' ('Accusant'). Perhaps the measles accused, or perhaps the sum of the evidence gathered became probatory evidence of plague. Catelano's further description of these measles, including their character (black and corrupted), abundance and bodily distribution, was useful and important evidence. The cadaver testified; Catelano, the expert, evaluated its appearance and reported the evidence in writing; the Health Office, via its commissioner and deputies, carried out a judgment.[5]

The second illustrative case, on Tuesday 23 March 1479, illustrates how a College physician's clinical narrative of signs and symptoms observed at a patient's bedside struggled to offer a clear, definitive cause of death.[6] As I have published a full translation of this text elsewhere, I recount only a summary of the initial report, focusing on the 'autopsy' that Catelano performed.[7] The deceased, a sixty-five-year-old man named Donato Giochario, had sought medical attention from Master Matteo dei Busti on the previous Saturday,

4 On the 1447 proclamation obligating heads of household to report to parish 'anziani', in writing, any illness occurring within their house, see G. Albini, *Guerra, fame, peste: crisi di mortalità e sistema sanitario nella Lombardia tardomedioevale* (Bologna, 1982), pp. 89–90.

5 In an exceptional letter from 4 June 1468, the health deputies reminded the new duke of Milan, Galeazzo Maria Sforza, that they were the ones who decided which households would be confined or sent out of the city. The duke had heard rumours that Catelano and the health commissioner, Hector Marchese, were shutting up houses that were not infected, hoping to profit. The deputies responded, 'this is news to us, and we are in better position to know because we are here.... They do nothing without our judgment.' A French translation of the Latin text can be found in M. Nicoud, *Le Prince et les médecins: Pensée et pratiques médicales à Milan, 1402–1476* (Rome, 2014), pp. 466–7. I, too, used this letter in my 'Contagion Theory and Contagion Practice in Fifteenth-Century Milan', *Renaissance Quarterly* 44 (1991), 213–56 (pp. 245–6, n. 70). The letter is found in ASMi, *Miscellanea Storica* [hereafter *Misc. stor.*], c. 2, n. 70.

6 ASMi, *Pop. p.a.*, c. 75, 5 May 1479.

7 I translate this report in full in my 'Epidemics and State Medicine in Fifteenth-Century Milan', in *Medicine from the Black Death to the French Disease*, ed. R. French, J. Arrizabalaga, A. Cunningham and L. García-Ballester (Aldershot, 1998), pp. 221–47 (pp. 229–30, and n. 29, p. 245). The report is found in ASMi, *Misc. stor. 2*, n. 420, 23 March 1479. Alas, I no longer possess a full transcription of the original Latin text of this letter.

after he suffered a fainting spell and diarrhoea. The physician, university educated and a member of the city's prestigious College of Medicine, applied cordials to quiet Donato's stomach distress and returned to visit the bedridden man twice a day. Matteo wove together a chronology of his own therapeutic interventions and evolving diagnosis of the man's illness with the sequence of Donato's symptoms or complaints. He analysed Donato's urine on Sunday morning, which to him raised no suspicion, and noted that his patient had eaten and was now resting comfortably. Two days later, however, Donato was dead.

In the official death report, Matteo embarked on a tortured defence of each step he had taken to manage the man's rapidly worsening condition. On Sunday night, Donato's fever had risen sharply. Urinalysis on Monday morning showed worrisome signs and Donato struggled to retain any morsel of food. Matteo called in a colleague, Master Absalom, and the two men together decided that Donato had now begun to show measles or other signs of plague.[8] From such evidence they reported the case to the deputies and chancellor of the Health Office, who then sent Catelano to see Donato before he died. Suspicion surrounded the case now, leading to a quite defensive explanation of the swelling they saw in one axilla. Multiple members of the household claimed that Donato had had that swelling for a decade or more, and it appears that Master Matteo trusted them. When Catelano visited the moribund Donato Giochario he, too, took a colleague with him, the recently appointed Health Office surgeon Master Dionigi.[9] These men found the patient restless and in terror of death ('cum inquietudinibus et accidentibus terroris et mortis'), with violet and black measles all over his body, 'from heel to head' ('ac morbilis violaceis et nigris per omnem fere ponum a calce usque ad capitem').[10] To them, Donato's case was not at all ambiguous, for he had a 'notable bubonic swelling in his left axilla and it was both blackened and corrupted' ('cum eminentia notabile bubonica denigrate corruptaque in sub asella sinistra'). They returned three hours later, finding the man in even worse condition ('Iterato post tres horas in morte revisus apparuerunt peiora prioribus'). Then they considered Master Matteo's diagnosis of a choleric-bilious fever that began on the previous Saturday, four days before Donato's death. Such diagnosis could not 'absolve' the death, the

8 This is Master Absalon dei Capitaneis of Bergamo (or Absalon Pergaminis), a senior College physician. See A. Bottero, 'I più antichi statuti del Collegio dei Medici di Milano', *Archivio storico lombardo* n.s. vol. 8, year 70 (1943), pp. 72–112 (p. 112); and F. Vaglienti, '*Noluit ire ad visum*: I segreti dei *Mortuorum Libri* di Milano da Francesco Sforza a Leonardo da Vinci (1452–1485)', in *La popolazione di Milano dal Rinascimento: Fonti documentarie e fonti materiali per un nuovo umanesimo scientifico*, ed. G. G. Merlo (Milan, 2013), pp. 25–59 (p. 30).

9 On both Catelano and Dionigi as diagnosticians for the Health Office, see the section below entitled 'A man called *Catelano*'.

10 This phrase usually found in medieval 'practica' (practical) texts is head-to-heel ('a capite ad calcem'), referring to the organization of pathological conditions discussed. See L. Demaitre, *Medieval Medicine: The Art of Healing, from Head to Toe* (Oxford, 2013) for an authoritative and accessible study of this genre of medieval medical texts.

Health Office examiners said, because choleric fever 'is deceitful and wicked' ('nec potuit fallax et impia febris ab istis absolvi').[11] This was a death from plague.

It is striking that the Health Office certifiers of cause of death could override the collaborative diagnosis of two elite College physicians and even put the reporting physician in a defensive position.[12] Similarly, the death of a servant in a household of the powerful Visconti clan could not be attributed to what Galenic medicine called 'accidents' – the succeeding events of an underlying internal pathological cause, such as a long-standing fever that led to wasting and, at the end, 'measles'. Accustomed to following the progress and progression of an illness, the College physicians read the patient's steadily more concerning condition in a way that saw rashes and swellings as visible evidence of hidden humoral disturbances. Where the attending physician saw signs that guided treatment, masters Catelano and Dionigi, acting as very early medical examiners, saw what medieval Italian jurists would call 'indicia' – manifest, even if only circumstantial, evidence offered in partial proof of a criminal's guilt. With an extreme reformulation of this epistemological divide, plague becomes the perpetrator of a crime against the community, but no one could actually 'see' or arrest the culprit. I will not carry the argument to that length.

I will argue that Milan's records were forensic: they carried both medical and legal authority. The administrative reporting practices and legal context that underlay these unusual cause-of-death reports offer a specialised forensic gaze, a cultural response to the high anxiety caused by recurring plague epidemics. But credit for my approach should go to Folco Vaglienti and Cristina Cattaneo, who first observed that Milan's fifteenth-century registers could be distinguished from comparable civic mortality rosters in other northern and central Italian city states because they showed 'the *intention of public authorities* to register all deaths (both natural and suspicious) with a specific medical report'.[13] Their striking two-part claim – that Milan's public authorities had the power to command medical reports on the deaths of all but the very youngest residents and that they intended to register all residents' deaths individually – led me to this study. Why and how the Milanese selected a medico-legal response to the unpredictable threat of recurrent plague outbreaks relates to relevant north Italian legal traditions and the expectations placed on physicians and surgeons in the control of urban violence. The unusual forensic approach to plague control used in Milan unintentionally exposed weaknesses in traditional Galenic diagnostic practices.

Resituating Milan's mortality registers within the history of forensic medicine begs some background review that is not standard fare in medieval medical history. Italian juridical

[11] ASMi, *Pop. p.a.*, c. 75, 23 March 1479.

[12] Nicoud, *Le Prince*, pp. 444–53, provides an extraordinarily detailed account of conflicts between prominent College physicians and the diagnoses that Catelano provided during the 1468 plague outbreak.

[13] F. Vaglienti and C. Cattaneo, 'A Medieval Contribution to the History of Legal Medicine: The First European Necroscopic Registry', *International Journal of Legal Medicine* 124 (2010), 669–70 (p. 669, emphasis added).

practices were established in the communal era (before 1250 CE or so) consequent to a 'medieval legal revolution'.[14] In the two case examples offered above, reporting physicians and surgeons, whether or not they worked for the Health Office, literally testified to their causal assessments: their names followed the word 'Iudicio' (by the judgment of). Each record offered a sworn report to the Sanità, which was in turn a kind of municipal court. I will thus summarise research on the thirteenth-century origins of forensic medicine and the judicial framework that led judges and other municipal authorities to use medical practitioners as expert witnesses. Most authoritative research on medieval forensic medicine has been written by legal historians, while the usual focus of historians of forensic medicine emphasises the slow development of a distinctive medical specialisation in the early modern era.[15] Law and medicine are epistemologically distinct ways of determining evidence that will guide subsequent action. In other words, they are working to separate ends and purposes. Physicians want to diagnose and cure; when the court asks experts for informed responses to their questions (which are not the same questions as those asked by the physician or even the patient), they want answers that the court understands as evidence that could be used toward the exoneration of an accused person, or instead towards proof of guilt.

Before turning to a brief summary of medieval juridical history relevant to my record set, it is useful to explain how the documents analysed in this study differ from the better-known, but significantly later, London *Bills of Mortality*. Both documents depended on information gathered at the parish level, but in other respects the London *Bills* contrast significantly with the Milanese *Books of the Dead* (*Libri mortuorum*). London's *Bills* were 'public' documents in the sense that we use that word today, as media, news or commentary readily available to those in the public sphere, subsequently discussed or analysed by persons who did not compile or witness the information at first hand.[16] The *Bills* had no legal authority, however, being broadsheets compiled weekly for the readers' unspecified uses. The causes listed in the London *Bills* also offered accessible, common English disease terms that conveyed assessments made by persons who possessed no medical expertise. Because the *Bills* essentially were a commercial venture, any reader with the means to purchase weekly *Bills* could also use their contents in ways that the producers could not control. The processed (or mediated) death data that they offered were published by private printers

14 K. Pennington, 'The "Big Bang": Roman Law in the Early Twelfth Century', *Rivista internazionale di diritto comune* 18 (2007), 43–70.

15 See C. Crawford, 'Legalizing Medicine: Early Modern Legal Systems and the Growth of Medico-Legal Knowledge', in *Legal Medicine in History*, ed. M. Clark and C. Crawford (Cambridge, 1994), pp. 89–116; A. Pastore, *Medico in tribunale: La perizia medica nella procedura penale d'antico regime (secoli xvi–xviii)* (Bellinzona, 1998); S. De Renzi, 'Medical Expertise, Bodies, and the Law in Early Modern Courts', *Isis* 98 (2007), 315–22; J. Duffin, 'Questioning Medicine in Seventeenth-Century Rome: The Consultations of Paolo Zacchia', *Canadian Bulletin of the History of Medicine* 28 (2011), 149–70.

16 J. Wernimont, *Numbered Lives: Life and Death in the Quantum Media* (Cambridge MA, 2018), pp. 22–9.

and sold individually or by subscription to interested members of the public.[17] They were not official (i.e., legal or governing) documents.

London's *Bills* offered death counts rather than registrations, tabulated from individual (and exclusively Anglican) parish mortality records, then aggregated at the city level by cause and by parish. Users of the *Bills* boldly trusted their own assessments of culled parish-level data, much as did Daniel Defoe's narrator in *A Journal of the Plague Year*: if you were clever, 'H. F.' tells us, you could see which parishes were affected early on, even when a parish reported only non-plague causes of death. You then could take steps to protect yourself and your family. Some Londoners pored over the weekly numbers as they would do with their account books, seeking productive guidance or trends in the numbers, then speculating how this information could guide public policy. Thus in 1663, the so-called 'father' of modern demography, London haberdasher John Graunt, believed that from tabulated counts of annual *Bills* and a comparison of normal with epidemic years he could determine annual mortality patterns.[18] But when Graunt reflected on causes of death, he dismissed any absolute claims one could make from the *Bills* because illiterate female parish searchers had supplied that information. They were the weak link in a chain of evidence that he was interpreting for the public's benefit.

In aggregate, even imperfect counts of causes and locations of deaths acquired medical and political significance. Yet, while the *Bills of Mortality* foreshadowed modern approaches to public health surveillance, they do not contribute directly to our understanding of the development of forensic medicine. The reported numbers in the *Bills* carried no individually identifying information about any recently deceased persons. The Milanese *Books of the Dead*, by contrast, relate to the history of forensic medicine, a field of scholarship that dates the earliest appearance of specialised forensic medical treatises to around 1600.[19] This study looks at practices in place more than a century earlier than this learned medical literature.

The wider temporal context of the Milanese records furthermore connects us to modern views of personhood and state registration, in that recording individual deaths and causes of death has become fundamental to our notions of what competent states do.[20] Dante Zanetti's comparison of annual registers from 1503, 1616 and 1783 showed a reduction in the complicated explanatory reports that can be found in 1503. The Office increasingly

17 W. Slauter, 'Write Up your Dead: The Bills of Mortality and the London Plague of 1665', *Media History* 17 (2011), 1–15.

18 A. A. Rusnock, *Vital Accounts: Quantifying Health and Population in Eighteenth-Century England and France* (New York, 2002), pp. 15–39.

19 Crawford, 'Legalizing Medicine', pp. 89–116. By 1600, each court had its own practices in reading and applying the law – the '*usus fori*'. Thus, the earliest textbook of forensic medicine, Paulo Zacchia's, compiled cases in Roman civil courts. See P. Stein, *Roman Law in European History* (Cambridge, 1999; Kindle edition 2012), chapter 4, section 9: 'Court Practice as a Source of Law'. On Zacchia, see Duffin, 'Questioning Medicine'.

20 S. Szreter and K. Breckenridge, 'Recognition and Registration: The Infrastructure of Personhood in World History', *Proceedings of the British Academy* 182 (2012), 1–36.

streamlined diagnoses to identify those few that required government and/or public health actions. Registers in the eighteenth century were more complete in a bureaucratic sense, because by then all recorded deaths included a certification of cause.[21] Other research on the activities the Health Office in the era of Spanish domination (1535–1706) shows how Milan's public health department became a model of early modern medicalised health management.[22]

Milan's early forensic approach to investigating worrisome deaths fell away, but an extraordinary public record endured. Every person who died and was buried in Milan was identified by name, surname, age, parish and sometimes occupation. Across the 287 years from 1503 to 1806, most annual death registers survive, gathering all Milanese into one great, inclusive paper cemetery.[23] By that time, Milan's elite medical personnel had no routine involvement in the certification of citizens' causes of death, no traces of the earlier era other than the books themselves and the local nickname given to the principal surgeon of the Health Office: the 'catelano'.[24]

Medieval legal tradition and the origin of European forensic medical cultures

The objectives of any forensic system differ from a society's concern with the general wellness of its citizens. In matters of health and medicine, the word 'public' referred to both urban sanitation and gratis healthcare; both were established medieval traditions. In Milan, as in other northern Italian polities, it was fundamentally the responsibility of government to protect its citizens from hazards to their health and safety; these are documented in statutes that pre-date the Black Death by a century or more. Guy Geltner's recent research lays out in astounding detail how urban Italians implemented aggressive public health legislation and mechanisms for enforcement in frequently updated urban

21 D. Zanetti, 'La morte a Milano nei secoli XVI–XVIII: appunti per una ricerca', *Rivista Storica Italiana* 88 (1976), 803–51; and G. Alter and A. Carmichael, 'Studying Causes of Death in the Past: Problems and Models', *Historical Methods* 29 (1996), 44–8.

22 A Visconti, *La pubblica amministrazione nello stato Milanese durante il predominio straniero (1541–1796)* (Milan, 1972 [1911]), pp. 179–301, reviewing the Office and its publications from the 1530s to the Napoleonic reforms. More recently, L. di Giammatteo and J. A. Mendelsohn, 'Reporting for Action: Forms of Writing between Medicine and Polity in Milan, 1580–1650', in *Civic Medicine: Physician, Polity and Pen in Early Modern Europe*, ed. J. A. Mendelsohn, A. Kinzelbach and R. Schilling (London, 2020), pp. 135–60.

23 Zanetti, 'Morte a Milano', estimating over 1.5 million deaths reported. By the eighteenth century, every death carried a diagnosis, although most causes were perfunctory and formulaic and were reported by the Health Office surgeon. See also A. Carmichael, 'Registering Deaths and Causes of Death in Late Medieval Milan', in *Death in Medieval Europe: Death Scripted and Death Choreographed*, ed. J. Rollo-Koster (London, 2017), pp. 209–36.

24 See the section below: 'A man called *catelano*'.

statutes.[25] Each city or town for which we have surviving medieval records configured its own approaches to public health maintenance, as well as the personnel who monitored health threats affecting public spaces and thoroughfares.

While the objectives and principles of public health were universally accepted, the particulars and personnel were locally inflected.[26] In many cities, health-promoting interventions extended to hiring public physicians ('medici condotti'), who are sometimes called 'medici plagarum' (wound doctors), and can thus be confused with those practitioners who had forensic authority. We have evidence of itinerant medical and surgical men contracted for limited terms of service as early as the 1220s and 1230s.[27] Some cities and towns publicly funded the provision of medical care to citizens along with enacting statutes relevant to urban sanitation.[28] For example, Milan's earliest surviving statutes contain chapters relevant to both traditional public health sanitation and healthcare and provide the names of each of the city's public hospitals.[29] The general health-promoting interventions made in response to novel plague outbreaks thus largely related to the enforcement of legislation long (and literally) 'on the books'. Plague treatises offered traditional medical advice that was oriented toward collective health, teaching authorities how to manage recurring urban epidemics, spelling out the complex environmental sources of risk to individuals and to cities.[30]

Forensic medicine instead pertained to public safety and criminal justice more than it did to public health, even though it was also predicated on the municipality's obligation to provide for the common welfare of citizens ('cives'). All flowed from the eleventh-century recovery of ancient Roman legal compendia known as the *Corpus Iuris Civilis*.[31] Because

25 G. Geltner, *Roads to Health: Infrastructure and Urban Wellbeing in Later Medieval Italy* (Philadelphia, 2019).

26 Geltner, *Roads to Health*, pp. 85–130. See also J. Coomans, 'The King of Dirt: Public Health and Sanitation in Late Medieval Ghent', *Urban History* 46 (2019), 83–105.

27 V. Nutton, 'Continuity or Rediscovery? The City Physician in Classical Antiquity and Mediaeval Italy', in *The Town and State Physician in Europe from the Middle Ages to the Enlightenment*, ed. A. W. Russell (Wolfenbüttel, 1981), pp. 27–8; and G. Pomata, *Contracting a Cure: Patients, Healers, and the Law in Early Modern Bologna* (Baltimore, 1998), pp. 37–42 and 157–8.

28 See R. Palmer, 'Physicians and the State in Post-Medieval Italy', in *Town and State Physician*, ed. Russell, pp. 47–61; I. Naso, 'L'assistenza sanitaria negli ultimi secoli del Medioevo. I *medici condotti* delle comunità piemontesi', in *Città e servizi sociali nell'Italia dei secoli XII–XV* (Pistoia, 1990), pp. 277–96; and di Giammatteo and Mendelsohn, 'Reporting for Action', p. 137, who see general civic physicians in the early modern era as the latter-day 'medici condotti' in Milan, because these practitioners had no noble pedigree.

29 A. F. La Cava, *Igiene e sanità negli statuti Milano del sec. XIV, Codice inedito* (Milan, 1946). Sanitation and healthcare regulations are found in the *Extraordinaria* section. Statutes relevant to forensic medicine are instead found in the *Criminalia* part of the statutes – public safety, not public health, but still the government's responsibility for maintaining the common good.

30 M. Nicoud, *Le Prince*, pp. 383–7.

31 The multipart *Corpus Iuris Civilis* was sponsored by Emperor Justinian around 530 CE. On its organization see Ascheri, *Laws*, pp. 9–19 and Stein, *Roman Law*, chapter 3, section 12.

Roman law was flexible across jurisdictions, it was useful in drafting contracts, property exchanges, inheritance disputes and so forth. It steadily replaced older customary laws by facilitating commercial transactions.[32] The transformative power of new Roman law in urban governance stemmed from the creation of a 'Societas populus', a corporate body. This particular medieval juridical device put communes on equal legal footing with territorial lords. Thus establishing their autonomous jurisdiction, early communes created a bureaucratic, institution-based governance that fused citizen interests and the obligations of a 'bonum commune' (public good).[33] An ideal of participatory governance became the hallmark of north Italian communes by the thirteenth century, and through it the safety, security and prosperity of all citizens was amplified in the novel rhetorical writing that we find among a rapidly expanding notariate.[34] The production and preservation of judicial and legislative documents vastly accelerated with the adoption of paper record keeping.[35]

Communes further created the 'podestaria' (mayoral office), a novel criminal justice apparatus that had no direct Roman precedent. By the thirteenth century, contemporary with the reinvention of 'medici condotti', many municipalities recruited foreign aristocratic executives, the 'podestà', to enforce their local communal statutes. Urban statute regulations and practices were quite local and specific and did not fully conform to Roman law. The 'podestaria' responded to ubiquitous, militarised violence among aristocratic clans that spilled into city streets and markets.[36] Ideally, these itinerant noblemen had no connections to any of the locally powerful families, but most communes put safeguards in place, limiting their terms of office and subjecting them to review by communal auditors at the conclusion of their contract. Many 'podestà' brought their own retinues of enforcers,

32 For the jurisdictional mosaic, see A. Gamberini, *The Clash of Legitimacies: The State-Building Process in Late Medieval Lombardy* (New York, 2018), pp. 17–29.

33 Gamberini, *Clash of Legitimacies,* pp. 40–6, emphasizes the rhetorical appeal of an ancient lexicon of 'libertas' (liberty), 'cives' (citizen), 'res publica' (public affairs), 'iurisdictio'(jurisdiction) and so forth, in the creation of a profoundly different structure to urban self-governance. In the *Societas Populi*, crimes against individual 'cives' (citizens) became crimes against the 'popolo' (populace). On the novel procedural manuals, see Aschieri, *Medieval Italian Law*, pp. 86–90; and Gamberini, *Clash of Legitimacies*, p. 59. Most earlier law codes specified person-based rights; 'ius novum' (new law) instead applied to territories.

34 R. G. Witt argues that manuals of 'ars dictaminis' (the art of letter-writing), which trained notaries in the art of composition and letter writing, were the most influential aspect of the twelfth-century legal revolution, in *The Two Latin Cultures and the Foundation of Renaissance Humanism in Medieval Italy* (New York, 2012), pp. 253–66, 359–62.

35 J.-C. Maire Vigueur, 'Révolution documentaire et revolution scripturaire: le cas de l'Italie médiévale', *Bibliothèque de l'École des chartes* 153 (1995), 177–85 and J. Bloom, *Paper before Print: The History and Impact of Paper in the Islamic World* (New Haven, 2001), pp. 209–11.

36 Aschieri, *Medieval Italian Law*, pp. 86–90; and Gamberini, *Clash of Legitimacies*, p. 59.

judges and notaries, all of whom were well positioned to aid the diffusion of knowledge and 'best practices' in urban government from one commune to another.[37]

Communal statutes in 1260s Bologna relevant to street crime provide the earliest documentation of evolving Italian forensic practices. When the 'podestà' was informed that an act of bodily violence had occurred, the magistrate dispatched a court notary to count and record the number of wounds that he thought were lethal, as well as the number that were not lethal. If the victim was still alive, the notary asked him to name the perpetrator, who could then be arrested by the law enforcement staff of either the 'podestà' or the commune. The objective, unstated in the relevant statute, was to prevent widening violence through reprisals or vendettas.[38] To modern eyes, the effort to link discrete wounds to individual assailants seems an odd approach, but under Roman civil law judges needed to assess the severity of each wound before assigning primary culpability, then align the legally allowed punishment to the degree of each perpetrator's guilt. Street brawls often involved multiple assailants, yet the law allowed no more than one guilty party per lethal wound. Building the case against a culprit, one or more office notaries elaborated a trial narrative, which was retained locally, not by the magistrate. By 1288, Bolognese statutes show that the 'podestà' in Bologna relied on a list of trusted resident physicians and surgeons who operated through a service lottery, renewed every six months. For each reported blood crime, two men on the list were called (and paid) to make a count of lethal vs. non-lethal wounds on the body of a recently injured person.[39] Only practitioners who were at least thirty years old, native Bolognese or long-term residents, who owned property and who had taken an oath to serve the commune faithfully were eligible legal experts.

In the 1300s, medical expert witnessing in criminal trials became a civic responsibility across much of north and central Italy, as well as in many towns and cities of Provence and eastern Iberia. Accusations brought to the 'podestà' or comparable judicial magistrate called for a surgeon's report on a wounded patient or recently deceased individual, although the routine involvement of physicians and surgeons was uncommon before the early fourteenth century.[40] Guido Ruggiero's classic study of early forensic medicine in Venice documents the active involvement of physicians with state police forces by at least

37 See M. Vallerani, *Medieval Public Justice*, trans. S. R. Blanshei (Washington, 2012), pp. 78–9, 115; T. Dean, *Crime and Justice in Late Medieval Italy* (New York, 2007), p. 11; and G. Geltner, 'Fighting Corruption in the Italian City-State', in *Anti-Corruption in History: From Antiquity to the Modern Era*, ed. R. Kroeze, A. Vitória and G. Geltner (New York, 2017), pp. 103–29.

38 As early as 1265, Bologna's 'podestà' involved physicians and surgeons in the assessment of wounds. See E. Dall'Osso, *L'organizzazione medico-legale a Bologna e a Venezia nei secoli XII–XIV* (Cesena, 1956), pp. 15–41; and Ascheri, *Laws*, pp. 232–3.

39 A. Simili, 'The Beginnings of Forensic Medicine in Bologna', *International Symposium on Society, Medicine and Law*, ed. H. Karplus (New York, 1973), pp. 91–100.

40 J. C. Vitiello, *Public Justice and the Criminal Trial in Late Medieval Italy* (Leiden, 2016), pp. 44–5, 65–81. Vallerani, *Medieval Public Justice*, offers an extensive and detailed case study of later thirteenth-century Bolognese law without ever mentioning the 'podestà's' use of local physicians to examine and assess the wounds on a victim of violent crime.

1281.[41] Within two days after he consulted with a wounded patient, a physician or surgeon needed to report that person's injuries to the main police agency, the 'Signore di notte' (men-of-the-night). Police even expected some of the city physicians to perform a partial dissection of a murder victim to look for internal damage when the severity of the victim's injuries was greater than appearance suggested. A few surviving police reports show that Venetian authorities wanted surgical experts to count and measure all wounds, identifying which particular lesions were likely to have been lethal blows. Carmel Ferragud, using Valencian archives, and Joseph Shatzmiller, with Provençal archives, document the broader guidance that medical testimony provided to the court, including details that helped to exculpate or condemn a known assailant in a violent crime.[42]

Physicians who provided expert testimony in service to judicial proceedings typically bolstered their professional reputations. Learned physicians also adapted the legal literary genre of 'consilia' (consultations/case studies) and, over the later Middle Ages, produced a new and dominant form of medical writing and pedagogy.[43] Nonetheless, medical expertise could not decide the fate of an accused. That was the responsibility of the judge, whether the 'podestà' himself or his criminal court judge. These basic power and knowledge relationships and reporting practices are reflected directly in the Milanese death registers and help to show how the documents are more juridical than medical. Milan's fifteenth-century *Magistrato alla Sanità* (Health Magistracy/Office) became comparable to a court of criminal justice, even though its juridical autonomy in epidemic crises can be documented only later on, in statutes of the Sanità published in 1534.

41 G. Ruggiero, 'The Cooperation of Physicians and the State in the Control of Violence in Renaissance Venice', *Journal of the History of Medicine and Allied Sciences* 33 (1978), 156–66 offers new archival research to Dall'Osso, *L'organizzazione*, pp. 45–68.

42 Both scholars further place their analysis in the context of medicalization. C. Ferragud, 'Expert Examination of Wounds in the Criminal Court of Justice in Cocentaina (Kingdom of Valencia) during the Late Middle Ages', in *Medicine and the Law in the Middle Ages*, ed. S. M. Butler and W. Turner (Leiden, 2014), pp. 109–32 and J. Shatzmiller, 'The Jurisprudence of the Dead Body', *Micrologus VII* (1999), pp. 223–30. M. McVaugh, *Medicine before the Plague: Practitioners and Their Patients in the Crown of Aragon, 1285–1345* (New York, 1993), pp. 209–10 also describes the Catalan practice of an expert determining when the victim of a crime is out of danger, a process that freed the assailant from further prosecution.

43 See C. Crisciani, 'Consilia, responsi, consulti: i pareri del medico tra insegnamento e professione', in *Consilium: Teorie e pratiche del consigliare nella cultura medievale*, ed. C. Casagrande, C. Crisciani and S. Vecchio (Florence, 2004), pp. 259–79. 'Consilia' constituted a new genre of medical writing that evolved rapidly during the fourteenth century, initially modelled on legal 'consilia' and offered as formal consultations written from one physician to another, the recipient seeking advice about a patient under care.

Medieval forensic cultures

Medical historian Christopher Hamlin offers the framework of 'forensic cultures' as a way to compare forensic practices across spatial, temporal or legal divides.[44] Criminal law based on local statutes and the *Corpus Iuris Civilis*, on the one hand, and the involvement of approved medical practitioners, on the other, are only two components of medieval forensic culture in northern Italy. For Hamlin, 'forensic facts' are the 'guts of rights' that include the often-unseen operational habits of institutions, technologies and legal frameworks, including how they operate in practice to identify crimes and criminals before rendering justice. Forensic cultures can be further described by what adjudicators see as fact and what persons are deemed capable of testifying to such facts; this, in turn, reveals how polities define authority and assign expertise in matters of justice. Beyond knowing the persons and networks involved with reporting practices, describing a forensic culture involves determining the parameters that a society uses to determine how 'facts' corroborate or are established independently of personal testimony. A framework of 'forensic culture' invites appreciation of commonalities in forensic practices, objectives and the acquisition of 'forensic facts'.

Medieval English forensic practices provide a useful contrast, by highlighting the coroner, who, like the *Bills of Mortality*, is more familiar to Anglophone scholars. This contrast can also sharpen our understanding of systems of justice in medieval Italy. Sara Butler's influential study of late medieval coroners and the practices of death investigation in England has encouraged an outsized attention to the coroner's role in the general study of medieval forensic medicine, although her purpose was to redress commonplace negative assessments of late medieval coroners when compared to the recruitment of expert medical-surgical witnesses on the Continent.[45] In England, from 1200 on, we find a forensic culture centred on a police official (the sheriff), a judicial official (the coroner) and the jury that the coroner empanelled, together guided by English common law rather than Roman law.[46] Juries established actionable 'facts' from evidence presented at a trial, facts that were usually restricted to the sworn testimony of those with first-hand knowledge of the crime or criminal. Some diligent early coroners – the office was established more than a half century before comparable practices were first documented in Bologna – probed and measured a victim's various wounds, presumably with

[44] C. Hamlin, 'Forensic Cultures in Historical Perspective: Technologies of Witness, Testimony, Judgment (and Justice?)', *Studies in History and Philosophy of Biological and Biomedical Sciences* 44 (2013), 4–15; Hamlin, 'Forensic Facts, the Guts of Rights', in *Global Forensic Cultures: Making Fact and Justice in the Modern Era*, ed. I. Burney and C. Hamlin (Baltimore, 2019), pp. 1–33.

[45] S. M. Butler, *Forensic Medicine and Death Investigation in Medieval England* (New York, 2015).

[46] P. Brand, 'The Beginnings of the English Common Law (to 1350)', in *The Oxford Handbook of European Legal History*, ed. H. Pihlajamäki, M. D. Dubber and M. Godfrey (Oxford Handbooks Online, 2018), pp. 442–8.

the same impulse to establish the severity of individual wounds. A corpse could not be buried until their work was complete.[47]

Even without invoking the larger framework of 'forensic cultures', we find convergences between English and Continental legal practices, especially in the ecclesiastical use of inquisitions. Pope Innocent III's decretals leading to the fourth Lateran Council of 1215 outlawed older trials by ordeal, which he expressly forbade because it was inconsistent with Roman law.[48] While English common law and coroners' juries did not admit expert witnesses, English jurists and prelates well understood inquisitorial procedures from canon law.[49] Church or canon law governed many behaviours and infractions not judged by local juries and it applied across Christendom. The earliest and foundational legal compendium in England, Bracton's *On the Laws and Customs of England* (1230), 'clothed' non-Roman customary laws and practices in a Roman legal garb.[50] Forensic practices in continental Europe and the British Isles thus diverged according to the body of law and legal experts consulted in adjudicating crimes, but shared traditions in their community reporting structures, their insistence on sworn testimony and their reliance on community reputation to determine which witnesses to a crime or interpreters of evidence could be trusted.

Innocent III introduced the 'inquisitio' (inquiry/inquisition) as a way to extract truth or facts when circumstances surrounding a crime lacked a clear accuser or accused. The Church's primary concerns were with crimes that did not involve the shedding of blood, such as heresy, adultery and clerical malfeasance, but ecclesiastical judges could initiate such inquisitions 'ex officio', by virtue of their power and office. By the mid-thirteenth century, Italian civil courts adopted similar judge-directed inquisitions as a powerful way to deter urban crime, revising their own local statute laws and procedures for enforcement. The 'podestà' tasked men in their retinues ('famiglia') to do investigative work, just as coroners shunted fact-finding investigations to their assembled juries of men of high social status. Italian communes transferred the establishment of 'forensic facts' to trained judges or other officials who more or less adhered to a 'ius commune' (late medieval common law, so called because canon and civil law conformed along procedural lines). Communal courts adopted a basic inquisitorial framework that echoed denunciations from parishioners, initiating proceedings with a rumour or '*clamor* … that reached the ears of the *podestà*'.[51] Those familiar with medieval England immediately recognise the 'hue and cry'

47 Butler, *Forensic Medicine*, pp. 45–7.

48 F. McAuley, 'Canon Law and the End of the Ordeal', *Oxford Journal of Legal Studies* 26 (2006), 473–513.

49 The importance of the Fourth Lateran Council to medical history was the impetus it gave to the collection of post-mortem findings in order to demonstrate sanctity. See J. Ziegler, 'Practitioners and Saints: Medical Men in Canonization Processes in the Thirteenth to Fifteenth Centuries', *Social History of Medicine* 12 (1999), 191–225. See also K. Park, 'The Criminal and the Saintly Body: Autopsy and Dissection in Renaissance Italy', *Renaissance Quarterly* 47 (1994), 1–33.

50 Stein, *Roman Law*, chapter 3, section 11: 'Civil Law and Local Laws of the Thirteenth Century'.

51 Vallerani, *Medieval Public Justice*, p. 51.

of English common law. News came to a sheriff when a crime was committed, prompting him to summon the crown's man – the coroner – to the scene of the crime and the investigation of the body seemingly dead from an 'unnatural' cause.[52]

English and Italian forensic cultures further resembled each other in their community-level crime-reporting practices, even though the underlying prosecutorial systems diverged. Moreover, localism in urban statute legislation and customary law ensured the existence of multiple forensic systems across later medieval Italy, France and Spain, despite the increasing reliance on 'ius commune'. While English common law did not wrest local power away from the peers of the realm, the forensic forum, a coroner's jury trial, similarly operated at the local level. In regions conforming to Roman law, trials allowed testimony by expert witnesses (permitted in Roman law) and decided cases by rational examination of documentary and testimonial evidence.[53] But both the English coroner and the Italian municipal judge responded to violent and accidental deaths, 'collecting and interpreting information about circumstances and causes of deaths'.[54] To contain violence, and especially 'blood crimes', northern Italian city dwellers and people of English shires alike appealed to persons that society had invested with forensic authority, who then personally or through their proxies focused on the externally visible injuries to a corpse. It is not surprising that some diligent thirteenth-century English coroners shared the very concern that motivated the Bolognese 'podestà' to gather specific bodily evidence by viewing a victim's mortal remains.

Milan's divergent path, 1360–1460

How did Milan alone arrive at a form of civic mortality registration that can be characterised as the 'first of its kind in Europe', its principal street-level actors performing as roving medical examiners, its health department serving as a court that decided the fate of a household when one of its members died of plague? A partial explanation requires consideration of two fundamental disruptions to the exercise of communal public justice that influenced local Milanese forensic practices: the transfer of ultimate judicial authority to a territorial lordship or 'signoria' and recurring plagues. Neither driver of change was particular to Milan, as both altered urban experience in most northern and central Italy city-states by the mid-fourteenth century.

52 Butler, *Forensic Medicine*, pp. 42–4.

53 For what follows here, see Ascheri, *Laws*, pp. 228–9, who points out that written proceedings opened the door to the appeal of a decision.

54 U.S. Institute of Medicine, 'Preface', in *Medicolegal Death Investigation System: Workshop Summary* (Washington DC, 2003), p. vii. See especially 'Comparing Medical Examiner and Coroner Systems', pp. 23–8. Stable URL: https://www.ncbi.nlm.nih.gov/books/NBK221919/pdf/Bookshelf_NBK221919.pdf.

From the early 1360s, catastrophic, multi-year plague outbreaks convulsed the duchy of Milan. Somehow Milan escaped the full assault of the initial Black Death, but Milan's losses in its first plague (1361–63) were staggering. Plagues returned in quick succession (1371–73; 1384–88; 1399–1402).[55] Throughout these decades, Visconti lords habitually surrounded themselves with prestigious physicians recruited from across Italy, incrementally grafting new plague-related governing practices onto old administrative structures.[56] But these court physicians could not easily exercise social and political power within Milan itself, because they were not residents or members of the commune's medical establishment. Prerogatives of communes, especially in the administration of justice, were defended wherever municipal autonomy remained intact.

Outside Milan, the Visconti lords asserted their 'plenitude' (or 'fullness') of power, reserving to themselves the 'control over the punishment of criminals, the imposition of fines, hearing of civil cases and appeals which normally went to the emperor, the power to raise taxes and punish rebels'.[57] Visconti lords in the fourteenth century systematically replaced the 'podestà' of subject cities with their own chosen candidates and mandated revisions to existing statutes in each and every subjected city, town, village or territory. But the extent to which a remote prince could summarily, top down, reorder a pre-existing local forensic system may have been limited. Joanna Carraway Vitiello analysed how such sweeping powers affected court procedures in Reggio Emilia, which fell under Visconti control from 1371 to 1404. She found evidence for medical expert witnessing with wound and crime records; she also showed that Visconti lords and their agents could, and did, interfere with court decisions at will, overriding cases that involved prominent landowners and their retainers.[58] Yet, when petty urban violence concerned persons in whom the Visconti had little interest, communal courts operated as before and educated physicians continued to weigh in as expert witnesses.[59]

In the capital city of Milan, where the stakes for the dynasty's stability were higher, the Visconti exerted control indirectly. They personally selected the 'podestà', but at street level forensic reporting practices remained with the district prior ('anziano') of each parish.[60]

55 Albini, *Guerra*, pp. 17–20.

56 Ibid., p. 10.

57 The transformation involved the acquisition of sweeping judicial authority. See J. Black, 'The Visconti in the Fourteenth Century and the Origins of their *Plenitudo Potestatis*', *Reti Medievali Rivista* 5 (2004), 1–20 (p. 7), http://www.rmoa.unina.it/2271/.

58 J. C. Vitiello, 'Forensic Evidence, Lay Witnesses and Medical Expertise in the Criminal Courts of Late Medieval Italy', in *Medicine and the Law*, ed. Butler and Turner, pp. 133–56.

59 Such protections and privileges for university-trained physicians and surgeons were widespread by the late fourteenth century, as shown in Ferragud's particularly detailed case study from the archival records of a Valencian mountain town 'Expert Examination of Wounds'.

60 E. Verga, 'Le sentenze criminali dei podestà milanesi, 1385–1429', *Archivio Storico Lombardo* 3rd s. 16 (1901), 106–11, shows that the vast majority of cases brought before the 'podestà' or his judges involved accusations of injured parties or the denunciations brought by parish 'anziani'

However powerful they became, Visconti and (later) Sforza lords relied on the smooth functioning of traditional city services and amenities for the vast majority of residents. The earliest civic statutes to survive were a 1396 redaction of documents compiled before the Black Death; they were still consistent with urban statutes published a century later.[61]

Plague threatened local law enforcement as well as the Visconti duchy's viability.[62] Territorial lords, different in status and obligation from even the richest communal citizens, had to ensure the overall security of their states, including protection of the state's border and safe passage along all commercial thoroughfares. Both urban and seigneurial administrators began to craft novel policies and appoint plague-specific personnel. Some new plague management ideas appeared in Milan before the 1399–1401 epidemic, but only from that outbreak can we document the appointment of a ducal plague commissioner. With the duke's interventions, a different sort of neighbourhood crime reporting took shape. Duke Giangaleazzo Visconti named jurist Johannes de Roxellis, a man in his entourage in charge of the Visconti office for bills and certificates (the 'officiali delle bollette'), to oversee 'the preservation of the health of the city and 'ducato' (jurisdiction) of Milan'.[63] Heads of household were to obligated report those who fell ill to the neighbourhood 'anziani', who then had to make written daily reports of illnesses and deaths, together with full information about their causes and details about the affected households.[64]

Neighbourhood officials and countryside consuls were pivotal to a centralised seigneurial management of plague in both city and territory, but did not involve Milan's College of Medicine directly. Indeed, as Marilyn Nicoud points out, during the plague outbreak of 1399–1401 Duke Giangaleazzo Visconti deliberately bypassed the College, commanding his special commissioner to recruit physicians and surgeons from outside Milan if the ill had insufficient access to medical care. As a corporation, the College of Medicine was accorded exercise of judicial oversight of its members, the right to elect officials without the duke's approval, as well as to set meetings, fees and matters pertaining to the ethical-professional expectations of all College physicians. The College also claimed the privilege of

---

and consuls in the countryside. On the long association of 'anziani' with denunciations to public authorities, see Vaglienti, '*Noluit ire ad visum*', pp. 38–44.

61 L. F. Zagni, 'Osservazioni sulle *subscriptiones* nei testament nuncupative a Milano dagli statuti cittadini del 1396 sin dopo le *Constitutiones dominii Mediolanensis* (1541)', *Studi di storia medioevale e di diplomatica* 1 (1976), 263–74.

62 In 1395, Giangaleazzo Visconti purchased the title and feudal privileges of 'duke' from the Holy Roman Emperor.

63 Albini, *Guerra*, pp. 20–2, 56–8, 88–9. The 'officiali delle bollette' was an innovation of Giangaleazzo Visconti from the mid-1380s and its offices appeared in every city under his control. It normally tracked both letters and persons that entered or left the duchy; thus refugees during plagues, famines and wars significantly complicated the officials' work and led to the appointment of special plague commissioners.

64 Ibid., p. 21, 84–6. By 1450, College physicians did not have to report to the 'anziano' and surgeons caring for an ill person for more than three days not only had to report to the 'anziano', they also had to consult with a College physician.

legitimating non-College practitioners within the city and its suburbs. Serving the court as a sworn expert witnesses was prestigious and a privilege that the College guarded jealously. In fact, no practitioner other than a member of the College could give an official (courtroom) judicial opinion on a wound. These aristocratic privileges, conceptualised in the pre-plague era, now carried novel risks that College physicians were slow to deal with in their revisions to statutes.[65] As a recent study has shown, a complex bureaucratic structure that preserved the privileges and allowed the physically safe participation of College physicians during plague times emerged much later, after 1535, with the recreation of the office as the 'Tribunale di Sanità' (Health Tribunal) of Spanish Milan.[66]

Medical care to the plague-stricken and the security of Milan were more important to the duke than the privileges he granted to the College.[67] The bits of evidence that we have suggest that the elite medical community hoped to offer its considered advice on plague to the duke and his commissioners but did not want to assume tasks related to the direct care of the plague-stricken. They were not eager to attend or consult on the care of acutely ill patients in order to decide which ones showed clear and convincing signs of pestilence.[68] Recurrent plague outbreaks prompted existential fear among all urban officials with each new outbreak. What risks did they assume by staying to serve? Under what circumstances were those holding communal posts legally obligated to remain in the city? The first juridical treatises to address these and other plague-predicated questions systematically did not appear until the 1510s.[69]

I argue, therefore, that ducal plague commissioners became comparable to the court of the 'podestà' acting ex officio, with notaries collecting and compiling street-level information during plague outbreaks. Decisions may not have been taken within that local office. How and where the duke's special commissioner actually performed his obligations is not clear, for he simultaneously oversaw plague surveillance and control in Pavia.[70] His primary responsibility was to enforce or implement each new ducal order, issued in a series of letters.

65 Bottero, 'Statuti', p. 104: 'et quod nullus alius possit dare aliquam sententiam super aliquo vulnere nec super aliqua infirmitate coram aliquo iustenente vel deputato nisi sit associatus cum aliquo phisico dicti Collegii Mediolani' ('and that no [physician or surgeon] offer a judgment on any wound or any other infirmity in the presence of the sergeant or deputy unless he is associated with some physician of the said College of Medicine of Milan').

66 di Giammatteo and Mendelsohn, 'Reporting for Action'.

67 Nicoud, *Le Prince*, p. 58.

68 Albini, *Guerra*, pp. 95–6, including the duke's general orders. Nicoud, *Le Prince*, p. 390, isolates the obligations of physicians and surgeons, arguing that the commissioner consulted with members of the city College of Medicine.

69 M. Ascheri, *I giuristi e le epidemie di peste (secoli xiv–xvi)* (Siena, 1997).

70 Albini, *Guerra*, p. 88 and A. Pasi Testa, 'Alle origine dell'ufficio di Sanità nel Ducato di Milano e Principato di Pavia', *Archivio storico lombardo* s. 10 102 (1976), 379–80. De Roxellis, Giangaleazzo's 'vicar general' was appointed in 1399.

To summarise the legal aspects of change from 1272 to 1447, Visconti lords steadily expanded their dominion over much of Lombardy, ruling with claims of unrestricted power and authority. But here as elsewhere, intervals of catastrophic loss of life and wealth threatened dynastic stability. Because the commune of the twelfth and thirteenth centuries had established its own jurisdictional boundaries within its walls and over its legal district, even Visconti assertions of unbridled seigneurial power could not override traditional social and political power within Milan proper. However powerful they became, Visconti and Sforza lords had to rely on the smooth functioning of traditional city services and amenities for the vast majority of Milanese residents. Outside Milan, especially in conquered towns and cities, the Visconti lords could reserve to themselves 'control over the punishment of criminals, the imposition of fines, hearing civil cases and appeals and the power to raise taxes and punish rebels'.[71]

Second, a politically hybrid approach to governance in plague years emerged within Milan by 1400. Communal-era neighbourhood officials remained pivotal to a centralised seigneurial management of plague in the city. (Indeed, we find significant structural continuities in death reporting up to the arrival of Napoleon![72]) The powerful, elected leaders of each parish had to collect all 'facts' pertaining to blood crimes ('i fatti di sangue') and denounce those details to the 'podestà' within two days, facing substantial penalty if they failed to comply.[73] Under the Visconti they were tasked with plague reporting as well.

Sforza-era reform

By the 1420s, during the regime of Duke Filippo Maria Visconti, we can see the vestiges of a newer epidemic reporting policy.[74] Filippo Maria likely created a permanently operating local Health Office separate from the earlier duchy-wide 'Offitio delle bollette', because Milanese aristocrats who created the 'Ambrosian Republic' at his death continued that Visconti policy, appointing a commissioner to receive written reports of illnesses and deaths from 'anziani' and medical practitioners throughout the city, suburbs and nearby countryside.[75] In October 1448, the former ducal official's title became 'Commissioner

71 The transformation involved acquisition of sweeping judicial authority. See Black, 'Visconti in the Fourteenth Century', p. 7.

72 A. Visconti, *La pubblica amministrazione nello stato Milanese durante il predominio straniero (1541–1796)* (Milan, 1911), pp. 295–7.

73 E. Verga, 'Le sentenze criminali dei podestà milanesi, 1385–1429', *Archivio Storico Lombardo* 3rd s. 16 (1901), 106–11, shows that the vast majority of cases brought before the *podestà* or his judges involved accusations of injured parties or the denunciations brought by parish *anziani* and consuls in the countryside. See also E. Welch, *Art and Authority in Renaissance Milan* (New Haven, 1995), pp. 38–40; and on the adaptation of the communal neighbourhood reporting system to ducal plague controls see Albini, *Guerra*, pp. 84–6.

74 Pasi Testa, 'Ufficio di Sanità', 376–86.

75 *Acta Libertatis Mediolani. I registri n. 5 e n. 6 dell'Ufficio degli Statuti di Milano (Repubblica Ambrosiana 1447–1450)*, ed. A. R. Natale (Milan, 1987), pp. 214–16, a proclamation from 7 September

for the Office of the Preservation of the Health of Milan'.[76] 'Anziani' continued to track strangers and visitors in the city by making inquiries ('inquisitioni') surrounding the circumstances of anyone coming from an area suspected of plague; they reported the details – who made an accusation, who circumvented the regulations.

As the would-be Republic faltered in 1449, plague cases were discovered in the suburban zone. Ordinary Milanese received few updates on the danger but remote facilities were readied to isolate plague-infected households. Ambrosian oligarchs hired plague doctors to serve in emergency isolation areas, giving temporary contracts and salary inducements comparable to traditional arrangements with 'medici condotti'.[77] None of the surgeons, barbers, apothecaries and the occasional physician sent to extramural isolation facilities was involved with identifying new cases of plague inside the city.

Because the Sanità archive has not survived,[78] we are left to speculate how, when and why a local civic agency, a properly Milanese (as opposed to a ducal) office with judicial powers to judge and sentence plague cases, took its distinctive form. It is clear that some changes were made by the Ambrosian Republic, which also successfully wrested control of hospital resources away from ecclesiastical managers.[79] Explicitly embracing the old communal ideal of serving the public good, the Republic's 'Deputati (or Officialis) super peste' (Deputies concerned with plague, sometimes called Officials) essentially became Sforza's 'Officio Sanitatis Mediolani' (Office of the Sanità in Milan; its formal name changed multiple times across the fourteenth through eighteenth centuries).[80] Sforza retained the network of 'anziani' to perform urban plague surveillance, as well as the commissioner position. He resided in Milan, reporting to the duke, his chancery and his Privy Council. Francesco Sforza's Health Office explicitly retained notaries, service personnel (including a person to carry the lists of the dead) and a 'medico fisico' (a university-educated

1447, 'Pro morbo et infirmis civitatis et Ducatus Mediolani' ('For the sick and infirm of the city and Duchy of Milan'). 'Anziani' and medical practitioners were required to report ill persons to this office, which also issued burial permits. Numerous early bans on cities and territories from which plague was reported were all handled by the 'offitialis bullettarum Mediolani' (the Milanese office of *bollette,* or bills and certificates). E.g., *Acta Libertatis Mediolani*, 3 July 1448, 'Pro morbo citivatus Arimini, Fani, Pixauri, Urbani et Anchone', p. 378.

76 *Acta Libertatis Mediolani*, 'Pro Offitio super sanitatis conservando', 2 October 1448, pp. 438–40. On the unusually early establishment of permanent cause-of-death reporting see F. Vaglienti, '*Noluit ire ad visum*', pp. 38–9.

77 Decio, *La peste in Milano*, pp. 11–17.

78 A fire on New Year's Eve 1502/03 destroyed the fifteenth-century archives of the Sanità. See F. Vaglienti, '*Noluit ire ad visum*', pp. 25–7.

79 Vaglienti, '*Noluit ire ad visum*', pp. 44–5, who believes the official called the 'catelano' was created during the lordship of Filippo Maria Visconti.

80 Albini, *Guerra*, pp. 78–9 and 103–6. On use of this older communal rhetoric see A. Gamberini, *A Companion to Late Medieval and Early Modern Milan* (Leiden, 2014), p. 23.

physician).[81] In other words, the new Sforza office was likely the earliest to include a learned physician on staff, acting in more than a consultant's role.[82] His reports and judgments are mentioned in letters to the duke as early as 1451.[83] Once plague ended, the Health Office endured – another change from the Visconti past. Earlier magistracies of whatever composition and authority had focused only on plague years and those who died of plague. From this point forward, reporting causes of death in all years, for every individual over the age of three years at death, had become a 'consolidated and habitual practice' by the time Sforza died in 1466.[84]

The extraordinary success of Sforza's Sanità flowed from its politically melded governance and from the administrative decision to preserve an office record of the deaths of each and every Milanese citizen. 'Anziani' could supply social, physical and narrative detail about the last illness of most individuals, but the Sforza Health Office did not expect them to determine causes of illness or death. Reflecting the traditional communal ethic of inclusiveness that served the common good, they therefore supplied names, occupations, relationships and descriptions of illness that came from householders and the neighbourhood. The names of Milanese residents, fully provided even with stillborn babies in these registers, became a birth right for citizens. Without the 'anziani' and the larger civic purpose to record keeping, death reporting might have remained an undifferentiated count of deaths and plague cases only in epidemic years. The full names of prominent and propertied persons – the clients of those who could afford the services of College physicians and surgeons – would have dominated death lists.

Other striking non-medical features of these records include continuity in record-keeping practices across significant periods of regime change, a reflection of persisting staff loyalty to each other and to civic integrity, even during prolonged hostilities and occupation by foreign troops. Health Office personnel acted as citizens in service to a common mission. My overall data set includes 134,809 individually recorded deaths up to early 1525. One of the worst plagues that Milan ever faced reached its peak in the summer of 1524, crippling the routine collection of death reports by late May. But reports from early 1525 resume daily record keeping as before, the format and objectives unchanged.

A man called Catelano

From the earliest surviving mortality register (it begins in late July 1452) through to the end of the century, the subset I used here to illustrate the practices of an early medical

[81] Imitating the Visconti dukes, Sforza continued to receive daily death bulletins from this local office, even while relying on his 'Secret Council' to confirm their reports. See my 'Registering Deaths'.

[82] However, the office commissioner appointed in October 1448, Giovanni de Curteregina, was a College physician. See *Acta Libertatis Mediolani*, p. 440.

[83] Albini, *Guerra*, p. 90.

[84] Albini, *Guerra*, p. 160; Carmichael, 'Registering Deaths'.

examiner, we have surviving death reports for 59,363 individual deaths, 28.5 per cent of whom were infants and toddlers (requiring no causal diagnosis). Within extant fifteenth-century records, the primary certifier of causes of death was a particular university-educated physician named Master Giovanni Catelano, a foreign matriculate to Milan's College of Medicine on 19 April 1450.[85] He is first mentioned in 1450 in letters sent by the newly created Sforza Health Office to the new duke.[86] Other frequently reporting 'high certifiers' also appear, including the various surgeons who worked for the Health Office and the publicly funded physicians who served in Milan's hospitals.[87]

Giovanni Catelano's name may reflect a job description. Vaglienti claims that Milan had an official, called the 'catelano' in Milanese vernacular, before the Sforza came to power and that the word referred to a public, salaried official specifically tasked with establishing causes of death. Intriguing as well is the etymology Vaglienti provides for the term 'catelano:' a woollen overgarment commonly worn by persons serving in an official communal capacity.[88] Unlike some other areas of northern and central Italy, in Milan few judicial and municipal archives survive from the communal and Visconti eras and the archives of the Sanità were destroyed in a fire, as mentioned earlier. Thus Vaglienti's claims are, unfortunately, difficult to verify or reject with extant documentation.

The *Libri mortuorum* offer some disconfirming evidence concerning Vaglienti's secondary claim, that Master Giovanni Catelano, ironically, did not hold the position of 'catelano'.[89] I compared the many particularly wordy and detailed causal diagnoses attributed to someone referred to only as 'catelano' to those expressly attributed to Master Giovanni Catelano, finding no salient differences in pattern or word choice. For example, the complicated case of Lord Azzone Visconti's servant, Venturino, was attested by the

85 Bottero, 'Statuti', p. 112: Dominus Magister Iohannes Catelanus.

86 Nicoud, *Le Prince*, pp. 59–61.

87 For the term 'high certifier' see L. Prior and M. Bloor, 'Why People Die: Social Representations of Death and its Causes', *Science as Culture* 3 (1993), 346–74.

88 Vaglienti, '*Noluit ire ad visum*', pp. 36–46, 53–4 on the 'catelano's' garment. Vaglienti's argument referenced an entry in the death register, 10 August 1452, in which the cause of death was 'reported by the gravediggers because master Giovanni of Florence did not want to go to see her' ('relatum sepultorum eo quia magister Johannes de Florentia noluit ire ad visum'). The case was of a five-year-old girl who had died with 'black measles' and a bubo in her left groin. She argued on linguistic grounds that the phrase 'ire ad visum' indicated an obligation to see a dead person who was not the physician's own patient, thus ascertaining the cause of death with his own eyes – a necroscopy. Therefore, she argues, the position already existed under the Visconti and this Giovanni of Florence held the post. Alas there is no surviving document alluding to a 'catelano' before the Sforza era. As to master Giovanni's refusal to confirm a plague death: neither the Republican oligarchs nor Sforza administrators reliably paid civil servants in these chaotic years.

89 Vaglienti, '*Noluit ire ad visum*', pp. 45–7. On the death-related duties of *anziani* in the early modern era, Vaglienti summarizes and expands on the work of C. Tedeschi, *Origini e vicende dei cimiteri di Milano e del servizio mortuario* (Milan, 1895), p. 74, who claims, without specific documentation, that the surgeon of the (late seventeenth-century) *Tribunale della Sanità* was called the 'catelano'.

'catelano'. As with most of the other frequent certifiers of cause of death who emerge in the records, Catelano/catelano had favourite diagnostic practices, in his case a preference for multi-causal reports even when a death was not plague related.

Apart from the death reports and some administrative documents of the new Ospedale Maggiore (Great Hospital), one particularly interesting mention of Catelano to general plague management occurs in a long epic poem that Bettino da Trezzo dedicated to Ascanio Sforza. Bettino described the Health Office's inability to 'render rasone' (determine and record a cause of death) during the worst months of the 1485 plague. The poem clearly details the reporting procedures: parish 'anziani' were instructed to send hourly reports to the health deputies, who would then send out people to confirm the cause and take action if needed. When this process broke down, Bettino claimed that survivors in many residences had to bury their dead occultly. Thus, there were no notaries, no descriptions, no way to calculate the city's losses.[90] He crafted a poem to capture the magnitude of the catastrophe, the resilience of the city and the rare successes of urban governance. To this last point he offered that those in household isolation 'were visited by the catelano, / Expert physician in such matters' ('In farli visitar del cathellano / Medico expert in ciò'). This 'catelano' also connected the household with other medical services, while the 'anziani' and other municipal authorities provided food.

Nicoud further shows that Giovanni Catelano's predecessor in the Sforza Health Office was not called 'catelano' and thus the very word might be a linguistic legacy of Giovanni Catelano's long and dedicated service to Milan.[91] As the 'fisicus epidemie' (plague doctor) to the Sanità for thirty to forty years, Catelano was especially prominent as the primary certifier of cause of death during crisis years, beginning with the plague outbreak of 1451–52, through its return in 1468–69, during the famine and non-plague epidemic of 1476–79, during the catastrophic plague outbreak of 1483–86 and in its aftermath. He was active until the mid-1490s, reporting on average 37.5 per cent of all diagnoses of cause of death in all years and months that can be retrieved from still-extant death registers and daily death reports.[92] If the Health Office practices were indeed similar to those of the commune-era 'podestà', a notary accompanied one or both men as they canvassed neighbourhood 'anziani'.

Plague diagnosis by 'autopsy', 1452–99

Catelano worked alongside a series of surgeons who served with him in the Sforza Health Office. They literally performed autopsies, in that they directly viewed both persons acutely ill and/or studied the cadavers of individuals who had not been in the care of a College of Medicine physician. Autopsy did not yet have its modern meaning, a post-mortem

90 Bettino da Trezzo, *Letimologia* (Milan, 1488).

91 Nicoud, *Le Prince*, pp. 59–62.

92 Of the 42,433 diagnoses for whom a cause of death was required, Catelano provided 15,909, or about 36 per cent.

dissection. Meanwhile, College of Medicine physicians performed their preferred role, directly advising the Health Office through the appointment of two members, every four months, to serve as deputies on the Sanità governing board.[93] However, none of the extant administrative documentation specified criteria for making post-mortem diagnoses of plague. Some illustrative case reports and a tally of the criteria that the Health Office actually used will thus be offered to show the epistemological gap that opened between elite College physicians and Health Office personnel. What the Collegians could confidently assert about plague and its management did not address the practical street-level challenges that Health Office personnel faced when determining whether a person did or did not die of plague.[94] Collegians offered advice that centred on environmental challenges, an approach exceedingly difficult to implement when epidemic mortality surged.

Deaths with a single suspicion-raising component could summon multiple diagnosticians, as we saw with both debated cases presented at this chapter's outset. So, too, could non-plague diagnoses from College physicians that the Health Office physician found problematic prompt a review. The level of suspicion was heightened when plague was already feared or identified within the city or its suburbs. In these cases, the larger urban context for assessing causes of death changed, and even prominent households could be held in quarantine for a few days to determine whether further cases would appear. After 1500 the procedures became somewhat routine, with many records indicating the temporary closure of a residence ('separatur/separantur per aliquos dies'). In Giovanni Catelano's era, the bureaucratic shorthand was more often the term 'suspected' ('casus suspectus'). Post-mortem signs, both visual and verbal, constituted a warning that could lead to temporary isolation.[95] Enforcing these epidemic protocols required collaboration between central-city and hyper-local authorities, not a programme of street-cleaning and waste removal in the potentially affected street.

In a non-epidemic year, here early July 1472, we can see that post-mortem appearances enhanced interrogation of household survivors. Thirty-year-old Antonia, wife of Jacobo

[93] *Statuta & Ordinationes Dominorum Phisicorum Collegii Mediolanensis* (Milan, 1517), unnumbered pages, chapter 34: 'Statutum de duobus prefectis sanitatis per collegium elligendis: Singulis quattuor mensibus habeat plenam auctoritatem collegium elligendi duos collegiatos qui sedeant deputati ad officium sanitatis Mediolani habeantque omnimodam potestatem auctoritatem & baliam agenda praecipiendi et scrutiniandi sicut habent alii praefecti dicti offitii sanitatis' (Statute on the two prefects elected by the College to the Sanità: Every four months the College has full authority to elect two colleagues to be seated among the deputies of the Office of the Sanità of Milan, and they shall have all power and authority to prescribe and scrutinize the actions of the magistrate and officials of the said Health Office.)

[94] Nicoud, *Le Prince*, pp. 402–7.

[95] Thus, the death report of twenty-seven-year-old Sister Eufemia de Magnis at the monastery of S. Magdalena. She died within six days and was examined post-mortem. 'Nothing was found that made a diagnosis of plague certain to us [Catelano and Dionigi]', but they, or perhaps the Deputies, flagged this a possible plague death: 'propter acutas conumeretur animadvertendum est consecutessus considerat pro mayori cautela'. ASMi, *Pop. p.a.*, c. 76, 2 April 1483.

Confaroneri, fell suddenly ill with 'collerica passione' (choleric affliction, caused by excess or corrupted yellow bile), vomiting and a variety of other symptoms attributed to her diet and mind-set. 'There was, however, a certain pustule in her right breast that has erupted, which we saw together with her husband and brother' ('Erat tamen quedam pustula in mamilla dextra iam excicata ... similes vidimus cum marito et fratre'). Three experienced practitioners contributed to the report: Master Sillani de Nigris, Catelano and Giovanni Pirovano. Sillani was a member of the College, very probably one of the deputies to the Health Office at the time of this report; he was as well a ducal physician. Master Giovanni Pirovano, nicknamed 'Scanzete' possibly for a wry demeanour in the face of serious situations, was a surgeon who worked for the Sanità.[96]

In years when confirmed plague deaths had already cropped up, post-mortem scrutiny intensified. A death reported on 20 January 1483 indicated that Jacobina, the twenty-four-year-old daughter of Cristoforo Scarlati, had been ill for at least fifteen days. She lived in San Babila parish in the East Gate sector of the city.

> But last Tuesday [the death report appeared on a Monday], she relapsed, taken ill with fever and colicky abdominal and iliac pain, with fecal and menstrual retention. Seen again in death she had some various measles, from which so much [can] proceed; it will be better to consider what happens [going forward]. In the judgment of masters Catelano and Dyonisio.[97]

Indeed, the two Sanità physicians kept attention on the household. Then on Thursday, 13 February, the death of Bernardina, daughter of Giovanni Petrobonello, eighteen years old, living near the Scarlati household, confirmed earlier suspicion about Jacobina. Bernardina fell ill on the previous Saturday with pestiferous ('accidentibus pestiferis') symptoms, subjugated urines ('urinis subiugalis') and vomiting, a known plague case that connected to a death three weeks earlier.

Rumours of plague in multiple areas inside the city walls quickly changed the diagnostic landscape. Jacobo of Intrania's wife, Domenica, aged thirty, fell ill, which led masters Catelano and Dionigi to visit her together, a reflection of the Sanità's high alert. Inspecting

96 Bottero, 'Statuti', p. 112 (Dominus Magister Syllanus de Nigris, who matriculated as a foreign member on 23 March 1458) and p. 111 (Dominus Magister Nicolaus de Arsago, who joined as a Milanese member of the College on 9 February 1450). Scanzete was explicitly named as a plague surgeon: Johannes de Pirovano dicte Scanzete, 'ciroyci nostri super pestem' (ASMi, *Misc. stor.*, 1, n. 457) who worked for the Health Office. He died at age eighty, from senility and a continuous fever, 12 November 1477, the diagnosis reported by Gabriel de Pirovano. A Magnificus dns. Gabriel Pirovanus died 5 August 1504, at age sixty-three, and thus may have been Giovanni Pirovano's son.

97 'Jacobina fila Cristofori Scarlati ... infirma iam 15 dies et plus die tamen Jovis proxima preterita per viam recidua male cepit infirma cum febre et doloribus ventris colicis et yliacis cum retention stercoris et mestruorum. Rivisa tamen in morte aparuerit quidam morbilli varii quia tante procedendum mediocriter considerabitur sequela. Iudicio magistrorum Catelani et Dyonisii.' ASMi, *Pop. p.a.*, c. 76, for all 1483 deaths.

her body pre-mortem, Dionigi noted an 'elongated uterus' and burning fever ('Inventa est cum causa et elongatione matricis').[98] On Tuesday 18 February 1483, Master Dionigi, the Health Office surgeon, returned and found her in terror of death. Domenica died within the hour and the diagnosis of plague seemed clear. He diligently inspected her body post mortem and interviewed those around her. Some of her neighbours declared that she had fallen ill just the previous Saturday, with pain on both sides of her groin from an inguinal swelling that they called a 'dragonzello',[99] ('visa per horam ante decessum eius cum accidentibus terroris et mortis; habita notitia a quodam sibi astantium quod cepit infirmari die sabati proxima passata et quod dolebat in altero inguinium ex dragonzelo ut dixit'). Although I cannot determine from this odd term precisely what a 'dragonzello' looked like, the salient issue is that the Health Office certifiers differentiated glandular swellings by post-mortem appearances rather than Galenic pathophysiological categories.

Domenica did not live in the affected Eastern Gate area, belonging instead to the parish of San Giorgio, near the large parish of San Lorenzo inside the walls. Suddenly, with this death and at this point, the earlier death of a twenty-year-old woman on 2 January occasioned a wider Health Office review. That woman was Helena, daughter of Matteo Rosati who lived in San Lorenzo parish, the porta Ticinese district, in the city's south-western sector.[100] Her death had been attributed to strenuous exertion in especially foggy air. She had returned home before succumbing to a fainting fever, pains in her entire chest region and the inability to bring up foul matter by coughing. Because she died within four days of the onset of illness, Catelano and Dionigi together had examined her cadaver as well as the urine she produced when still alive, finding at the time no certain signs of plague.

Here we see an epidemiological case-tracing approach that Catelano seems to have invented during the 1468 plague outbreak while trying to respond to the concerns of the very young Duke Galeazzo Maria Sforza, Francesco Sforza's firstborn son. The duke, like all the Visconti and Sforza princes before him, held plague to be contagious. Through case tracing, the path of plague could be found out.[101]

98 ASMi, *Pop. p.a.*, c. 76, 18 February 1483, a Tuesday.

99 The term may come from the French 'la dragonne', which refers to a wrist strap used in holding a sword or epée securely, a suggestion made by F. Cherubini, *Vocabolario Milanese-Italiano*, v. 2 (Milan, 1814), p. 57.

100 ASMi, *Pop. p.a.*, c. 76: Jacobina Scarlati lived in San Babila parish, porta Orientale district, inside the walls. So, too, did Bernardina, whose death was reported on Thursday, 13 February: 'Bernardina filia Johannis de Putheobonello, annorum xviii, infirma a die sabeti citra cum accidentibus pestiferis ut urinis subiugalis, vomitu, et cum glandula in inguine sinistro quod de occulta falatam aliarum defunctarum ut que decessit in 4ta die 2a Januarii et Christofori Scarlati que decessit 20 Januarii'. (Bernardina, daughter of Giovanni of Puteobonello, 18 years old, fell ill around Saturday with pestilential signs and subjugated urines, vomiting, and with a glandular swelling in the left groin, dead within 4 days and thereby linking to [literally, here, showing secrets of] other deaths on 2 January and Cristoforo Scarlati, who died 20 January.)

101 See my 'Contagion Theory and Contagion Practice in Fifteenth-century Milan', *Renaissance Quarterly* 44 (1991), 213–56.

Even ambivalent 'indicia' (indications or marks) of plague on a cadaver prompted further inquiry, and in this way were similar to the collection of evidence for crime investigations. Verifying plague resembled crime investigations in the public sphere. Process-oriented accounts of a last illness, those lacking description of visible bodily lesions, were instead typical of reports made by Galenic physicians. For example, on 10 March 1480, Master Niccolò Arsago, himself a College physician, died suddenly at age fifty-four. Another prominent practitioner, Gabriel Pirovano, reported that he had seen the doctor's cadaver. According to Niccolò's wife, the doctor had dined before suddenly experiencing a burning stomach affliction, vomiting enormously such that he died in the process. 'Arbitror' – 'I judged', Gabriel said in his report – that the doctor had suffocated from the descent of catarrh ('descensus catarri', usually understood as generated in the brain) and the ascent of food ('assensu cibi') or other substance in his stomach; as such, the death was 'not suspected' ('sine suspectu'). Similarly process-driven, even as plague was taking hold of Milan in 1483, on Thursday 7 June, Giovanni Cusano, aged 74 years, had a continuous fever for fourteen days, with chills and tremors. In the fourth day he emitted violet measles, but without any other suspect signs except thirst. At the end of the seventh day, a rash attributed to excess black bile appeared on his back, testicles and one tibia, such that the whole tibia was swollen as well as the testicle and penis. Thus, 'And I, Antonius Cusanus, physician, visited him together with other physicians.'[102] Although Antonio Cusano did not diagnose plague, he allowed reason for caution. His approach to the task of reporting a cause of death was to chronicle the sequence of changes to the old man's condition. He neither specified on which day the team of doctors saw the man nor offered a description of his post-mortem findings.

Said another way, plague diagnoses provided by Health Office practitioners privilege the evidence of visible lesions on a cadaver. Consider a Catelano report on 29 June 1483 of an eleven-year-old boy who died of pestilential fever with a hard swelling ('petracia') in his left axilla and two carbuncles, one on the bony back of the neck and the other four digits to the left.[103] Or, instead, a domestic servant, fourteen years old, who on 22 July 1483 fell ill after lunch with continuous vomiting. Catelano viewed her body four days later and found a carbuncle in the area over the spleen and a bubo in the groin on the same side. Black measles disseminated from the bubo.[104] This too was a plague death. The exacting standard of physical diagnosis post mortem, at least with the first or index cases within a given

[102] 'in fine septima supervenit colera in dorso et testiculis et in una tibia ita quod tibia tota que alias prout facta et testiculi et verga devenerunt ad extiomenum … Et ego Antonius Cusanus phisicus ipsum visitatum unam cum aliis phisicis, iudicio magistri Antonii de Cusano.' ASMi, *Pop. p.a.*, c. 76, 7 June 1483.

[103] 'cum petracia in subassella sinistra et carbonibus duobus altero supra spondalem cinguli et altero parte distante per iiij digitos ad sinistra'. ASMi, *Pop. p.a.*, c. 76, 29 June 1483.

[104] 'infirma a die Jovis citra post prandium, cum vomitu quasi continuo et secessu ut constat per matrem astantis ei … Considerata tamen mortua reperta est cum carbone circha regionem splenis et Bubone in inguine eiusdem partis cum morbilis nigris hinc inde desiminatis in fine 4te, iudicio Catelani.' ASMi, *Pop. p.a.*, c. 76, 22 July 1483.

household, rose during the subsequent outbreak, even in 1485 when the Office could no longer manage all the formal record keeping. Their clerical priority became the daily letters listing deaths and new cases, dispatched to the acting duke, Ludovico Maria Sforza.[105]

The criteria Sanità physicians and surgeons used to establish a diagnosis illustrate forensic purposes, especially where the consequences of the diagnosis to surviving household members gradually stabilised. Analysis of the observed 'indicia' or signs visible on bodies underpins my claim that Health Office medical and surgical practitioners supplied what served the process of justice. Most records further documented testimony from witnesses or neighbourhood authorities, just as courtroom trials required. In some death reports, we see both elements and more, such that they resembled the initial crime narratives composed by notaries since the thirteenth century and retained as public records.[106]

Table 2.1 summarises evidence from plague deaths related to the post-mortem physical findings. Only twenty-nine (1.5 per cent) of the newly found cases of plague reported no relevant clinical or physical sign that led to the diagnosis. Making a diagnosis of plague prompted the Health Office physician or surgeon to record forensic facts or evidence verified from a literal autopsy – viewing the cadaver. In many cases, the side of the body (e.g., a left-side bubo) was also specified, a seemingly gratuitous medical detail but highly important if the diagnosis is seen as evidence in a juridical context. There was, as well, an alternative basis to support a plague diagnosis involving a short course of illness. In 513 (27.1 per cent) of these cases, the report noted the number of days the victim had been ill; in 456 (88.9 per cent) of these 513 reports, the last illness played out over four or fewer days, evidence that required close watch on the health of individual households.

Two hundred and nineteen death diagnoses were explicitly made by inspecting the cadaver of a deceased person, thus by the testimony of the diagnostician. I included neither the reports made by gravediggers (not medically authoritative), nor the formulaic reports that appeared in records between 1479 and 1482: 'visus mortuus s[ine] s[uspicione]' (seen dead, without suspicion). In other words, although in those cases the formula confirmed that a particular death was or was not due to plague, they did not offer an alternative cause of death. The testimony of the body was crucial in resolving doubt: 37.9 per cent of the 219 reports were made by two or more physicians/surgeons. An example of this kind of explicit, but plague-negative, minimalist report is one from Dionigi [of Nuremberg, who frequently worked with Catelano]: a fifteen-year-old youth 'erat culpatus secundum relatione' (those reporting the death blamed plague). The report exonerated him, however, saying that the boy was seen in death without other suspicious findings ('visus in morte absque suspitione aliquo apparuent').[107]

105 Carmichael, 'Registering Deaths'.

106 See Vallerani, *Medieval Public Justice*, p. 129, on the medieval judicial-notarial innovation, the 'writing of the crime'.

107 ASMi, *Pop. p.a.*, c. 75, 15 August 1479. The Master Dionigi who worked with Catelano at the Health Office is surely Dyonisius de Norimbergo. He seems to have joined the Health Office after the 1477 death of Giovanni Pirovano, the Sanità's surgeon dealing with plague cases in the

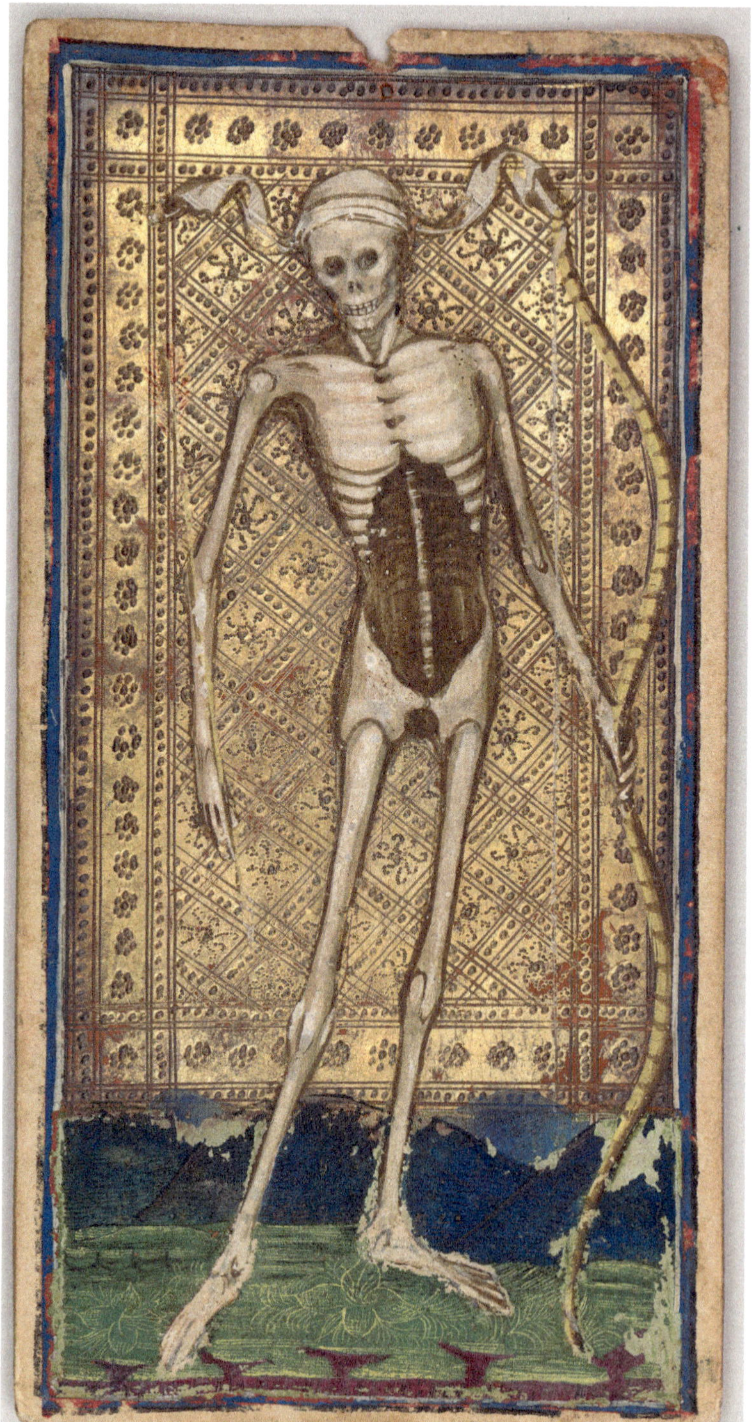

Fig. 2.1. Visconti-Sforza tarot card, Death (Skeleton), Milan, Italy, c. 1450–80. The Morgan Library and Museum, New York, Manuscript M.630.12.

Table 2.1. Milan Health Office Evidence for New Cases of Plague: Physically Visible Lesions Seen Post-mortem, n=1,891.

Primary basis of diagnosis	**Reported diagnoses by bodily region**	**No. of cases**
	measles, red measles, erysipelas, red 'signs'	34
	black or purple measles, black 'signs', blackened body	121
Rash	'pestilential measles'	450
	pustules	13
	'anthrax'	11
	inguinal bubo	317
Bubo	axillary bubo	137
	cervical bubo	19
	no location noted	4
	inguinal *glandula*	87
Glandula	axillary *glandula*	44
	cervical *glandula*	9
	no location noted	1
	inguinal *aposteme*	120
Aposteme (abscess)	axillary *aposteme*	47
	cervical *aposteme*	76
	no specified location	18
	inguinal region	44
Swelling (*eminencia*) or tumour	axillary region	5
	cervical region	38
	other specified location on body	2
Carbuncle (eschars)	*carbone* or *carbunculli*	115
Dragonzello	inguinal region	8
Non-specific plague evidence	pestilential 'signs' or pestilential fever	29
	pestilential 'accidents' (i.e., symptoms)	52

But compare this plague-confirming report, involving more than one physician, a new case of plague on Wednesday 8 October 1483:

> Apolonia, wife of Giovanni Leuco, 40 years old, fell ill on Sunday, at around 20 hours; the doctor who was caring for her did not know what killed her, but diligently contemplating in death, which can better determine, she was found with an oblong eminence in her right inguinal area, radiating and reddened toward the centre with purplish measles disseminating from it. She died at the end of three days, six days' time altogether; neighbours fled and servants were in fear at this sentence, which confirms [the cause]. In the judgment of masters Catelano, Stefano Triviglio, and Dionisio.[108]

While this example suggests that the Health Office considered post-mortem 'autopsy' more reliable evidence for diagnosing plague than the diagnosis based on an attending physician's report, the court of the Health Office also appealed to the length of time the person had been ill, the behaviour or testimony of neighbours and the response of persons in the household of the deceased.

In Milan, many other diagnoses also seem to have been made from direct view of a nude cadaver, providing opportunity to locate observable lesions anatomically. On which side of a body, or in what specific location, a wound or injury was visible was often medically gratuitous information, because the cause of death did not vary according to the side of the body affected. With 1,045 deaths reporting one or more wounds as the cause, less than half (42.2 per cent) noted the bodily location. Unsurprisingly, head, thorax and abdominal wounds comprised two-thirds of this subset and over 92 per cent were male. In 60 per cent of deaths attributed to breast cancer, the record specified right, left or both-breast involvement and/or whether the area was ulcerated. With breast cancer reports, 83.6 per cent of all victims were persons over age forty at death.[109]

A surprisingly common observational habit that Catelano and Dionigi adopted during the plague wave from 1483 through 1486 is fascinating, but speculative to formulate and tedious to analyse. In individuals whose bodies evidenced 'carbunculi' (carbuncles) or plague eschars ('carboni'), as well as glandular swellings, both men tended to note the side of the eschar and the side of the swelling. In other words, it is possible that they

---

city. Dionigi became the highest certifier after Catelano either retired or died in 1495 (only a handful of death reports between 1495 and 1503 have survived). He died in April 1504, at age eighty. Confusingly, there was a different Master Dionigi in earlier records: 'Dionysius de Cerutis', who died in 1483 at age sixty.

108 ASMi, *Pop. p.a.*, c. 76, 8 October 1483: 'Apolonia uxor Johannis de Leuco, annorum xl.ta, cepit infirma die dominico hora quaxi xx.a nescio qua labe defecirt /constat Iudicio Medici curantis. Sed contemplate in morte diligenter quod Melius Potuit, reperta est cum eminentia oblonga in Inguine dextro irradiante cum rubedine in parte domestica cum morbiis vyolaceis hinc Inde deseminatis. Terminata in fine iii.o completo sextus tempus vicinitas fuga et Pauer domesticorum hanc sententiam Aliqualiter confirmat. Iudicio M. Cat., Stefani de Triviglio & dyonisij'.

109 Before 1500, 183 deaths were attributed to breast cancer; 3.8 of whom were male; 8.7 per cent were younger adult women, aged twenty to forty at death.

suspected the two different-appearing physical lesions were related, a view that contemporary Galenists did not advance. In 1485, Catelano further expressed within death reports his own conclusion that pleurisy could be viewed as a different contagion even in time of plague.[110] This, too, was not the common view.

Conclusion

Historians of forensic medicine highlight the judges' power when referring to a 'Continental system', but no such system existed before the time of the *Constitutio Criminalis Carolina* of Habsburg Emperor Charles V, first published in 1532.[111] Based on a slightly earlier compilation (the Bamberg Code, 1507) that used late medieval Italian penal law as a framework, the *Carolina* outlined judicial procedures for determining guilt, especially the use of torture in investigation and the application of severe corporal punishments if sufficient evidence existed of guilt.[112] Early specialised texts and judicial proceedings pertaining to forensic medicine appear much later, outside the temporal scope of this study, and have led to valuable recent studies of forensic medical practices in early modern Italy.[113] But there has been little in-depth consideration of evolving Italian legal traditions on which the *Carolina* was based and nothing whatsoever that speaks to a broadened state forensic interest in certifying causes of deaths that were not subject to the criminal court.

Forensic cultures were local and specific. They offer a framework that shifts our historical attention to social practices and priorities. In general, the forensic or legal medicine that was invented in medieval Italian communes built upon the expectation that, as citizens, physicians and surgeons were expected to serve the 'common good'. Yet in many towns and cities this kind of medico-legal work became a privilege, a source of income, honour and status that divided rather than united urban practitioners.[114] Brutal and recurrent plague outbreaks reordered the structures of risk for university-trained practitioners. Municipalities and territorial states could no longer rely on the original purpose of forensic

[110] ASMi, *Misc. stor.*, 4, n. 739: '14 February 1485: Reynaldo of Bergamo, forty-seven years old fell ill with true pleurisy on the left side, struggling and in danger of contagion and death [because he was in a plague-suspected house]. His wife and one of his daughters had died of pleurisies in the previous ten days, such that pleurisy should be considered another epidemic or pestilence': 'Reynaldo de Pergamo, annorum xlvii ... infirmatur a die veneris citra pleuresi vera lateris sinistra satis difficilis et periculosa de contagia, et morte decesserunt [sic] hac causa et uxor et quedam sua filia ut predie dixi huius pleureses altera epidimia pestilencia considerabitur Chatelani'.

[111] P. Oestmann, 'The Law of the Holy Roman Empire of the German Nation', in *Oxford Handbook*, ed. Pihlajamäki, Dubber and Godfrey, pp. 738–40. An article by R. P. Brittain, 'Origins of Legal Medicine: *Constitutio Criminalis Carolina*', *Medico-Legal Journal* 33 (1965), 124–7, may have solidified the view among Anglophone historians of forensic medicine that the *Carolina* code marks the beginning of Continental legal medicine.

[112] See Crawford, 'Legalizing Medicine', pp. 89–116.

[113] A. Pastore, *Medico in tribunale*; De Renzi, 'Medical Expertise'; Duffin, 'Questioning Medicine'.

[114] Crawford, 'Legalizing Medicine', pp. 92–4.

consultants: deterring street violence through legal action against aggressors. Larger cities and towns made temporary contracts with foreign itinerant plague doctors to meet emergencies and minimise risk to local 'civic physicians'.[115] The non-noble practitioners who performed the lion's share of community healthcare between 1500 and 1800 were full members of the community, working in all years.[116]

Milan offers a unique, local case study of continuity in expert forensic medicine that followed medieval ideals while transferring forensic authority and civic trust to a novel Health Office. Medical and surgical professional men working for the Office rather than private clients performed work consistent with the objectives of modern medical examiners. But their experiential learning was not the approach common in academic medicine. Their learned contemporaries were proud of a reason- and theory-based understanding of human pathology and would come to write treatises of forensic medicine only much later, in the 1600s, when reason could win the day and pathological anatomy had advanced a new set of questions about disease processes.[117]

115 Di Giammatteo and Mendelsohn, 'Reporting for Action', pp. 137–8, use 'civic doctors' as a collective referring to non-college physicians and surgeons working in Milan during the Spanish era.

116 Palmer, 'Physicians and the State'.

117 S. De Renzi, 'Witnesses of the Body: Medico-Legal Cases in Seventeenth-Century Rome', *Studies in the History and Philosophy of Science* 33 (2002), 219–42.

3

Epidemic Illness in the Last Book of Giovanni Villani's *New Chronicle*, 1345–48: Warfare, Sin and the Heavens

NICOLE ARCHAMBEAU

In her essay 'Universal and Particular: The Language of Plague, 1348–1350', Ann Carmichael looked at a large collection of chronicles and physicians' texts to see how writers described plague as an epidemic illness.[1] This chapter adapts Carmichael's approach to explore ideas of epidemic illness before the Black Death arrived. This approach helps modern scholars to consider how contemporaries revised previous ideas of the causes of epidemics when faced with the first wave of the Second Plague Pandemic.

Rather than study an array of texts as Carmichael did, this chapter focuses instead on one influential chronicle – the last book of Giovanni Villani's *New Chronicle* – to unpack this author's complex understanding of the interconnectedness of warfare, sin and the movement of planets as causes or indicators of epidemic disease.[2] My intention here is neither to investigate what actually transpired on the ground nor to take a broad approach to how the mechanics of warfare generated and spread disease.[3] Rather, my interest is in teasing apart the perceptions of one influential writer in fourteenth-century Italy to see how disease was linked to warfare through the lens of sin, astrology and natural disaster

1 A. G. Carmichael, 'Universal and Particular: The Language of Plague, 1348–1350', in *Pestilential Complexities: Understanding Medieval Plague*, ed. V. Nutton (London, 2008), pp. 17–52.

2 I use the translations found in *The Final Book of Giovanni Villani's New Chronicle*, trans. R. I. Diakité and Matthew Sneider (Kalamazoo, 2016). The standard modern critical edition is Giovanni Villani, *Nuova cronica*, ed. G. Porta, 3 vols. (Parma, 1990–91), but the Italian text cited in this chapter is from the *Cronica di Giovanni Villani: A miglior lezione ridotta coll'ajuto de'testi a penna*, IV, ed. I. Moutier and F. G. Dragomanni (Florence, 1845), which has been in more general use in modern scholarship on the history of medicine and is easily available online.

3 The scholarship on battleground disease and its spread is significant. Among many others covering a broad time period, see P. Mitchell, 'The Spread of Disease with the Crusades', in *Between Text and Patient: The Medical Enterprise in Medieval and Early Modern Europe*, ed. F. E. Glaze and B. Nance (Florence, 2011), pp. 309–30; S. Govaerts, *Armies and Ecosystems in Premodern Europe: The Meuse Region, 1250–1850* (Amsterdam, 2021), pp. 183–98; V. J. Cirillo, 'Fever and Reform: The Typhoid Epidemic in the Spanish–American War', *Journal of the History of Medicine and Allied Sciences* 55 (2000), 363–97; M. O. Humphries, 'Paths of Infection: The First World War and the Origins of the 1918 Influenza Pandemic', *War in History* 21 (2014), 55–81.

in the years and months leading up to the Black Death. In other words, Villani did not make the kind of direct association between warfare and epidemic disease that we might immediately recognise; rather, to him the two were the linked results of an unfortunate entanglement of aristocratic sin in the shadow of a malevolent planetary conjunction.

Villani's *New Chronicle* and epidemic disease: setting the stage

Giovanni Villani came from a banking family in Florence. Born in 1280, he died in 1348 during the Black Death. For more than twenty years, he worked on the *New Chronicle*, a universal history whose final book covers the early to mid-fourteenth century. Scholars consider Villani's text to be an important example of Florentine historical writing in the vernacular.[4]

As it was for many writers of his time, for Villani the political and natural worlds were not separate. Famines, floods and earthquakes were equally devastating as military defeat, and each reflected God's judgment on the affected parties. A strong thread of morality, linked to Fortune's wheel and God's punishment, runs through Villani's book as it explores the activities of political leaders in the city of Florence and far beyond. Laurence Moulinier has shown the value of using the *New Chronicle* to explore contemporary views of disasters, both natural and human. Moulinier's work focused on the chronicle's account of the 1333 flood in Florence, pointing out Villani's attempt to understand a range of causes for disaster, including human, celestial and supernatural. Of special interest to Villani was the intertwining of these causes and their cascading effects on each other.[5]

The same range of diverse causes can be seen in Villani's views of epidemic illness. Although he died during the Black Death and so could not write about it specifically, he does mention pestilence and mortality fourteen times in the chronicle, frequently using the words 'pestilence' and 'mortality' together to strongly suggest that people died (and did not just become ill for a time) from whichever epidemic illness(es) were present.[6] He also provides a contemporary understanding of sickness and 'why' pestilence and mortality happened, based on the widespread acceptance that moral, natural and astrological influences worked together.[7]

4 P. Clarke, 'The Villani Chronicles', in *Chronicling History: Chroniclers and Historians in Medieval and Renaissance Italy*, ed. S. Dale, A. Williams Lewin and D. Osheim (Philadelphia, 2007), pp. 113–27 (pp. 113–15); L. K. Morreale, 'French Literature, Florentine Politics, and Vernacular Historical Writing, 1270–1348', *Speculum* 85 (2010), 885–93.

5 L. Moulinier, 'L'Inondation de 1333 à Florence: Récit et hypothèses de Giovanni Villani', *Médiévales* 36 (1999), 101–2.

6 Since all but a few of these references occurred before plague had reached the Italian peninsula, the word pestilence rarely could have referred to plague. Villani did mention symptoms when he spoke of plague, however. See Carmichael, 'Universal and Particular', p. 35. Many epidemic illnesses would have had similar symptoms, so he may not have found it necessary to specify.

7 G. Zanella, 'La peste del 1348: Italia, Francia, e Germania', in *La Peste Nera: dati di una realta et elementi di una interpretazione: atti del XXX Convegno storico internazionale, Todi, 10–13 ottobre 1993* (Spoleto, 1994), pp. 49–60.

Yet for Villani the most common cause of pestilence and mortality was warfare.[8] Seven references to pestilence and mortality occurred in relation to sieges and extended raiding across the peninsula. Many of his chapters focus on specific moments of fighting that resulted in a local epidemic, including a discussion of how displaced people, fighting for months at a time, encountered epidemic illness in military camps. Especially problematic in this context was the summer heat.

Like his contemporaries, Villani saw mercenary warfare as akin to a natural disaster. Similar to a flood or an earthquake, the violence of war could make a powerful, sinful ruler weak, thereby revealing God's judgment.[9] As many educated individuals did, he saw a strong, if not necessarily predictive, relationship between the heavens and the earth.[10] Just as plague treatise writers soon claimed, Villani's chronicle points to the March 1345 conjunction of Saturn, Jupiter and Mars in the sign of Aquarius as a malevolent astrological moment that signalled a danger that God might punish sinful behaviour on Earth. Two of his references to epidemic disease were celestial, including a detailed account of the conjunction of 1345 that explains how the dire position of planets and stars created a sense of impending doom that could manifest as weather extremes, disrupted harvests and famines, along with pestilence and mortality.[11] Yet Villani was very clear that human fortunes were not at the mercy of the stars, insisting that human actions and choices mattered. Rather, God could and would intervene if people made immoral choices.[12] Several chapters discussed how rulers and royal families were making dangerously immoral decisions at a time when the heavens suggested a moral reckoning was at hand. Ultimately, those decisions were also linked to the spread of epidemic disease.

The Angevin royal family of Naples, which was an ally of the city of Florence, was one of those families making dangerous decisions. Two of the most dramatic for Villani were Queen Johanna's assassination of her first husband, Andrew of Hungary, in 1343 and her remarriage to his rival, Louis of Taranto, shortly thereafter.[13] Villani provided a detailed account of the assassination, which implicated Queen Johanna and Louis of Taranto,

8 Another common cause was food scarcity. Five of Villani's thirteen references to mortality and pestilence described events that explicitly mentioned food shortage, sometimes in conjunction with warfare. Caferro discusses the strategy of attacking a region during crises in W. P. Caferro, 'Warfare and Economy in Renaissance Italy, 1350–1450', *The Journal of Interdisciplinary History* 39 (2008), 167–209 (p. 173).

9 Clarke, 'The Villani Chronicles', pp. 121–3.

10 Carmichael, 'Universal and Particular', pp. 31–2. This view was common among authors at the time. Zanella, 'La peste del 1348', pp. 49–135. J. Arrizabalaga, 'Facing the Black Death: Perceptions and Reactions of University Medical Practitioners', *Practical Medicine from Salerno to the Black Death*, ed. L. García-Ballester, R. French, J. Arrizabalaga and A. Cunningham (Cambridge, 1994), pp. 237–88.

11 A. Campbell, *The Black Death and Men of Learning* (New York, 1966), pp. 34–47.

12 Carmichael, 'Universal and Particular', pp. 22, 32.

13 Although Villani was convinced, not everyone at the time believed that Johanna was involved in Andrew's assassination. See E. Casteen, *From She-Wolf to Martyr: The Reign and Disputed Reputation of Johanna I of Naples* (Ithaca, 2015), pp. 29–66.

repeatedly noting that Christians found their marriage deeply scandalous because of their purported participation in the assassination.

The final chapters that Villani wrote before his death followed King Louis of Hungary's response to the death of his brother and the loss of the Crown of Naples for the Hungarian branch of the family. Over the course of four years, Louis prepared for an invasion of the kingdom of Naples. He tried to take the port city of Zadar from the Venetians, which he could use as a base to move supplies and soldiers from Hungary into the Italian peninsula. He supported other lords' attacks against Queen Johanna and her supporters, destabilising the peninsula politically and increasing mercenary activity. Finally, in 1347, he invaded the kingdom of Naples, hiring mercenaries as he moved through and conquered the region. When plague subsequently emerged in Mediterranean port cities, much of the peninsula was busy dealing with the mercenaries who swelled King Louis's ranks or, worse, attacked communities after he moved on.

To understand how a contemporary like Giovanni Villani thought that mercenary warfare contributed to pestilence and mortality on the eve of the Black Death, I will begin with an example of local fighting. This example is not related to King Louis of Hungary's campaign, but it uses Villani's chronicle to build a picture of what mercenary warfare looked like in the mid-fourteenth century and how it could create the conditions that cause epidemic illness, especially for the mercenaries themselves. I then briefly consider Villani's broad sense of how the heavens opened the way for God to punish immoral behaviour. Finally, the chapter brings these various threads together by briefly describing Andrew of Hungary's assassination and then follows the stages of King Louis of Hungary's invasion on the eve of the Black Death. Throughout his chronicle and for years before plague arrived, Villani wove pestilence and mortality into his description of the events taking place on the Italian peninsula, providing valuable insights into contemporary views of warfare, moral behaviour, deadly natural phenomena and humans' place in the observable world.

Epidemic illness and mercenary warfare

Although he makes seven references to pestilence and mortality in relation to warfare, Villani is relatively terse in his actual description of illness. Most references do not describe signs or symptoms, leaving it unclear whether he meant a specific disease when he spoke of pestilence.[14] He is more specific about the conduct of mercenary warfare. Although each instance of warfare he described was different, overall, mercenary warfare was not a series of large pitched battles; instead, it was an occupation by decentralised military companies.[15]

[14] All of the references considered events before 1347, so Villani clearly is not referring to plague.

[15] For an overview, see W. Caferro, *John Hawkwood: An English Mercenary in Fourteenth-Century Italy* (Baltimore, 2006), pp. 63–4.

To get a sense of the contours of mercenary conduct as they related to health and illness, I will analyse Villani's description of an attack on the 'contado' (county) of Pisa in 1344. I will start with a brief summary of the events and then analyse this example of mercenary warfare in terms of how this type of fighting might cause epidemic illness.[16] This example helps us to see some of the common elements of fourteenth-century mercenary warfare that could generate epidemic illness and death.[17] For example, mercenaries were displaced people. They lived far from home in camps of hundreds or thousands of men and their animals. They frequently lived in proximity to the newly dug earthworks that formed their camps or local defence efforts. Their eating habits, hygiene and camp sanitation could be unpredictable and unorganised. In short, mercenary warfare created conditions in which epidemic diseases could flourish among the attackers.

According to Villani, during fighting among rival city states Lord Luchino Visconti brought his forces against the Pisans in early April 1344. (Although Villani does not provide the number of these mercenary troops, later references suggest the number was over 2,000 men and perhaps as many as 3,000.) He concentrated his attack in the area of Versilia, on the western coast of Italy just north of Pisa. Prior to Visconti's arrival, the Pisans had constructed a defensive trench with palisades from the seashore, inland to Castello di Montegioli. They guarded the trench day and night with what Villani described as 'a very large army of horsemen and foot soldiers'.[18] Visconti's troops broke through the Pisan defences, capturing and killing many in the Pisan army. News of the Pisan defeat spread through the region. One mercenary leader, Lord Benedetto Maccaioni, whom Villani described as a 'rebel against Pisa', responded by bringing his 300 soldiers, who had been wintering nearby, to join Visconti's troops.[19] This added more displaced men and horses to a region already facing the strain of invasion.

Visconti and Maccaioni took advantage of the failure of the Pisan defences and made a circuitous tour through Pisan territory. The Pisans had not been idle, however, and the main body of the invading troops was ambushed by 500 mounted Pisan soldiers and crossbowmen waiting near a bridge. Many Visconti and Maccaioni forces were killed or captured; the rest fled into the nearby hills. This created yet another displaced community, one comprised of men who used violence to survive in a potentially hostile countryside.

When the leader of Visconti's rear guard in Versilia heard about this ambush, he led roughly 1,500 horsemen through the region to meet up with the remaining Visconti

16 For a consideration of what made a mercenary, see S. Morillo, 'Mercenaries, Mamluks, and Militia: Towards a Cross-Cultural Typology of Military Service', in *Mercenaries and Paid Men: The Mercenary Identity in the Middle Ages*, ed. J. France (Leiden, 2008), pp. 243–59.

17 For other studies that consider mercenaries and disease, see B. Campbell, *The Great Transition: Climate, Disease, and Society in the Late-Medieval World* (Cambridge, 2016), pp. 267–27 and W. Caferro, *Petrarch's War: Florence and the Black Death in Context* (Cambridge, 2018).

18 *Final Book*, p. 71. Italian: 'e quelle fortezze si guardavano di di e di notte con loro gente assai grossa a cavallo e a piè'; *Cronica*, IV, 56.

19 *Final Book*, p. 71. Italian: 'rubello di Pisa'; *Cronica*, IV, 56.

troops. The combined forces camped near Santa Gonda. These soldiers stayed in the region for months, attacking and capturing Pisan towns and castles and harassing Pisan cities and roads.[20] About 1,000 Pisan horsemen chased the army, which included Maccaioni's remaining men, but did not catch them.

As the weather warmed in July and August – and as Pisan soldiers continued to track and follow Visconti soldiers – life for men on both sides may have become even less orderly. The Visconti soldiers would have had to keep moving in order to avoid both an extended siege in enemy territory and a decisive battle. They moved through a hostile region, taking or buying the food and other supplies they needed, camping or staying in hostile towns. Life for these men would have been one of repeated disruption. By July and August, for the thousands of men who camped together in the Valdera and the Maremma, the food and hygiene disruptions – not to mention periodic fighting – would have weakened the group, leaving the men vulnerable to illness.[21] According to Villani, the Visconti army only left the 'contado' of Pisa in August because 'the excessive heat and discomfort brought about a sickness, and many took ill and died'.[22] Villani did not specify how many died of illness, but the dead included Maccaioni. According to Villani, 'because of the mortality and pestilence, the host departed',[23] while the survivors returned to Versilia, the first place that they had captured. They wintered there, keeping hostages from Pisa to ensure their safety. In February, Visconti led 500 men on a raid to the walls of Pisa, 'doing great damage – burning and taking great plunder in men, animals, and goods'.[24] They only left the region when Luchino Visconti's brother-in-law, the backer of the expedition, died. Luchino Visconti made peace with the Pisans, who paid him and his men 100,000 gold florins to return the hostages and leave the region entirely.

In this brief chapter of Villani's chronicle, we see many elements that made warfare a source of epidemic illness. The clearest for Villani was heat and discomfort caused by large groups camping together and raiding in July and August. Villani uses the word 'disagio', which, translated as discomfort, suggests a lumpy campsite.[25] But in thinking through what an extended, if small, military campaign like this entailed, we can dig into a general word like discomfort and explore the elements that would spread epidemic illnesses.

Villani's description of this extended raid began with the building of a trench and palisades near Versilia. It is difficult to know how long or wide this trench might have

20 In their circuitous movement through the 'contado' of Pisa, they also threatened Florence, which is likely why Villani includes the event.

21 *Final Book*, p. 72.

22 Ibid., p. 71. Italian: 'se non fosse che per lo soperchio caldo e disagio vi si cominciò una corruzione, onde assai ve n'ammalarono e morirono'; *Cronica*, IV, 57.

23 *Final Book*, p. 72. Italian: 'Per la mortalità e pestilenzia si parti la detta oste con quegli ch' erano iscampati'; *Cronica*, IV, 57.

24 *Final Book*, p. 81. Italian: 'faccendo grande danno d' arsione, e levando grandi prede d' uomini e di bestie e d'arnesi'; *Cronica*, IV, 67.

25 *Cronica* IV, 96.

been, but for it to deter an invading army it would have had to be a significant undertaking. A large Pisan army that included horsemen and foot soldiers manned the trench and palisades. Villani does not give us the number, but, based on the size of the attacking forces, one might assume that this included at least 3,000 men and horses. There may have been a camp with supplies, but these men were defending Pisa, so local communities may have been willing to sell them supplies.[26] At the very least, however, we see substantial dislocation of men and animals living near extended earthworks and new construction.[27]

In addition to the large Pisan army and the disruption of earthworks and palisade construction, the invading Visconti troops and Lord Benedetto Maccaioni's men added to the number of mounted and foot soldiers in the region. Again, Villani does not give specific numbers, but his estimates give a sense of the number of fighters attacking the trench and palisades; added to this would be supply and support efforts for this invading force. We get a better sense of numbers after Visconti's troops were ambushed. According to Villani, although Visconti took his main force into Pisan territory, the company left in Versilia was large enough to send about 1,500 into Pisan territory after the ambush and still protect Versilia. Using Villani's estimates, roughly 7,000–9,000 people – attackers and defenders – could have been fighting in this region for several months.

Without careful planning and management, this area of dislocation and disruption would be a prime place for epidemic illness to emerge and spread. Although military medicine rarely appears in general studies of medieval warfare, there is evidence that military leaders were aware of the problems inherent in military camps and the mercenary experience.[28] Historians of medieval medicine have explored the military experience through surviving medical treatises. Guy Geltner and Michael McVaugh, for example, show that medieval writers advised avoiding, whenever possible, the construction of camping sites near marshes or stagnant water.[29] They considered how to assess water sources.[30] And

26 For military hygiene, see M. McVaugh, 'Arnald of Villanova's *Regimen Almarie* (*Regimen Castra Sequentium*) and Medieval Military Medicine', *Viator* 23 (1992), 201–14; G. Geltner, 'In the Camp and on the March: Military Manuals as Sources for Studying Premodern Public Health', *Medical History* 63 (2019), 44–60.

27 For cases of co-infection of louse-borne trench fever (*Bartonella quintana*) and plague (*Y. pestis*) in a late medieval mass-burial site in France, see T. N. T. Tran et al., 'Brief Communication: Co-detection of *Bartonella quintana* and *Yersinia pestis* in an 11th–15th Burial Site in Bondy, France', *American Journal of Physical Anthropology* 145 (2011), 489–94.

28 McVaugh, 'Arnald of Villanova's *Regimen Almarie*', p. 205. As Michael McVaugh points out, 'probably because military medicine did not produce a genre of technical writing, nothing is ever said about it in modern accounts of armies, war, and military practice in the Middle Ages'. He cites the work of historians such as Philippe Contamine, Ferdinand Lott and Hans Delbrück as examples.

29 Geltner, 'In the Camp', p. 49–51.

30 McVaugh, 'Arnald of Villanova's *Regimen Almarie*', p. 211.

there is evidence that some companies had access to physicians and apothecaries.[31] Troops forced to move and react rapidly, however, would have had few opportunities to consider the location or water quality of a campsite. Smaller companies or those recovering from ambush, like those of Lord Luchino Visconti, may not have been able to employ physicians.

Another aspect that can help modern audiences to imagine the structure of mercenary warfare is political affiliation. Loose political affiliation, if any, could create a situation in which soldiers acted with little oversight or top-down control. In other words, no one could disband them or order them to stop fighting. Instead they lived off a region until they chose to leave. Villani's chronicle is actually a bit misleading here. He referred to the majority of troops by the political entity they supported, as if each side had a united army of men drawn or conscripted from their own political and cultural region. By the middle of the fourteenth century in the Italian peninsula, however, this was profoundly unlikely. There might have been a relatively small group of soldiers with strong political and cultural ties to lord and city, but it is more likely that each side was primarily comprised of groups of hired soldiers who had little political or cultural affiliation to their leaders or even to each other.[32]

By the late thirteenth/early fourteenth centuries, many military and powerful city leaders began to use professional soldiers more frequently and their employ and the defence against them were a large part of every city and regional lord's budget.[33] Pisa was no exception. These professional soldiers came from all over Europe. The men fighting for and against Pisa may have come from Germany, England, Spain, France or other Italian regions. As professional soldiers, they were much better trained, better armed and had more experience than local citizen militias. Not surprisingly, they were quite successful, and by the middle of the fourteenth century most leaders had to use them.[34]

Professional soldiers tended to work in small groups of between fifty and one hundred, with a leader who negotiated contracts and led the group. Men followed successful leaders, regardless of their political or cultural background. This meant that an army of 5,000 men actually consisted of many small groups, likely speaking different languages and with different weaponry and supplies. With so many leaders, each of whom likely had different expectations about setting up camp, hygiene would not have been consistent. Soldiers from other regions, like England and Germany, would have brought their diseases or

31 Ibid., p. 206. For an earlier time period, see P. Mitchell, *Medicine in the Crusades: Warfare, Wounds and the Medieval Surgeon* (Cambridge, 2004).

32 P. Contamine, *La vie quotidienne pendant la guerre de cent ans: France et Angleterre, XIVe siècle* (New York, 1978).

33 M. Mallett, *Mercenaries and Their Masters: Warfare in Renaissance Italy* (Totowa NJ, 1974), pp. 6–24; D. Waley, 'Condotte and Condottieri in the Thirteenth Century', *Proceedings of the British Academy* 61 (1975), 337–71; Caferro, 'Warfare and Economy'.

34 L. Green, 'Changes in the Nature of War in Early Fourteenth Century Tuscany', in *Medieval Warfare 1300–1450*, ed. K. DeVries (Farnham, 2010), pp. 69–92 (pp. 70–2).

dispositions with them, alongside their weapons. Overall, this was not a uniform deployment but, rather, a loose group effort, perhaps even among the defenders.[35]

After breaking through the Pisan trench near Versilia, the invaders likely did not stay neatly together in a group as they made their way through the 'contado' of Pisa. The movements of Maccaioni's men give us a glimpse of the fluid and unpredictable nature of these military groups. Three hundred soldiers under Maccaioni were already 'making war' in the area before they joined the successful Visconti attack.[36] If we think about warfare at the time, this meant groups of fifty to one hundred professional soldiers working together under one or two leaders. They were initially spread out, moving unpredictably. After the reserve Visconti forces arrived, however, Villani describes a more cohesive group. This group captured towns and castles and raided cities and roads. Considering the behaviour of other mercenary companies, they may have stayed in captured castles and looted the towns.[37]

Although it is not the focus of this chapter, it is easy to see how mercenary activities made life difficult for people living in the area. Planting, harvesting and transportation all became significantly more dangerous.[38] As Guy Geltner has shown, officials in the region of Lucca and Bologna actively sought to protect the health of the people in their cities and in surrounding regions.[39] They inspected and repaired roads, bridges, canals, watermills and city walls. They also monitored industries like tanning and butchery to make sure that certain polluting tasks happened outside city walls and did not contaminate city waterways and air. Active mercenary companies in the region made infrastructure difficult to repair and extra-mural work more dangerous, perhaps forcing livestock sales, butchery and tanning inside the city walls. At the same time, as invading mercenaries made food production and distribution difficult, they also competed with local communities for food and livestock.

This example of fighting in Pisan territory shows Giovanni Villani's world, one in which many small groups of armed men lived on the Italian peninsula from one contract to another. Sometimes they remained in small groups loosely attached to city-states or powerful leaders. Sometimes they broke away from local leadership and joined together into their own companies. For example, in 1342, following another truce that Pisa negotiated, Villani describes how a group of 2,500 mounted and foot soldiers, mostly German, formed

35 K. DeVries, 'Medieval Mercenaries: Methodology, Definitions, and Problems', in *Mercenaries and Paid Men*, ed. France, pp. 43–60.

36 *Final Book*, p. 71. Italian: 'a guerrigiare'; *Cronica*, IV, 56.

37 For examples from nearby regions, see N. Archambeau, *Souls under Siege: Survival Stories of War, Plague, and Confession in Fourteenth-Century Provence* (Ithaca, 2021), pp. 81–94.

38 Caferro, 'Warfare and Economy', p. 173.

39 For an overview of polluting activities that officials might try to curb, see G. Geltner, *Roads to Health: Infrastructure and Urban Wellbeing in Later Medieval Italy* (Philadelphia, 2019), p. 113.

an independent company. The soldiers did not go home or leave the peninsula. In order to keep the company from attacking them, the Pisans paid it to attack their neighbours.[40]

These were professional soldiers for hire. They lived in a part of Europe where they were likely to be hired and rehired frequently by warring city-states. During a contract, they might travel significant distances, build earthworks, camp for months on end and engage in skirmishes, pitched battles and sieges. And all of this might take place far from the places they called home. When not employed by a lord, they needed to support themselves until they were hired again.[41] In many ways, mercenary companies were a permanent, if fluctuating, invasion force. While this semi-transient population might not introduce new diseases in the same ways that long-distance trade could, their activities added strain on local resources and created an environment in which epidemic illness, what Villani called pestilence and mortality, could thrive.

1345: a dangerous time to sin

In March 1345, there was a long foreseen conjunction of Saturn, Jupiter and Mars in the sign of Aquarius. Astrologers knew that this conjunction brought dangerous stars into alignment, which they – and Villani – believed created a time of significant potential change. Villani described the conjunction in detail and then explained its potential impact:

> According to what is said and what is written in the books of the great ancient masters of astrology this conjunction, with aspects of the other planets and signs, signifies, if God consents, great things in the world: battles; murders; great lordships and sects; the appearance of prophets and of new errors in the faith; the coming of new lords and of new peoples; famine and mortality in those climes, kingdoms, countries, and cities over which the said signs and planets have influence … We do not say that this is by necessity, but more or less by the pleasure of God, who disposes the heavenly bodies through his justice and mercy, according to the merits and sins of nations, kingdoms, and peoples to cleanse and to reward.[42]

40 *Final Book*, p. 40. This behaviour was not uncommon and was very costly for regional leaders. See Caferro, 'Warfare and Economy', p. 176.

41 Green, 'Changes in the Nature of War', pp. 69–92.

42 *Final Book*, p. 85. Italian: 'Questa congiunzione co' suoi aspetti e degli altri pianeti e segni, secondo il detto e scritto degli altri ne' libri degli antichi e grandi maestri de strologia, significa, Iddio consenziente, grandi cose al mondo, cioè battaglie, omicidi, e grandi commutazioni de' regni e de' popoli, e morte di re, e traslazione di signorie e di sette, e apparimento d'alcuno profeta e di nuovi errori di fede, e nuova venuta di signori e passamento di gente, e carestia e mortalità appresso in quelli climati, regni, e paesi e cittadini, la cui influenza a' detti segni e pianeti è attribuita … Questo non diciamo che sia di necessità, ma fia il più e il meno al piacere di Dio di provvedere a' detti corpi celestiali mediante la sui giustizia e misericordia, e secondo I meriti e peccati delle genti e de' regni e de' popolo per punire e remunerare'; *Cronica*, IV, 71–2.

Most historians studying plague are familiar with texts about this conjunction written during and after the Black Death. Perhaps the most familiar example is the plague tract produced by the Paris Medical Faculty in October 1348.[43] As Carmichael points out, the tract considered the conjunction part of what made the pestilence universal. It paired a celestial cause with a terrestrial cause and impact.[44] This text, and others influenced by it, emphasised that the conjunction, especially the effects of Mars, created a deadly corruption of the air that then gave rise to the great epidemic of plague.[45]

For Villani, writing before the arrival of plague, pestilence was only one possible disaster that might follow this conjunction. In the autumn of 1345, immediately following the conjunction, a series of natural disasters struck Florence and other cities on the Italian peninsula. According to Villani, two earthquakes hit the region. More importantly, unseasonably heavy rain fell from the end of July to the beginning of November. This disrupted harvesting and planting and caused floods, which destroyed roads, bridges and property. For Villani, 'the recent conjunction had begun to show its effects'.[46]

Villani's view of the conjunction reflects what medieval astrologers had written about it, both before and as it happened.[47] One example that Carmichael highlights includes three scholars advising Pope Clement VI in Avignon who wrote about the conjunction in 1344 and 1345.[48] They included the Jewish astrologer Levi ben Gerson and two Christian scholars, Firminus de Bella Valle and Johanne de Muris. Pope Clement VI, who worked with astrologers because of his interest in calendar reform, requested their assessment of the conjunction.[49] Levi ben Gerson describes the relationship between humans and the heavens in a way that helps us better contextualise Villani's view. According to ben Gerson,

> It is necessary to look at the implications [of stellar influences] for the future so that [this investigation] will direct men to take counsel concerning evil so that it will not occur, and concerning good so that it will occur … in this way it is possible for a man to change

43 Carmichael, 'Universal and Particular', p. 22.

44 Ibid., p. 18.

45 Arrizabalaga, 'Facing the Black Death', 252–54; see also L. Jones, *Patterns of Plague: Changing Ideas about Plague in England and France, 1348–1750* (Montreal, 2022), pp. 127–9, 171.

46 *Final Book*, p. 97. Italian: 'E la congiunzione passata cominiciò a monstrare le sue influenzie'; *Cronica*, IV, 87. For more on this flood and floods in earlier time periods in Villani's chronicle, see Moulinier, 'L'Inondation de 1333 à Florence', pp. 93, 101–2. Even though the 1333 flood happened long before the 1345 conjunction, there are astrological, supernatural and moral explanations for its occurrence and effects.

47 For an overview of the history of the study of great conjunctions, see J. D. North, 'Astrology and the Fortunes of Churches', *Centaurus* 24 (1980), 184–85; B. Goldstein and D. Pingree, 'Levi ben Gerson's Prognostication for the Conjunction of 1345', *The American Philosophical Society* 80 (1990), 1–60 (p. 3). Goldstein and Pingree mention a Jewish scholar writing about this particular conjunction as early as 1136.

48 Carmichael, 'Universal and Particular', p. 22.

49 Goldstein and Pingree, 'Levi ben Gerson's Prognostication', pp. 3–7.

> what is implied by the decree of the stars, namely, [first,] things related to free will and, second [things dependent on] divine providence.[50]

For ben Gerson and most contemporary scholars, the heavens did not curtail human free will. They instead revealed a moment of potential for extraordinary good or evil.

Villani held a similar view of how the heavens and human actions related to each other. Conjunctions like the one in 1345 opened moments when significant change could happen, if God so chose.[51] If people lived in accordance with Christian faith, then the changes could be positive. If people sinned, the events could be devastating. It is important to note that, for Villani, the sins of leaders were not individual sins. Nations, kingdoms and peoples committed sins or accrued merits and were treated accordingly. This put a burden on leaders to live up to Christian ideals. When they did not, both they and their kingdoms suffered. For Villani, two of the most egregious sins committed at this dangerous time were the assassination of Queen Johanna of Naples' first husband, Andrew of Hungary, and her remarriage to Louis of Taranto shortly thereafter.

In his construction of the events, Villani dovetailed what transpired in the kingdom of Naples with the 1345 conjunction and natural phenomena. He ended his chapter on the conjunction and its impact with these words:

> the floods were a sign and a cause of the bad harvests and food shortages the next year, which we will later describe. We will leave for a while matters in our Florence and tell, in the following chapter of the scandalous and wicked sin and act of treason committed among the heirs and relatives of King Robert.[52]

For Villani, this was a dangerous moment to sin, and the royal family of Naples had really sinned. Villani narrated the entire story of Andrew of Hungary's assassination immediately following his description of the conjunction of 1345. He described the earthquakes, rain, floods and bad harvests, then directly linked those events to the dangerous conjunction of the heavens that he had explained in an earlier chapter. In the next sentence, he turned to the wicked sin of the assassination of Andrew of Hungary, thereby linking that specific event for the reader to both the conjunction and the natural disasters. If this were a horror movie, half the audience would be watching the screen through their fingers.

Since Villani saw this event as a moral cause of disaster, it is worth looking at in detail. There are many surviving narratives of the assassination of Queen Johanna's first husband,

50 Ibid., p. 11. This is their translation. For the original Hebrew, see p. 10.

51 For this passage, see Carmichael, 'Universal and Particular', pp. 31–2 and L. Green, *Chronicle into History: An Essay on the Interpretation of History in Florentine Fourteenth-Century Chronicles* (Cambridge, 1972), pp. 37–8.

52 *Final Book*, p. 97. Italian: 'E fu segno e cagione che avvenne il seguente anno di male ricolte e carestia di vittuaglia, come innanzi faremo menzione. Lasceremo alquanto de' nostri fatti de Firenze e racconteremo d' uno screpio, e scellerato peccato e tradimento commesso per le rede e congiunti del re Ruberto tra loro, come diremo nel seguente capitolo'; *Cronica*, IV, 86–7.

Andrew of Hungary, and each contains its own interpretation of what transpired.[53] Villani claimed to have heard the story from one of Andrew's bailiffs and his version of events emphasised the guilt of Queen Johanna and the Taranto and Durazzo branches of the Angevin royal family.[54] On the night of 18 September 1345, Andrew was called out from his sleeping apartment to receive important news. Johanna urged him to go hear it, directing her chambermaid to lock the door behind him. In the hall, many important counts waited for Andrew. They grabbed him, put a noose around his neck and hanged him out of the window above the garden. Men waiting in the garden pulled on his feet to strangle him. They had hoped to hide his body in the garden, but a Hungarian chambermaid saw what was happening and screamed. The men in the garden fled and Andrew's body was taken down by others and eventually buried in Naples. For Villani, Queen Johanna expressed very little grief, causing rumours that she had assisted with – and possibly even instigated – the assassination.

The local investigation quickly found and executed an assassin, but few were satisfied with the investigation.[55] Many, including Villani, suspected the chamberlain. He was eventually publicly tortured and executed.[56] Pope Clement VI also had doubts about the local investigation. According to Villani, the pope and cardinals condemned this murder and excommunicated everyone involved. The pope sent the count of Andri to 'take revenge against whoever was guilty'.[57] He had two cartloads of Queen Johanna's supporters stoned and then burned.

The conjunction of 1345 was showing itself not just in horrendous natural disasters, but through political and moral disasters as well. In Villani's words, 'the death of King Andrew threw the entire kingdom of Puglia [i.e. Naples] into disorder'.[58] The people of Naples then revolted. King Louis of Hungary and his family accused everyone in the Angevin royal family of complicity and began preparations to invade the Italian peninsula.[59] The various lords of the kingdom of Naples sided with different claimants to the throne. Each

53 Casteen, *From She-Wolf to Martyr*, pp. 29–66.

54 *Final Book*, pp. 97–100.

55 The initial investigation was mainly carried out by Charles of Artus, who was King Robert of Naples's bastard son and count of Saint Agata. See É.-G. Léonard, *Les Angevins de Naples* (Paris, 1954), p. 335.

56 É.-G. Léonard, *Histoire de Jeanne 1re, reine de Naples, Comtesse de Provence (1343–1382)*, 3 vols. (Monaco, 1932–36), I, 486–7. Villani points out that the chamberlain's tongue was pierced with a hook so that he could not speak and therefore name anyone else during public torture.

57 *Final Book*, pp. 99–100. Italian: 'e facesse giustizia di chiunque de ciò fosse colpevole'; *Cronica*, IV, 88.

58 *Final Book*, p. 100. Italian: 'Per la morte del detto re Andreasso si scompigliò tutto il regno di Puglia'; *Cronica*, IV, 89.

59 Among those accused were cardinal bishop Talleyrand, related by marriage to the duke of Durazzo and an associate of Pope Clement VI. See Norman Zacour, 'Talleyrand: The Cardinal of Périgord (1301–1364)', *Transactions of the American Philosophical Society* 50 (1960), 1–83 (p. 35). Villani shared this view.

claimant hired his own men-at-arms to protect against others and against the King of Hungary, who also threatened to take the throne from Johanna. According to Villani, 'for this reason, the entire kingdom was divided, disunited, and fearful, the roads were infested with thieves, and there was no justice'.[60]

According to some sources, Pope Clement VI sent diplomats to the Hungarian and Neapolitan courts to negotiate peace. Soon afterwards, he declared an official investigation into Andrew's murder.[61] The ongoing papal investigation sought to question Johanna and members of the other two branches of the Angevin family that were contending for the throne, including the princes of Taranto and the dukes of Durazzo. In this way, the pope hoped to assuage the anger expressed by the Hungarian branch of the Angevin family and stave off invasion.

Pope Clement VI couched the investigation in the language of pastoral care. He instigated the investigation, he said, on behalf of '[those things] which pertain to the health of their souls', by which he meant not just Andrew, but anyone involved in the violent act, which itself was a serious sin and could lead to damnation or worse at this profoundly inauspicious moment if the guilty parties did not repent.[62] Queen Johanna refused to participate in the papal inquest, however. Her choice for a second husband, Louis of Taranto, also refused; he was a contender for the Crown of Naples and had remained close to Johanna for years.[63]

Villani presented Johanna's behaviour as particularly sinful: 'All Christians who heard of [this decision for Johanna's second husband] condemned it; all who knew of it were horrified and predicted that such an abominable sin would have evil consequences.'[64] For Villani, since people's moral choices – especially those made by political leaders – had political and even environmental repercussions, this sinful behaviour had the potential to seriously harm the entire kingdom of Naples. Under the influence of the malevolent conjunction, the repercussions would be amplified.

Over the subsequent chapters, Villani recounted the events of 1345–48, clearly framing them for the reader as the direct result of Andrew of Hungary's death and of Johanna and Louis' immoral behaviour. To drive the point home, Villani recounted historical stories of the political losses faced by other immoral leaders, such as the royal family of Tunisia; in doing so, he was making clear what happened to immoral leaders.[65] He also repeatedly

60 *Final Book*, p. 100. Italian: 'Per la qual cosa tutto il regno stava sciolto e scomunato e in tremore rubandosi i comuni sanza niuno ordine di giustizia'; *Cronica*, IV, 89.

61 For the beginning of the pope's inquest, see Léonard, *Histoire*, I, 533–4.

62 'que salutem animarum ipsorum respiciunt'. Ibid., I, 514.

63 Ibid., I, 645–9.

64 *Final Book*, p. 152. Italian: 'Onde fu ripreso da tutti i cristiani che lo sentirono, e ciascuno che'l seppe ne significò e disse, che sarebbe con mala riuscita sì abbominevole peccato'; *Cronica*, IV, 149.

65 *Final Book*, pp. 155–6.

linked the conjunction, natural phenomena and sinfulness to his overview of the political turmoil of these years.

The King of Hungary's slow, disastrous invasion of Naples

More than half of the final book of Villani's *New Chronicle* explores King Louis of Hungary's invasion of the Italian peninsula. Since this violent invasion occurred on the eve of the Black Death, affected the entire peninsula and was coupled with unseasonable rain and famine, it is worth tracking its various stages. These years ultimately became just as devastating as Villani had predicted, based as they were on sinful behaviour undertaken under the influence of the dangerous astrological conjunction.

According to Villani, upon hearing of his brother Andrew's death in 1345, both King Louis of Hungary and another brother, King Stephen of Poland, were enraged. The Hungarian barons all wore black and demanded revenge. They had a black banner made that showed Andrew hanging from a noose. Other lords from the region, including those from Bavaria and Austria, vowed to help, forming, according to Villani, a league with the kings of Hungary and Poland. Representatives visited the pope in Avignon, demanding that King Louis of Hungary be crowned king of Naples. They were not, however, well received.

To open a path for his invasion of Naples, the King of Hungary worked to secure the city of Zara (present-day Zadar) on the Dalmatian coast. After rebelling from Venetian control, the city had been continually besieged by land and sea by the Venetians, who were 'paying well to send soldiers on horse and on foot from Lombardy, Romagna, and Tuscany'.[66] Villani wove his own city into these events by describing three men from Florence who led soldiers against Zara. Essentially, the three Florentines established an army from the small groups of professional soldiers in residence on the Italian peninsula, like the ones around Pisa in the events described above. They then joined the larger, predominantly mercenary, army built by the Venetians to attack Zara from August 1345 through May 1346.

The king of Hungary led an army from Slavonia that included, according to Villani, 'thirty thousand Hungarians and Germans, mostly horsemen'.[67] Before the king of Hungary's army could arrive, the Venetians made an assault on Zara. Villani described massive war machines on both land and sea. He listed 17,000 men at arms and 4,000 crossbowmen in a rare pitched battle that lasted a full day and night. The Venetians did not take the city before the Hungarian king arrived, however, so they pulled their forces back and fortified a nearby building with 'moats, palisades, and wooden towers'.[68] The king of Hungary freed

66 *Final Book*, p. 108. Italian: 'mandandovi soldati a cavallo e a piede di Lombardia e di Romagna e di Toscana con grande soldo'; *Cronica*, IV, 98.

67 *Final Book*, p. 108. Italian: 'trentamila tra Ungari e Tedeschi, a cavallo la maggior parte'; *Cronica*, IV, 98–9.

68 *Final Book*, p. 109. Italian: 'e quello come bastia afforzarono con fossi e steccati e torri di legname'; *Cronica*, IV, 99.

and provisioned Zara, but was not able to drive the Venetians out of their nearby fortress before he had to return to Hungary.[69]

The Venetians stayed in their fortress over the summer, but now they were the ones being besieged. According to Villani, they were able to refresh their troops but 'there began a great sickness and mortality and many men died'.[70] In this instance, as in the example of the 'contado' of Pisa discussed earlier, summer fighting, combined with large-scale earthworks and dislocated men, led to pestilence and death. Villani did not describe symptoms, but diseases like dysentery were common problems for soldiers; whatever disease it was, Villani wrote that the mortality was so aggressive that only a quarter of the men that the Florentine lords had led to Zara lived to return.[71]

This battle involved the movement of men who originated from many regions around the Adriatic coming to fight together for ten months in the hills and sea around Zara. The presence and availability of professional soldiers made for a constant stream of men, horses, galleys and war machines. Unlike the Visconti troops discussed earlier, who could move their camp, these men were living in a roughly fortified fortress. Hot summer weather, makeshift living conditions, the constant threat of attack and the ubiquitous presence of the rotting bodies of the fallen led to sickness and death.

Between the death of Andrew of Hungary in 1345 and Johanna's remarriage in early 1347, the king of Hungary threatened Naples but, according to Villani, was not able to invade, due to other military ventures and environmental difficulties in Hungary, Poland and Slavonia. The king did, however, successfully lay the groundwork for a later invasion. According to Villani, he backed those attacking the cities and people who supported Queen Johanna and Louis of Taranto. For example, he encouraged attacks against Milazzo in Sicily and towns near Gaeta – which was an important port for the Crown of Naples – as well as uprisings in the Abruzzi region.[72]

Villani particularly covers the uprisings in the Abruzzi region in the central peninsula; they were exceptionally violent and took place alongside a regional famine made worse by unseasonable rains. By May 1347, the disruption caused by famine allowed a local lord to take much of this territory away from the Queen of Naples. To support this lord, the King of Hungary sent officials to the region who 'brought a great quantity of money to sustain the inhabitants of L'Aquila and to hire men-at-arms on horse and foot'.[73] According to Villani, these officials hired more than a thousand men who then attacked towns and laid siege to cities in the region still loyal to the queen. To solidify King Louis of Hungary's

[69] According to Villani, a famine in Slavonia weakened the king of Hungary. *Final Book*, p. 135.

[70] Ibid., p. 109. Italian: 'E per disagi vi si cominciò grande infermeria e mortalità, e morivvi molta gente'; *Cronica*, IV, 100.

[71] Ibid.

[72] *Final Book*, pp. 124, 125, 141–3, respectively.

[73] Ibid., p. 142. Italian: 'grande quantità di moneta per mantenere quegli dell' Aquila, per soldare gente d'arme a cavallo e a piè per lo detto'; *Cronica*, IV, 138.

interests in the region, Hungarian and German soldiers arrived from Slavonia, swelling the numbers of fighting men.

Queen Johanna's forces then retaliated by laying siege to L'Aquila with their own host of over 2,000 men, a number that Villani claimed increased daily.[74] The Angevins did not pay well, however, so most leaders left with their troops when their required service to the Crown of Naples was finished. At this point the Hungarian forces arrived, freed L'Aquila and attacked towns still supporting the queen.[75] By October, the Hungarian leaders and local lords faithful to them controlled the region. When Queen Johanna and Louis of Taranto attempted to retake the region, they failed.[76]

Villani saw this failure as a surprising turn of events, since Johanna and her supporters had far more men and continually hired more. To explain their lack of success, he turned again to the framework of sinfulness and the lingering impact of the conjunction of 1345: 'When God wishes to punish lords and peoples for their sins, He takes away all their power and all their concord.'[77] The Angevin lords surrounding Queen Johanna subsequently began to fight amongst themselves and their advantage in the region disappeared.

Throughout 1347, officials and thousands of professional soldiers moved constantly between Hungary and the central Italian peninsula, engaging in battles, skirmishes and sieges. Villani did not link this particular activity to plague or pestilence, but the rains, famines and fighting described over several chapters reveal communities that were struggling. It is no surprise that the Hungarian officials arrived in the region with money, not just for troops but also for food to support themselves and people in the region. The king of Hungary's efforts, along with the infighting within the Angevin royal family, weakened royal authority in the kingdom of Naples. In 1347, a papal legate and his entourage arrived from Avignon to support Queen Johanna, but, as Villani put it, 'they were little obeyed or feared'.[78] Villani described a political situation in which 'the country was filled with corruption as everyone plundered as much as they could from [their] communes'.[79]

Over the course of the chapters in his final book, Villani constructed his story by dovetailing events. Sinful leaders, a dangerous conjunction in the heavens and destructive natural disasters had led a once-prosperous kingdom into disarray. Part of that disorder was the presence of groups of professional soldiers available for hire. As we have seen, the king of Hungary did not have to invade to wage a military attack on Queen Johanna and Louis of Taranto: the many disgruntled local lords and powerful members of the Angevin royal family still trying to secure the throne fought amongst themselves, using the

74 *Final Book*, p. 142.

75 Ibid.

76 Ibid., p. 157.

77 *Final Book*, p. 157. Italian: 'Ma a cui Dio vuole per le peccata giudicare, toglie a' signori e a' popoli la forza e la concordia'; *Cronica*, IV, 155.

78 *Final Book*, p. 125. Italian: 'ma poco furono ubbiditi e temuti'; *Cronica*, IV, 118.

79 *Final Book*, p. 125. Italian: 'e il paese tutto corrotto a rubare i cammini [communi?], e chi più potea'; *Cronica*, IV, 118.

mercenary troops on hand. The king of Hungary supported some uprisings, perpetuating the disruption. Villani's chronicle shows the complex yet rapid unravelling of a kingdom and the epidemic illnesses that emerged because of a lack of leadership and God's punishment of sinfulness.

After describing the king of Hungary's support of local uprisings, Villani once again reminded readers of the sins of the Angevins in Naples. In August 1347, Queen Johanna married Louis of Taranto. Villani linked their marriage back to the assassination of Andrew of Hungary and noted rumours of their affair while Andrew was alive. He ended the chapter with the sentence, 'From this followed much evil, as we shall tell ahead.'[80] This is one of many sentences that Villani used to directly link the perceived sinfulness of Johanna's marriage and Andrew's assassination to political turmoil in the kingdom of Naples in 1347 and 1348, providing the moral causation of the suffering that people were living through.

The chapters that directly precede and follow Villani's description of Queen Johanna and Louis of Taranto's marriage also link their sinful marriage to other devastating events. For example, in the chapter that immediately precedes the marriage, Villani remarks that a comet appeared in August 1347, bringing 'great mortality to the lands where the planet and sign [Taurus] rule'.[81] In the chapter that follows the announcement of Johanna and Louis's marriage, Villani describes how a great mortality came from the East and wiped out two-thirds of the population of Sardinia and Corsica, along with the Genoese who had just conquered the islands.[82] In this way, Villani layered Andrew's assassination, Johanna and Louis's marriage and the king of Hungary's attacks with experiences of famine, heavenly conjunctions, sinful behaviour, epidemic illness and natural disaster.

Eventually, the king of Hungary did invade the peninsula. According to Villani, King Louis left Hungary at the beginning of November 1347, just after his representatives and troops had secured Sulmona in the Abruzzi region. The king travelled overland through Slavonia rather than by ship, perhaps because he had lost control of Zara to the Venetians after the extended, repeated famines of 1346 and 1347.[83] Villani tracked Louis's movements through the Italian peninsula, putting the king in Udine on 26 November. From there, Louis travelled through Verona, Modena and Bologna down to Rimini, where he arrived on 16 December. From Rimini, he travelled to Foligno, arriving on 20 December.[84]

80 *Final Book*, p. 152. Italian: 'onde seguì molto male, come innanzi per noi se ne farà menzione'; *Cronica*, IV, 149.

81 *Final Book*, p. 151. Italian: 'e ingenerò assai mortalità ne' paesi ove il detto pianeto e segno signoreggiava'; *Cronica*, IV, 148–9.

82 *Final Book*, p. 152. This was likely a reference to plague, which hit Genoa at the end of 1347. For a reassessment of the dating the movement of plague, see H. Barker, 'Laying the Corpses to Rest: Grain, Embargoes, and *Yersinia pestis* in the Black Sea, 1346–1348', *Speculum* 96 (2021), 97–126.

83 P. Engel, *The Realm of St. Stephen: A History of Medieval Hungary, 895–1526*, trans. T. Pálosfalvi (London, 2001), pp. 159–61.

84 For these dates, see *Final Book*, pp. 160–2.

By 27 December, he was in Sulmona in the Abruzzi region, in the territory of the kingdom of Naples.[85] In less than a month, King Louis of Hungary had moved a small invasion force over half the length the Italian peninsula (figure 3.1).[86]

Villani provides some details about what King Louis's invasion looked like. The force immediately surrounding the king was a small, fast-moving group that Villani estimated comprised about 1,000 men.[87] With the number of military companies available for hire in the region and general dissatisfaction with Queen Johanna and Louis of Taranto, the king did not need to bring a full army with him.[88] Instead, Villani noted that the king brought treasure to buy supplies and hire men. Even so, the poor weather and famines meant that he could not assume that he would find all that he needed. Villani stated that the king of Hungary 'ordered that men-at-arms follow continually after him, [since he was mindful of] the shortages of the previous year, shortages which were still affecting the lands beyond the mountains and Italy'.[89] To put these events in the context of epidemic illness and the emerging Black Death, in late 1347 significant numbers of fighting men were travelling between Hungarian lands and the Italian peninsula when plague was already present in Genoa.[90]

As the king of Hungary travelled, he met with representatives of local governments who either offered safe passage or gave other evidence of their support against Queen Johanna and Louis.[91] Since he had a valid claim to the throne of Naples – through both primogeniture and his dead brother's rights – few lords chose to directly oppose Louis. Local political leaders of towns where the king and his invasion force chose to stay offered food, rest and even entertainment in some cases. According to Villani, they also provided troops to travel with and support the invasion force. Villani put the numbers of soldiers at between 150 and 500 at each major city the king visited. Since men were still coming from Hungary, the number of fighting men travelling with the king of Hungary grew constantly and significantly. Lords whose lands did not lie on the route the king chose to take sent ambassadors to meet him. Villani spends several chapters describing the ten ambassadors that Florence sent to meet the king in Rimini and offer Florentine support.[92] Even the ruler of Venice tried to send an embassy but, according to Villani, the king of Hungary

85 Léonard, *Histoire*, II, 1–5.

86 Map(s) created using ArcGIS® software by Esri. ArcGIS® and ArcGIS Pro™ are the intellectual property of Esri and are used herein under licence. Copyright © Esri. All rights reserved. For more information about Esri® software, please visit http://www.esri.com.

87 *Final Book*, p. 161.

88 W. Caferro, *Mercenary Companies and the Decline of Siena* (Baltimore, 1998), pp. 1–14.

89 *Final Book*, p. 161. Italian: 'e ordinò, ch' al continuo il seguissono gente d' arme, come sofferisse il tempo, per lo caro ch' era stato l' anno passato, et era ancora e di là da' monti e in Italia'; *Cronica*, IV, 160.

90 Barker, 'Laying the Corpses to Rest', p. 109.

91 Léonard, *Histoire*, II, 8–9.

92 *Final Book*, p. 163–8.

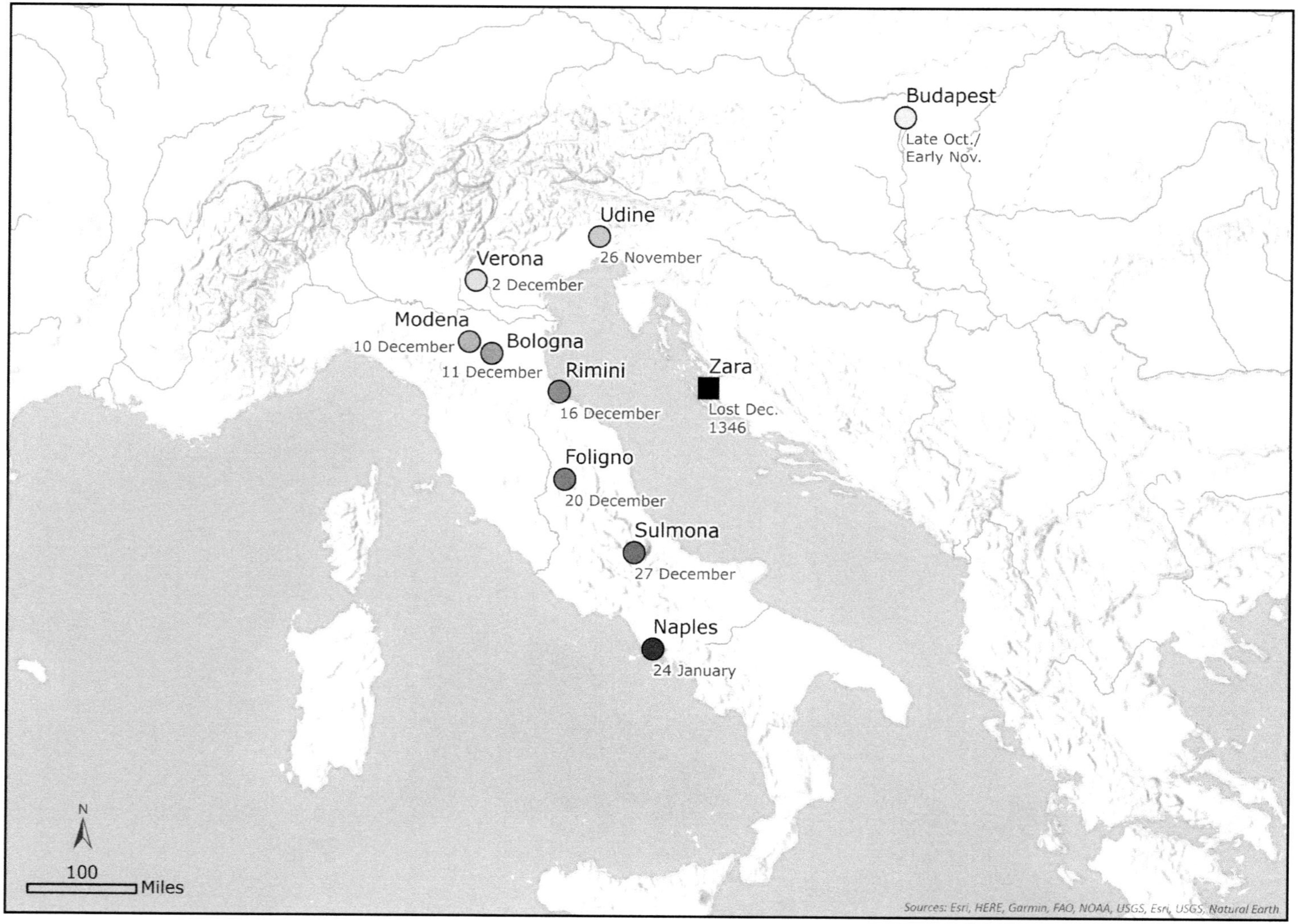

Fig. 3.1. Louis of Hungary's invasion of Naples, 1347. Map Sources: Esri, HERE, Garmin, FAO, NOAA, USGS, Natural Earth.

refused to receive it.[93] In early January 1348, the king of Hungary's force captured, plundered and burned the castles near Sulmona, where lords tried to stop his advance.[94] The king then travelled to Benevento to avoid Louis of Taranto's troops in Capua and was welcomed into the city.[95] When the lords of Naples, who were in Capua with Louis of Taranto, saw that the king of Hungary had a strong position and support in Benevento, they left Capua and travelled to meet the king. Having lost the support of the lords of the city, Queen Johanna and Louis of Taranto left the region. By the end of January 1348, then, the king of Hungary had essentially captured the kingdom of Naples without a siege and without a sizable pitched battle.

Louis of Hungary had expected a battle, however, and so he had accumulated an army. By the time he arrived in the environs of Naples, Villani estimates that he had 'over 6000 soldiers and a vast following'.[96] Not only had he gained soldiers from the cities he passed through, but the advance forces that had captured Sulmona and the Abruzzi region also joined him near Benevento. These soldiers were not his own men; they were hired men and he may have had little control over their actions. For many professional soldiers in the peninsula, joining the king of Hungary's invasion force, whether officially or unofficially, would have been profitable.

Villani gives the reader a sense of the instability of this invasion force and its impact on the regions through which it passed. Across multiple chapters, he noted that there were brigands who followed the king of Hungary's men and plundered the population.[97] For example, the people of Benevento feared that they might be attacked, since the king's men had harmed many through theft on their journey.[98] They closed the gates of Benevento until they saw King Louis of Hungary himself, his presence reassuring them. When the king left, however, the men of Benevento armed themselves and attacked the brigands who followed in the king's wake.[99] In another example from the city of Aversa, the king of Hungary ordered his Hungarian troops to protect the city and bring to justice the bandits and brigands following them.[100]

After King Louis established himself in Naples, the mass of professional soldiers that had built up around his invasion force became more of a danger than a support. According to Villani, King Louis heard that Queen Johanna and her supporters had bribed the leader of his troops that had captured Sulmona and the Abruzzi region. King Louis chose to dismiss the rumour, but paid his hired military leaders very well and had them swear an

93 Ibid., p. 161.

94 Ibid., p. 168.

95 The other branches of the Angevin family made a tenuous peace and raised armies in order to expel this invasion force. Léonard, *Histoire*, II, 24–6.

96 *Final Book*, p. 169. Italian: 'più di seimila cavalieri e popolo infinito'; *Cronica*, IV, 168.

97 *Final Book*, p. 169.

98 Ibid.

99 Ibid.

100 Ibid., p. 170.

oath not to fight against him or his allies.[101] The military leaders agreed and, according to Villani, formed a company of 3,000 mounted soldiers that moved into the region of Terracina, where they lived by plunder.[102]

Immediately after describing his negotiations with the military leaders, Villani states that King Louis of Hungary travelled to the outlying cities of the kingdom of Naples not only to confirm his lordship, but also 'to escape the pestilence of sickness which had already begun and was already great in Naples'.[103] For Villani, then, the king of Hungary's invasion and the thousands of troops and brigands in his wake were to be considered in the immediate context of plague in the Italian peninsula. The violence and theft perpetrated by these professional soldiers was spreading at the same time as the devastating first wave of plague, which had arrived via the Genoese grain-shipping network.[104]

Villani may not have made a causal link between the soldiers and plague, but the modern reader of his chronicle can see their joint movement: the disruption and dislocation surrounding these fighting men at least exacerbated, if not spread, plague and other epidemic illnesses. The fast-moving group of mounted soldiers surrounding King Louis of Hungary and the unknown number of 'brigands' following in his wake likely made conditions worse in cities and towns by keeping people within the walls and putting strains on the food supply.[105] And, as Ann Carmichael reminds us, other infectious diseases did not disappear when plague emerged.[106] The spread of other diseases may also have been influenced by this fast-traveling, disruptive group that moved into the area just as plague was taking hold.[107]

Plague certainly impacted on the southern Italian peninsula during the king of Hungary's invasion and was a major factor in his experience of ruling Naples. By the middle of May 1348, his occupation of the kingdom of Naples had turned popular support against King Louis. The severe punishments he meted out for the death of his brother Andrew, especially the beheading of Charles of Durazzo (the husband of Johanna's younger sister Marie), led to riots and uprisings against him and his troops. Fortune's wheel had turned. Louis of Hungary was forced to leave the Italian peninsula, which allowed Queen Johanna and Louis of Taranto to return to Naples. For Villani, the heavens were not responsible for experiences of political failure. Instead, God's wrath could be foreseen in those conjunctions, making it an even riskier time for people to act sinfully. That punishment was experienced through famines, military defeat and epidemic illness.

101 Ibid., p. 173.

102 Ibid.

103 Ibid. Italian: 'e per cessare la pestilenzia della mortalità, che già era cominciata a Napoli grandissima'; *Cronica*, IV, 173.

104 Barker, 'Laying the Corpses to Rest', p. 122.

105 *Final Book*, p. 169. Italian: 'malandrini'; *Cronica*, IV, 169.

106 A. Carmichael, *Plague and the Poor in Renaissance Florence* (Cambridge, 1986), pp. 10–26.

107 See Barker, 'Laying the Corpses to Rest'; O. Benedictow, *The Black Death, 1346–1353: The Complete History* (Woodbridge, 2004), pp. 72–3; Caferro, *Mercenary Companies*, pp. 25–35.

Conclusion

This chapter has analysed the last book of Giovanni Villani's *New Chronicle* to give modern audiences a contemporary perspective of the causes of epidemic illness on the eve of the Black Death. It reveals a complex relationship among warfare, sin and the heavens.

For contemporaries, mercenary warfare in particular was ubiquitous and could contribute to outbreaks of epidemic illness. These professional soldiers had little or no loyalty to city-states or leaders, could travel long distances and lived off the continual wars in the region; they are also an important context to the arrival of plague. These examples from Villani clearly show contact among displaced peoples, the disruption of thousands of mercenaries camping and moving through the region and the instability of military alliances. Their methods of fighting created contact, disruption and instability, which in turn generated a landscape fertile for the eruption and spread of disease. Clearly, their near-constant presence could destabilise towns and cities as they competed for food and destroyed infrastructure,[108] but, more importantly for this chapter, the mercenaries themselves – not just the local population they attacked – are an important community to consider in regard to the proliferation of disease-inducing environments.

Warfare appeared most frequently in relation to epidemic illness in Villani's chronicle, but his worldview also included a strong sense of the importance of moral conduct and the influence of the heavens. Villani characterised some behaviour of political leaders as egregiously 'unchristian', provoking God's punishment. During times of dangerous planetary conjunctions, God's punishment could appear in the form of surprising military losses, famines or epidemics. Villani stressed that the conjunctions of planets did not constrain or predict human behaviour, but they did create a moment of potential extreme punishment, with famines, floods and earthquakes serving as warnings.

Warfare, sin and the heavens came together in King Louis of Hungary's invasion in 1347, which took place on the eve of the Black Death. The mercenaries' activities, which were already in play, were heightened by the king of Hungary's invasion. They joined his invasion force in large numbers. Others followed in the wake of his army, looting and attacking. These men harassed southern regions of the Italian peninsula just as plague spread through its cities. By the time of the second wave of plague in 1360–61, contemporaries started to see that mercenaries could move disease from one region to another in supply ships, baggage trains and their own bodies.[109] Villani put this devastating invasion

[108] P. Contamine, *La vie quotidienne pendant la guerre de cent ans: France et Angleterre, XIVe siècle* (New York, 1978.)

[109] This more direct perception of links between plague and mercenaries emerges in the second wave of plague in 1360–1. See Carmichael, 'Universal and Particular', pp. 37–8. Carmichael notes that Gui de Chauliac, physician to the pope, described many mercenaries descending from northern lands as a precursor to the second wave of plague in Avignon in 1361. For the perceived influence of armed men during the second wave of plague, see also J. Glénisson, 'La Second Peste: L'épidémie de 1360–1362', *Annuaire-Bulletin de la Société de l'Histoire de France* (1968–9), 27–38 (pp. 30–1).

in the context of the sinful behaviour of Queen Johanna of Naples and Louis of Taranto and the extraordinary conjunction of 1345.

The fascinating and complex last book of Giovanni Villani's *New Chronicle* gives us a contemporary picture of epidemic that we can put in conversation with Carmichael's 'Universal and Particular' as well as other views of the Black Death. Villani's chronicle highlights the combined impact of heavy rain and famine, conjunctions of the heavens, sinful behaviour of lords and political instability. As he states,

> Observe, O reader, how many disasters occurred in this year to our city – hunger, mortality, ruin, storms, fires, and discord between citizens – because of the excess of our sins. May it please God that these signs correct our defects, that He not condemn us to greater punishments, fearsome punishments, for faith and charity have failed between citizens.[110]

To these we might also add plague, the pestilential disease from which Villani himself soon died, leaving his chronicle unfinished.

[110] *Final Book*, p. 145. Italian: 'E nota, lettore, quante tempeste occorsono in questo anno alla nostra città di Firenze, fame, mortalità, ruine, tempeste, folgori, fuochi, e discordie tra' cittadini, per lo soperchio de nostri peccati. Piaccia a Dio che questi segni ci correggano de' nostri difetti e peccati, acciocchè Iddio non ci condanni a maggiore guidicio, che paura ne fa, si è fallita la fede e carità tra' cittadini'; *Cronica*, IV, 141.

4

Colours of Disease and Death in the Early Modern Ottoman Cultural Imagination

NÜKHET VARLIK[1]

> And among His signs is the creation of the heavens and the earth, and the diversity of your languages and colors. Surely in this there are signs for people who have knowledge … And there are also Signs for those who take heed in the numerous things of various colors that He has created for you on earth.
>
> (*Qur'an*: al-Rum, XXX, 22 and al-Nahl, XVI, 13)

In the early days of the COVID-19 pandemic, it quickly became clear that this new viral disease displayed different symptoms on white and coloured bodies. Before mass testing became available, these clinical differences caused problems in diagnosis and at times slowed down, complicated, impeded or altogether compromised treatment, eventually aggravating the disproportionately higher infection and mortality rates among black and brown bodies in the United States.[2] The punishing discrepancy among different

1 This chapter could not have been completed without the constant encouragement, support and help of my co-editor and dear friend Lori Jones, whom I thank from the bottom of my heart. My thanks also go Seçil Yılmaz for her careful reading of the chapter and thoughtful suggestions. I would also like to thank the scholars of disease and death whose work continues to inform and inspire my own work. In particular, I thank Ann Carmichael, who was the first to make me think about the materiality of plague buboes and inspired me to think about their colours, and Monica H. Green, whose published research stressing the significance of race as an important theme in disease history was one of the inspirations for this chapter. Earlier versions of this chapter were presented at the conferences 'Visual Plague: Image, Imagination and Imaginary', held at the University of St Andrews on 12–14 July 2018, and 'The Worlds that Plague Made: Cultures of Disease in the Medieval and Early Modern Period', held at New York University on 13–14 April 2018. I thank Christos Lynteris and Karl Appuhn, respectively, for their invitations, and the audience at both conferences for their valuable feedback. *A note on translation and transliteration*: Ottoman Turkish is transliterated using the modern Turkish alphabet. Arabic transliterations omit diacritical marks as much as possible. Except as otherwise noted, all translations are mine.

2 For higher infection and case fatality rates among the racial and ethnic populations in the United States, see, for example, S. D. Romano et al., 'Trends in Racial and Ethnic Disparities in COVID-19 Hospitalizations, by Region – United States, March–December 2020', *Morbidity and Mortality Weekly Report* 70 (16 April 2021), 560–5; A. E. Iyanda et al., 'Racial/Ethnic Heterogeneity and Rural-Urban Disparity of COVID-19 Case Fatality Ratio in the USA: A Negative Binomial and GIS-Based Analysis', *Journal of Racial and Ethnic Health Disparities* (2021),

racial groups painfully exposed the existing socio-economic inequalities in public health and access to healthcare resulting from deep-seated systemic racism. One aspect of this poignant discussion involved medical diagnosis – in particular, how diagnosis was determined by skin colour.[3]

This should not be entirely surprising, as it was already well known that Western medical knowledge and practice has long favoured white bodies. Clinicians in the Global North are much better equipped to recognise and diagnose conditions as they appear on a white body than they are on a non-white body. For example, they are trained to diagnose skin lesions, rashes or blue lips in the manner those conditions appear on white skin. Since clinical research remains largely limited to diagnostic knowledge drawn from white skin, there exists a significant bias in knowledge and expertise among modern health professionals.[4] Moreover, since the majority of published medical research is produced in the Global North, whence it is distributed, there is the additional risk of disseminating that bias globally – even where it may not be applicable to the majority of cases.

The practice of medical knowledge being drawn from and offered to the service of white bodies at the expense of non-white bodies is not unprecedented. Modern history of medicine has preserved numerous painful memories of such moments, including the exploitation of non-white bodies as 'anatomical material' in medical education and research.[5] Here I use modern history as a critical moment to reflect on the longer evo-

---

https://link.springer.com/article/10.1007/s40615-021-01006-7 (last accessed 28 August 2021); V. R. Maritza, 'The Disproportional Impact of COVID-19 on African Americans', *Health and Human Rights* 22 (2020), 299–307.

3 S. Page, 'A Medical Student Couldn't Find How Symptoms Look on Darker Skin. He Decided to Publish a Book about It', *Washington Post* (22 July 2020) https://www.washingtonpost.com/lifestyle/2020/07/22/malone-mukwende-medical-handbook (last accessed 23 June 2022).

4 R. C. Rabin, 'Dermatology Has a Problem with Skin Color', *New York Times* (30 August 2021) https://www.nytimes.com/2020/08/30/health/skin-diseases-black-hispanic.html?surface=home-discovery-vi-prg&fellback=false&req_id=376443936&algo=identity&imp_id=923090689 (last accessed 28 August 2021). The lack of racial and ethnic diversity in medical research and clinical trials is well known. See, for example, L. Konkel, 'Racial and Ethnic Disparities in Research Studies: The Challenge of Creating More Diverse Cohorts', *Environmental Health Perspectives* 123, no. 12 (2015), A297–302.

5 For a recent reflection on the legacy of medical racism and violence in the United States, see A. Nuriddin, G. Mooney and A. I. R. White, 'The Art of Medicine: Reckoning with Histories of Medical Racism and Violence in the USA', *The Lancet* 396 (2020), 949–51. Historians of American medicine in particular have extensively studied how race and assumed racial differences have informed medical and public health policy for diagnosing, identifying and mitigating epidemic diseases. See, for example, J. Downs, *Sick from Freedom: African-American Illness and Suffering during the Civil War and Reconstruction* (New York, 2012); D. M. Oshinsky, *Polio: An American Story* (Oxford, 2005); E. Fenn, *Pox Americana: The Great Smallpox Epidemic of 1775–82* (New York, 2001); N. Shah, *Contagious Divides: Epidemics and Race in San Francisco's Chinatown* (Berkeley, 2001); S. M. Reverby, *Tuskegee's Truths: Rethinking the Tuskegee Syphilis Study* (Chapel Hill, 2000); H. Markel, *Quarantine! East European Jewish Immigrants and the New York City Epidemics of 1892* (Baltimore, 1997); J. W. Leavitt, *Typhoid Mary: Captive to the Public's Health*

lution of medical bias toward white skin, since it has much deeper roots in premodern medicine that made use of colours in myriad ways, from diagnosis to treatment. This, in turn, reinforced long-lasting associations between colours and diseases. Plague, for example, infamously acquired an association with the colour black (more on that later); other infectious diseases have also acquired close associations with particular colours. Cholera was associated with blue, while tuberculosis was sometimes called 'white plague'. Yellow fever is, of course, associated with yellow, and scarlet fever with red. In effect, diseases acquired colour associations beyond medical knowledge as their meaning and symbolism changed on the basis of historical and cultural contexts.[6]

Colours have been used in the service of medicine, science and statecraft, as well as to create meaning and build culture. To study the colours of disease and death in a premodern society, it is helpful to remember that cultural imagination was never necessarily limited to medical definitions. The clinical colours of plague and other infectious diseases mostly relied on visible symptoms of diseases, almost always observed, recorded and remembered on white skin. Beyond medical sources, however, we find a rich body of testimonies reflecting different experiences of disease and death. Here, colours that define life also define disease and death.

This chapter is a preliminary survey of the role of colour in the diagnosis and understanding of disease and death in the late medieval and early modern world, with a focus on early modern Ottoman history. In the main, it seeks to situate colours as they were imagined by those who experienced disease and death and as they were reflected in emotions and symbolism, as well as in the material realities that made sense of them. My goal here is not to trace the origins of the epistemic injustices of modern medicine as they pertain to race; rather, I hope to catch a glimpse of how different medical and non-medical traditions used colour to generate insight into disease and death, while simultaneously underscoring how colours and, especially, their medical manifestations are historically constructed – often anachronistically. To this end, I first explore the colour associations of death and disease (plague in particular) in historical epidemiology. Then, I shift the focus to Ottoman colour cosmologies to offer a closer reading of medical and non-medical meanings and symbolisms of colour. Next, I briefly survey the evolution of the use of colour in the service of medicine in the premodern world. This background helps to reconstruct the use of colour in association with plague in the Ottoman context, by tracing the genealogies of the various colours of plague in medical and non-medical traditions that informed the Ottoman cultural imagination.

(Boston, 1995); A. M. Kraut, *Silent Travelers: Germs, Genes, and the 'Immigrant Menace'* (Baltimore, 1994).

6 See, for example, the brilliant analysis of the cultural meanings of disease in S. Sontag, *Illness as Metaphor; and, AIDS and Its Metaphors* (New York, 2006).

What colour was plague?

What is the colour of plague?[7] Is there a colour universally associated with this infamous disease? Was it black, and, if so, why? Today, the term Black Death is accepted to be virtually synonymous with plague; the misnomer 'black plague' is often used in common parlance. A common etymology has it that the Black Death takes its name from the black spots and necrosis that appear on some plague victims' bodies, yet it is not clear where this false belief originates. It is evident that the term Black Death was not even used commonly until the nineteenth century, and only at this point did this medieval pandemic come to be associated with the colour black. Moreover, that etymology anachronistically assumes a purely medicalised definition of the pandemic, which clearly was not the case until the modern period. Whatever its genealogy, the term Black Death (and its equivalent in other European languages) is not a product of a medicalised thinking of plague. I discuss this question of why the Black Death is black elsewhere in greater detail, but suffice it to say that the Black Death was *not* black because plague caused black spots and necrosis on its victims' bodies.[8] On the contrary, the 'black' in the Black Death refers not to 'blackness' (nor to any specific colour, for that matter) of plague's clinical manifestations but, rather, reflects an exclusively nineteenth-century European historical imagination of past epidemics. That particular historical imagination has largely prevailed until the present.

In fact, plague had myriad other colour associations in premodern contexts. Such colour correspondences are important to situate plague and other diseases in larger cultural and cosmological contexts. Most of those who witnessed plague outbreaks (or other epidemic diseases) in the premodern world had their subjective experiences outside the limited framework of formal medicine. They heard rumours about it. They feared it. They prayed and hoped for protection from it. They lost their loved ones to it. Or they themselves were its victims or survivors. Historical sources offer ample evidence to trace those subjective experiences. For example, plague survivors showed the visible scars of buboes, likely common enough to be identified easily. An early seventeenth-century Ottoman register that contains physical descriptions of young 'devshirme' (child levy) conscripts indicates that 7.5 per cent of them were plague survivors with visible scars. Likewise, those with pockmarks on their faces also occupied a similar ratio in the same register.[9] This suggests that survivors of plague and smallpox, which amounted to 15 per cent of this one group of conscripts, were easily identifiable by the rest of society.

7 B. Gutiérrez-Rodilla, 'Les causes d'une couleur: la peste noire', in *Le corps polychrome: couleurs et santé*, ed. F. Collard and É. Samama (Paris, 2018), pp. 151–60.

8 See N. Varlık, 'Why Is Black Death *Black*? European Gothic Imaginaries of "Oriental" Plague', in *Plague Image and Imagination from Medieval to Modern Times*, ed. C. Lynteris (Cham, 2021), pp. 11–35.

9 The *devshirme* system involved the recruitment of Christian children from the Balkans to serve in the empire's military and administrative elite. See G. Yılmaz, 'The Devshirme System and the Levied Children of Bursa in 1603–4 A.D.', *Belleten* 79 (2015), 901–31.

It is fascinating for a historian to read the identification of an individual as a survivor of plague (or smallpox) or a physician's first-hand descriptions of a plague bubo, down to its exact shape, place, size and colour, but we are also humbled by the limitations of those accounts that fail to capture the full range of individual experiences about such bouts of epidemic disease in all of its colours. To fill in the gaps in our knowledge, it is important to listen to the testimonies of our historical actors as they expressed their experiences in various ways and to contemplate their imaginaries of disease and death. In what follows I offer a brief discussion of how colours figure in the Ottoman sources, not with respect to their medical characteristics but, rather, about how they were imagined. The colours mentioned here, unlike those that appear in medical texts, were not simply used for medical diagnostic precision or prognostic prediction; rather, they were invoked and recorded to *colour* imagination. They allowed those experiencing disease and death to engage in their own kind of personal and cultural diagnosis. As such, they improve our ability to connect to past actors and their stories, emotions and experiences as well as their attempts to explain or understand what was happening around them.

Colours in Ottoman plague imaginations

Mothers wore black, fathers blue,
Hearts solemn, eyes full of tears,
Some, yearning for their groom
Some, bidding farewell to their bride
Those narcissus-eyed, moon-faced brave warriors
Their cheeks are made of roses and Judas tree
Those mouths that become ant's burrow
Their lips full of blood-wine
Those white-faced, sweet-tongued brave warriors
Nights are the guests in the graveyard
Those with white skin lie down neatly spread out
It is right there, in black soil[10]

Such were the heart-wrenching lines written by the Anatolian mystic-poet Şeyyad Hamza (fl. 1348), who lost his children to plague during the Black Death, in the earliest known poem about plague in the Turkish language. The poet makes open references to the end of times and the signs of the impending apocalypse. By likening plague to a 'rain of death (ecel yağmurı)', he establishes it as something that comes down from the skies and pours

[10] Analar ḳara geymiş atalar gök / Yürekler başlu gözler ṭolu ḳandur / Kimi güyegücügi ḥasretinden / Kimi gelincüginden ayrılandur / Şu nerkis gözlü ay yüzlü yigitler / Yañakları gül-ile erġavāndur / Ḳarınca iñi olmış ol ağızlar / Ki bunlaruñ ṭudağı la'l ü kāndur / Ol aḳ yüzlü şirin sözlü yigitler / Guristānda giceler mīhmāndur / Ol aḳ tenler döşenüp şöyle yatur / Ḳara ṭoprak içinde dermeyāndur. M. Akar, 'Şeyyad Hamza Hakkında Yeni Bilgiler', *Türklük Araştırmaları Dergisi* 2 (1987), 1–14 (p. 4).

onto earth. He similarly likens plague to a 'wind of death (ölüm yili)'; whomever it touched 'fell down to the soil (düşer toprağa)', just like dead leaves falling on the ground in the autumn. Here plague 'picks people' (direr bu ẖalḳı)', 'ripe or unripe (ẖamı gögi dimez)', just as we harvest fruit from an orchard. To depict the burial scene by the graveyard, he turns to the bright colours of life (e.g., flowers, roses, narcissus and Judas tree), giving readers the sense of a rose garden, only to contrast it to the colours of death. The white faces of young victims of plague are then contrasted with the blackness and darkness of the soil, leaving a sense of an unreal, dreamlike quality; the reader sees the graveyard through the poet's eyes.

The same apocalyptic tone is also present in *Dürr-i Meknun* (The Hidden Pearl), a popular fifteenth-century encyclopaedic text, traditionally attributed to Ahmed Bican Yazıcıoğlu (d. after 1465).[11] Vividly describing the events associated with the Islamic millennial expectations of the apocalypse, the text refers to the appearance of plague as 'white death' ('mevt-i ebyaz'), alongside widespread famine and blood, which is designated as 'red death' ('mevt-i ahmer').[12] Here the colour white is used in association with plague; while rather unusual, it is worth noting that Islamic sources did assign different colours to death, perhaps drawing from the old Sufi tradition that maintained associations between death and colours. According to this tradition, there were four categories of death: white, red, green and black, each referring to the death of the self, the ultimate goal for mystics in their quest to reconnect with God by following different paths. Hence, white death meant the death of the self by means of fasting; black death, by means of suffering from other people's oppressive behaviour; red death, by means of fighting the self; and green death, by means of denying the appearance of the body, wearing old clothes and the like.[13]

A curious incident recounted by the fifteenth-century Ottoman chronicler Oruç describes how a poor wagon driver encountered two horsemen in black attire riding black horses as they raced toward him. In fear, the wagon driver hid under the wagon and watched them go by like lightning. Immediately after them, another horseman in green attire riding a pale horse and waving a lightning whip passed by. This latter horseman was Hızır, the renowned Prophet-Saint believed to miraculously appear to help those in need. He said that the horsemen in black were

> plague and pestilence. They live among people. God sent them. They obey the orders of God. I have received an order from God to expel them. They were eight in total; I killed six of them. If I can kill those two before they reach the seashore, there shall not be another plague for thirty years
>
> (Ol atlular öletdür, anlar tâ'ûnlardur. Bu halkuñ içinden çıkmazlar. Anlar dahı Hak ta'âlâ emriyiledür. Hak emrinden taşra çıkmazlar ve illâ kudret şimdi şöyle yüz gösterdi kim,

[11] On the question of the authorship of *Dürr-i Meknun*, see C. Grenier, 'Reassessing the Authorship of the *Dürr-i Meknūn*', *Archivum Ottomanicum* 35 (2018), 1–19.

[12] Y. A. Bîcan, *Dürr-i Meknun: Saklı İnciler* (Istanbul, 1999), p. 120.

[13] İ. Şener, 'Türk Edebiyatında Ölüm, Mezar, Fena ve Bekaa Temaları', in *Geçmişten Günümüze Mezarlık Kültürü ve İnsan Hayatına Etkileri Sempozyumu* (Istanbul, 1999), pp. 377–93.

> bu halkuñ içinden tâʿûn götürile. İmdi girü Hakk'uñ emriyile ben kulını bunlara havâle itdürdi. Bunlar sekiz kişiydi, altısını katl itdüm ikisi kaldı. Eger bu ikisini deñize girmedin katl idersem otuz yıl bu halk içinde tâʿûn olmaya).[14]

In this rather exceptional story, our chronicler portrays plague and pestilence in the form of 'black riders'. To add to the colour symbolism used in the story, it may be helpful to note that Prophet-Saint Hızır ('al-Khidr', the green one), without whose help plague could not be controlled, appeared riding a pale horse. Colours are embedded in rich layers of symbolism in this story; as we hear the story of a poor wagon driver, of his fear and frustrations, we also hear of his hopes for miraculous cures – all emotions coded in colour.

Another story with colour symbolism comes from the famous seventeenth-century Ottoman traveller Evliya Çelebi, in which a mystic encountered 'the soldiers of plague (tâʿûn askeri)'. While praying, the mystic found himself surrounded by countless numbers of soldiers, but the soldiers looked nothing like the ordinary soldiers he knew. They were divided into two encampments. In one camp were those dressed in white garments, living in white tents. In the other camp were those dressed in black, holding spears and living in black tents. Seeing this, the mystic conversed with members of the former encampment, who told him that they were good and benevolent spirits (ervah-ı tayyibe); when they pierced someone with their spears, the wounded contracted plague but would recover and ultimately survive the disease. Pointing to the encampment of soldiers in black tents, they told the mystic that those were the evil or malevolent spirits (ervah-ı habise); whenever they pierced someone with their spears, the wounded died of plague – if a Muslim, then as a martyr.[15] This story echoes some familiar themes in plague literature and art, such as the motif of the spear (also sometimes an arrow) or plague being inflicted by countless armies. It also includes the contrast between white and black and the symbolism that ensued.

As these examples show, Ottoman sources offer a rich array of materials through which to explore the use of colour in descriptions of visual, sensory and emotional experiences of disease and death, as different colours were used to elicit certain emotions. For example, mourning practices included wearing black, covering the tent of the deceased with black cloth (or moving to a black tent), sometimes covering the coffin with black or blue cloth, spreading a black pelt on the floor and cutting off the tail of the owner's white-grey horse (figures 4.1. and 4.2). Using a white cloth for shrouds was also conventional.[16] In a similar vein, descriptions of lived experiences of plague and suffering (at both the individual and

14 Oruç Beğ, *Oruç Beğ Tarihi: Giriş, Metin, Kronoloji, Dizin, Tıpkıbasım*, ed. Necdet Öztürk (Istanbul: Çamlıca Basım Yayın, 2007), pp. 163–5, facsimile 111a–12b. For a more detailed discussion of this story, see N. Varlık, 'From "Bête Noire" to "*le Mal de* Constantinople": Plagues, Medicine, and the Early Modern Ottoman State', *Journal of World History* 24 (2013), 741–70.

15 Evliya Çelebi, *Evliyâ Çelebi Seyahatnâmesi*, ed. Yücel Dağlı, Seyit Ali Kahraman (Istanbul: 2001), 4: 341–2. For a more detailed discussion of this story, see N. Varlık, *Plague and Empire in the Early Modern Mediterranean World: The Ottoman Experience, 1347–1600* (Cambridge, 2015), pp. 237–8.

16 E. Eldem, *Death in Istanbul: Death and Its Rituals in Ottoman-Islamic Culture* (Istanbul, 2005).

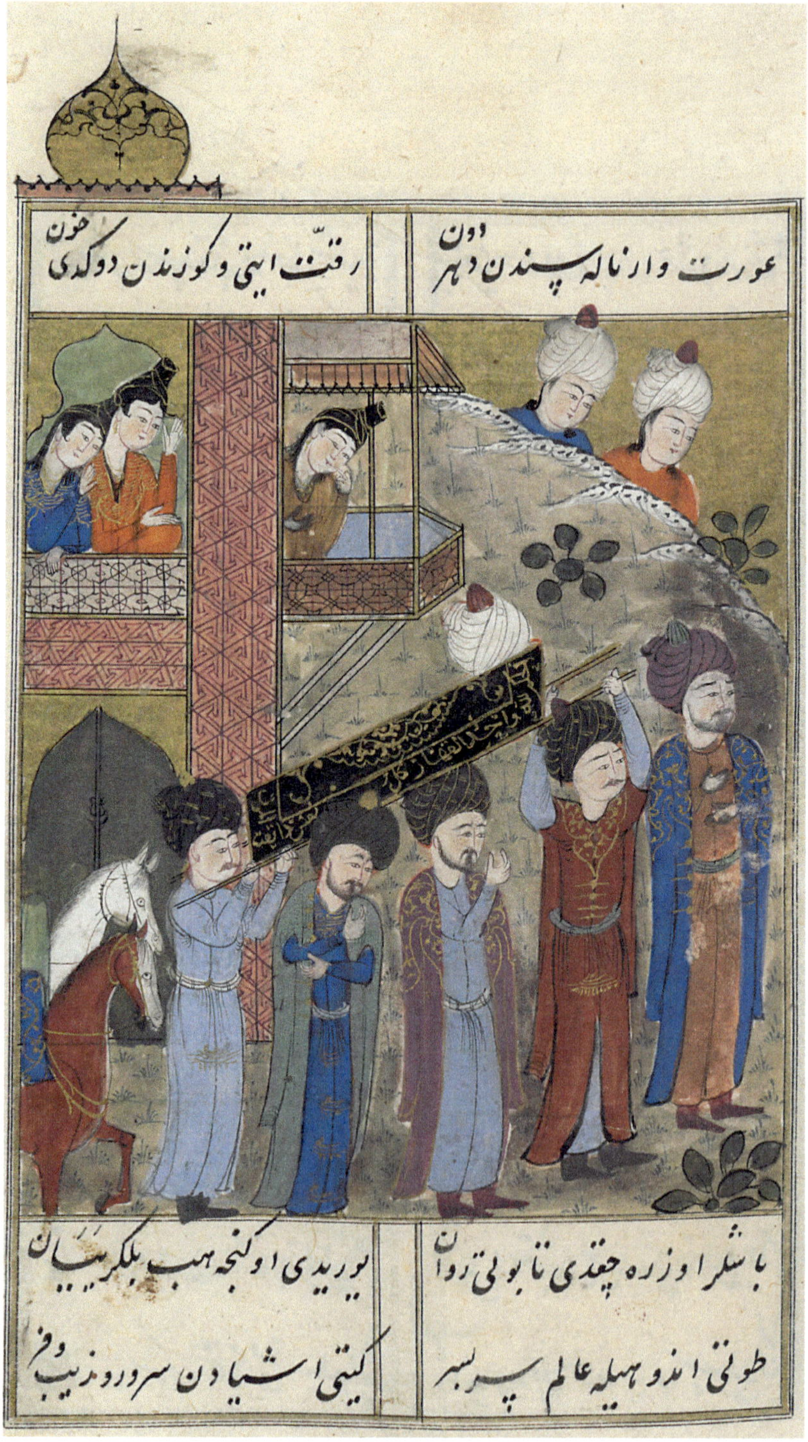

Fig. 4.1. Funeral of Bayezid II, Şükrî, *Selimnâme*, Topkapı Palace Museum Library MS H 1597–1598, fol. 62a.

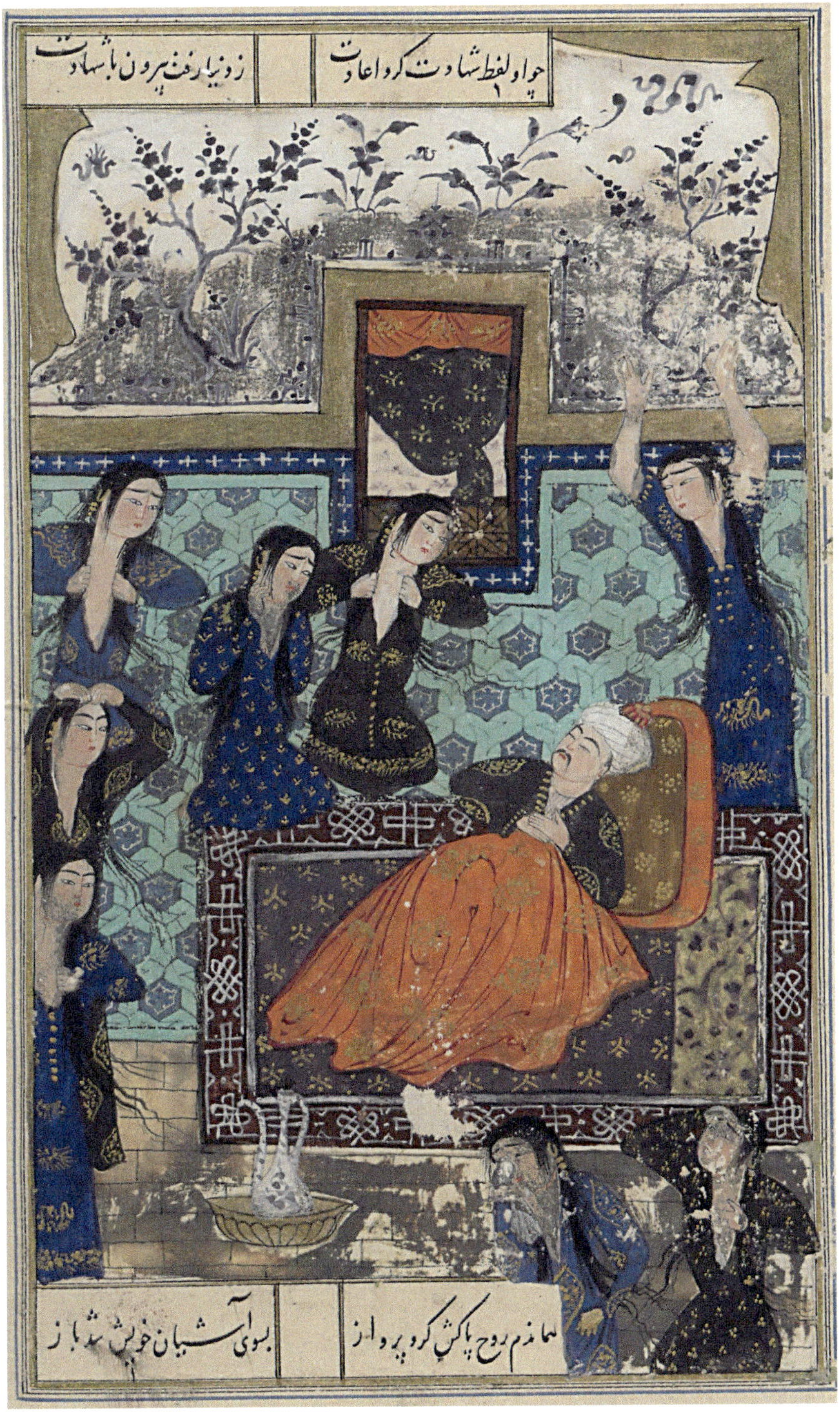

چو او لفظ شهادت کرد عادت
ز دنیا رفت بیرون با شهادت
همان دم روح پاکش کرد پرواز
بسوی آشیان خویش شد باز

Fig. 4.2. Mihr's Death, Tebrizî, *Mihr ü Müşterî*, Topkapı Palace Museum Library MS H 831, fol. 203b.

societal levels) include copious references to colours. In particular, it is interesting to note how different genres conjured up particular images and metaphors of plague, how they engaged colour symbolism used in the Ottoman cultural imagination and how plague represented the emotional landscape of suffering that underscored the anxieties of early modern Ottoman society.

Not unlike other premodern societies, the Ottomans cultivated a broad spectrum of knowledge, expertise and traditions around colours in conjunction with disease and death. Some of those had deeper roots in ancient medical traditions and cosmologies. Others were based on their own historical experiences, including medical and non-medical understanding of disease and death. What follows is a brief survey of the evolution of the use of colours in premodern medicine as a background to situate the Ottoman case in its larger historical context.

Colour in the service of medicine

Throughout the history of medicine, colours served myriad purposes. Since at least Antiquity, medical texts demonstrate that colours were used in diagnosing and predicting the course of diseases, in identifying, naming and classifying them (premodern nosology and nosography), in medical forensics and in various methods of treatment. Colours, like other visible markers of disease, offered visual clues and hence assisted healers to develop better insights to treat them. The idea that certain colours reflected certain signs of disease on one's body (or in the body fluids) is ancient. In ancient Mesopotamia, colours were used to assist medical diagnosis and prognosis: in Akkadian texts, for example, the term 'arqu' referred to the pale skin of a sick person or the yellowish skin of one infected by jaundice.[17] Different colours of 'pustules' likewise were associated with different health outcomes: while white pustules indicated that the patient would get well, black and red pustules indicated the opposite.[18]

Other examples from ancient medical traditions illustrate how colours served medical knowledge and practice as part of a systematic body of correspondences, in which colours were thought to correspond to certain key properties for health. Prominently in ancient Chinese medicine, the five elements (wood, earth, fire, water and metal) were believed to correspond to colours (red, white, black, yellow and green/blue), alongside directions (west, south, east, north and centre), taste, body parts, diseases and treatments. Recent scholarship has suggested that such elaborate correspondences had implications beyond what might appear as symbolic meanings; they likely had empirical foundations, such as those drawn

[17] S. Thavapalan, *The Meaning of Color in Ancient Mesopotamia* (Leiden, 2020), p. 74.

[18] U. Steinert, 'Disease Concepts and Classifications in Ancient Mesopotamian Medicine', in *Systems of Classification in Premodern Medical Cultures: Sickness, Health, and Local Epistemologies*, ed. U. Steinert (New York, 2021), pp. 140–94 (p. 170).

from observations of nature and reflections on sensory and abstract implications.[19] Likewise, ancient Greek medicine attributed a special place to colour in humoral medicine, in which each humour (blood, yellow bile, black bile and phlegm) was associated with a specific colour (red, yellow, black and blue/green, respectively). These correspondences were based on four elements (air, fire, earth and water) and four qualities (hot, dry, cold and wet), extending to four types of personality (sanguine, choleric, melancholic and phlegmatic), four seasons (spring, summer, autumn and winter), four stages of life (childhood, youth, adulthood and old age) and four internal organs (heart, gall bladder, spleen and brain/lungs), along with correspondences to planets, animals, minerals and many other categories that helped to contextualise health and that could be used for therapeutic purposes.

The humoral theory of ancient Greek medicine merits special attention here, as it was prevalent throughout western Eurasia during the medieval and early modern periods. The works of ancient Greek and Roman medical authors, such as those attributed to Hippocrates (d. c. 370 BCE) and Galen (d. c. 210 CE), helped to establish the foundations of a medical system that became the dominant medical paradigm for centuries. During the late antique era, Byzantine and Islamic medical authors further expanded on the earlier medical scholarship and contributed to the diversity of interpretations of this tradition. Islamic medicine, as heir to Greek humoral medicine, incorporated this medical paradigm and developed it further, while translations of the Islamicate medical corpus transmitted into the Latin tradition and were diffused into European vernacular languages starting in the late Middle Ages.

Central to this pervasive medical paradigm was the idea that the four humours had to be maintained in a state of balance for the preservation of health. Once that balance was disturbed, illness ensued. Not unlike other ancient medical systems, humoral medicine relied on a system of correspondences because the human body was considered to be a microcosm of the larger cosmos. Health and disease thus had connections to the world around it. By the same token, colours also had associations with other beings outside the human body, such as plants, animals and minerals, as well as with such distant entities as celestial bodies, planets and stars. Such associations were not only important for medicine, but also for astrology, physiognomy and alchemy. These correspondences also helped the development of pharmaceuticals that laid the foundations for early collections of 'materia medica' (medical material/substance).[20]

To better understand the importance of colour correspondences in all of this, it is critical to consider the principal disease theory in premodern medicine, by which the causes of diseases were not differentiated from the symptoms of diseases. Rather, how a disease manifested itself was considered key to its identity. This is particularly important

19 V. Bogushevskaya, 'Ancient Chinese "Five Colors" Theory: What Does Its Semantic Analysis Reveal?', in *Essays in Global Color History: Interpreting the Ancient Spectrum*, ed. R. B. Goldman (Piscataway NJ, 2016), pp. 225–44.

20 For one specific example of this related to the use of red coral and its assumed correspondences, see Nichola Harris's chapter 10 in this volume.

for infectious diseases. For example, most infectious diseases were considered to be 'fevers', since that was one of their primary symptoms. Similarly, coughing or headaches that are accepted as mere symptoms today were considered as diseases in their own right according to premodern medicine. Since premodern medicine identified and classified diseases based on their visible symptoms, colours received ample attention, since they allowed the identification of diseases as they manifested on a patient's body. In other words, colours mattered because symptoms on the skin became markers or identifiers of disease. By studying disease symptoms, and especially the visual expression of an infection on skin (it being among the most visibly important of all symptoms), one could identify, name and classify them. It was for this reason that some infectious diseases, such as leprosy, syphilis or smallpox, were long considered and classified as diseases of the skin, because they caused various types of visible rashes or lesions.

As colours acquired a broader range of correspondences, they served knowledge making in a number of disciplines, ranging from medicine to astrology and alchemy. Colours were one of the elements in the system of cosmological concordances – the hegemonic way of imagining the cosmos across premodern cultures. Colours were thus part of a larger epistemology that relied on cosmological correspondences, in particular the correspondence between the human body and the larger cosmos. The legacy of premodern medicine with respect to the importance of colours is illustrated in many disease names that include direct or indirect references to colours (and we continue to use them today). Disease names such as jaundice, yellow fever, scarlet fever and green sickness are largely vestiges of premodern nosology that used colours to identify and name diseases.[21] Today, we also use other medical prefixes of Greek origin that refer to colours, such as 'leuko-' (white, e.g., leukocyte: a white blood cell), 'melan-' (black or dark, e.g., melanoma: black tumour of the skin); 'cyan-' (blue, e.g., cyanosis: a blue discolouration of the skin due to the circulation of blood low in oxygen). Other diseases have also acquired colour associations in the public imagination or popular culture, sometimes because of how they are depicted in art and literature.

Contrary to common belief, however, colours are (and were) not fixed and universal ontological entities. Rather, they are drawn from subjective, phenomenal experiences – a form of biological, social and cultural consensus that is always in flux. Recent research on colours from a number of disciplines including philosophy, history and art history, psychology and cognitive science underscores the variability of colour perception in different populations across time and space.[22] Philosophers stress that colours are to be understood in their epistemic and phenomenological contexts, rather than as stable ontological entities. In other words, what we understand today as a consensus of what is accepted as 'blue' or 'red' showed variations in history. Like other visual and non-visual cues, colours are socially and culturally constructed in specific contexts. They both encapsulate and reflect

21 H. King, *The Disease of Virgins: Green Sickness, Chlorosis, and the Problems of Puberty* (London, 2009).

22 See for example J. Cohen and M. Matthen, ed., *Color Ontology and Color Science* (Cambridge MA, 2010).

cultural conventions, traditions and beliefs. Similarly, the meaning, symbolism and values of colours also change over time. While a certain colour is used to express a certain emotion in one society, it could mean something else in others. For example, the colour black is often associated with death, grief and mourning, but those associations are not timeless or universal. Thus, before discussing how colours were used in medicine, it would be helpful to briefly discuss how both colours and their meaning change over time and space.

Ottoman colour cosmologies

Ottoman colour cosmologies represent a hybridity of influences, featuring two distinctly identifiable, yet intertwined, lineages: ancient Turkish and Islamic. Both had well-established colour correspondences, embedded in deeper cosmological traditions and languages (Turkish and Arabic, respectively), but there were also overlaps, interactions and exchanges between them, suggesting that the premodern meanings attributed to colours in the Ottoman context were also hybrid. In fact, this indicates clearly how meanings pertaining to colours were also in flux.

Ancient Turkish colour cosmology was informed by the Shamanistic belief system that centred on the sky god Tengri. Common among the Turko-Mongol nomadic tribal groups in various iterations across a large swath of the Eurasian steppes, this animistic religion's cosmology is reflected in its colour correspondences. Even after the mass conversion of the Oghuz Turks to Islam during their centuries-long movement toward western Asia, this colour cosmology was preserved in one form or another. In the centuries following their arrival and settlement in Anatolia in the late eleventh century, this memory seems to have still been alive and well, as testified in their naming practices of their new surroundings. In this set of correspondences, colours were associated with directions (e.g., black–north, red–south, blue/grey–east and white–west) and with the geographic names (e.g., seas, rivers, mountains and winds) that were associated with those directions. An obvious example is the naming of seas according to this colour concordance; hence, to the north was the Black Sea ('kara-deniz'), to the west was the Mediterranean ('ak-deniz', literally white sea), to the south the Red Sea ('kızıl-deniz') and so on.[23] Similarly, colours were also used to name peoples inhabiting those places, such as the tribal confederation of the White Sheep ('Ak-koyunlu') and the Black Sheep ('Kara-koyunlu'), among others. As these examples show, colours had associations with geographic and topographic elements; directions and even notions of sovereignty and state building were sometimes embedded in them.

Ancient Turkish texts from the seventh century onward reveal a clear hierarchy of colours: white ('ak'), black ('kara'), blue ('kök/gök'), green ('yaşıl'), red ('al'), yellow ('sarıġ'),

[23] This is, however, controversial. For an argument that the etymology of the Black Sea can be traced back to its earliest uses in Hungarian, Khazar and Bulgar sources, which predate its usage in Turkish, see O. Karatay, 'On the origins of the name for the "Black Sea"', *Journal of Historical Geography* 37 (2011), 1–11. Karatay does, however, underscore the colour associations with directions used by the peoples of the Eurasian steppes (p. 2).

grey ('boz'), brown ('yağız'), purple ('yıpkın') and multi-coloured ('ala').[24] Anatolian Turkish seems to have mainly preserved this hierarchy and its set of meanings and symbolism. The five main colours were black, white, red, blue/green and yellow, which corresponded to north, west, south, east and centre, respectively. Black appears as an adjective in titles, place names and natural objects in ancient and middle Turkish, as testified in the Orkhon inscriptions of the early eighth century; it could mean great, holy, high or noble, but also 'brave and noble Turkic people or tribe'.[25] White symbolised light, purity and wisdom. Red represented hot and fire. Yellow often referred to disease, disaster and hate. Blue/green, which was the 'sky' colour, does not neatly correspond to a net colour category today; it could refer to blue, green or grey/pale.[26] And while similar colour correspondences appear in other cultures, it is important to note that they are not universal.

To understand the full spectrum of colour symbolism as it was used in the Ottoman Empire, it is helpful to consider the Islamic religious tradition, especially the Qur'an and the Hadith. The colours mentioned in the Qur'an are white, black, red, blue, yellow and green, with white and black being the most frequently mentioned for their symbolic and metaphorical power. For example, black is sometimes referred to as darkness of the night or as stain on the heart of disbelievers. But overall, black, white and yellow seem to have been the most important colours for the early Muslim community. Hadith collections underscore that certain colours were to be preferred over others. For example, white, with its positive associations with light and life, was considered to be the best possible colour to wear, likely based on its symbolic value as an expression of moral purity among the Arabs. The practice of using white cloth for shrouds is also often traced to this tradition. Black, however, and in stark contrast to its Turkic meaning, had negative associations, since it symbolised disbelief, evil, rage, grief and the Devil; in particular, it was associated with unbelievers. Interestingly, red is mostly absent in the Qur'an, being mentioned only with reference to the colour of mountain trails, and somewhat ambiguously in the Hadith. It appears in different contexts, which might suggest that it was not a fixed entity in the cultural world of Arabia in the seventh century. For example, it was used to refer to the Prophet's hair, to the redness of the sun, the heat of the fire in hell, drying or dying trees or an angry face. Some jurists argued that wearing a red dress (for men) was not acceptable, although there were differing interpretations. Yellow has associations with the transitory nature of life in the Qur'an, and is also somewhat ambivalent in the Hadith. Overall, red and yellow are seen as controversial colours in the Hadith. Green has associations with nature and heaven in both the Qur'an and the Hadith, and it is overall a favoured colour in Islamic culture. Blue, and especially blue eyes, has negative connotations.[27]

24 Z. Otyzbay, *Türk Kavram Sisteminde Renkler* (Ankara, 2019).

25 On 'kara', see H.-W. Choi, 'On the Shamanic Concept of Qara "Black" in Turkic', *Türk Dilleri Araştırmaları* (1992), 103–8.

26 Y. Kalafat, *Türk Halk İnançlarında Renkler* (Ankara, 2012).

27 For colours in Islamic history, see S. Gündüzöz, 'Renk', *Türkiye Diyanet Vakfı İslam Ansiklopedisi* (Istanbul, 2007), 34: 571–2; A. Topaloğlu, 'Renk' *Türkiye Diyanet Vakfı İslam Ansiklopedisi*

Together, the ancient Turkish set of associations and the Islamic influences informed Ottoman culture as it cultivated its own colour sensibilities and meanings. The heterogeneous vocabulary used for colours also testifies to this diversity. While ancient Turkish words for colours continued to be used, Arabic and Persian colour words were used alongside them, although each had a particular context. Generally speaking, while ancient Turkish words retained their symbolic expressions, loan words were more commonly used in the context of material culture and in textual traditions. For example, *The Book of Dede Korkut*, a collection of epic stories of the Oghuz Turks that circulated for centuries as part of the oral tradition and was written down in the late fifteenth or early sixteenth century, makes references to colours that demonstrate how those older symbolisms were still alive and accepted. The story of Boghach Khan tells of his father's humiliation at being put in a black tent (kara otağ) by Bayındır Khan. The latter had ordered that anyone who had a son was to be put in the white tent (ak otağ), anyone who had a daughter in the red tent (kızıl otağ), and anyone who had neither son nor daughter in the black tent. Having neither at the time, Dirse Khan was put in a black tent, a black felt mat was spread beneath him and he was offered mutton stew made from black sheep. The repeated black symbolism increased his sense of humiliation.[28]

The colour symbolism used here would have been fully legible to the story's Ottoman audience, not only as a story of a remote past, but as a lived experience in their own society in which colours essentially imposed social hierarchies. Colours were used as a tool for governance in Ottoman society to reinforce norms of social hierarchy. Certain colours in dress and headgear could be worn only by members of certain classes. For example, Jews were expected to wear red headgear and black shoes, while Christians were expected to wear black hats. Darker colours – those with negative connotations in the Muslim context, such as black or dark blue – were reserved for non-Muslims. Muslims, by contrast, were free to wear headgear of any colour, and yellow shoes were reserved for them.[29] However, repeatedly issued dress codes that tried to regulate colours suggest that, despite all efforts, those distinctions were not easy to maintain.[30]

(Istanbul, 2007), 34: 572–5; H. Akyüz, 'Hz. Peygamber'in Hadislerinde Renklerin Dili', *Atatürk Üniversitesi İlahiyat Fakültesi Dergisi* 41 (2014), 373–97. Blue eyes were seen as a disability in Mamluk Egypt. See K. Richardson, *Difference and Disability in the Medieval Islamic World: Blighted Bodies* (Edinburgh, 2014).

28 *The Book of Dede Korkut*, trans. and ed. G. Lewis (New York, 1974), pp. 27–8; M. Ergin, *Dede Korkut Kitabı* (Ankara, 2018), 78.

29 B. İ. Argıt, 'Clothing and Fashion in Istanbul (1453–1923)', *History of Istanbul* 4, https://istanbultarihi.ist/485-clothing-and-fashion-in-istanbul-14531923 (last accessed 28 August 2021).

30 The type and design of dress in Ottoman society was a perennial source of fascination for European travellers, who typically described them in their travelogues and illustrated them in costume albums. Ottoman dress has likewise been the subject of many studies in modern scholarship. See for example, E. Fraser, 'The Color of the Orient: On Ottoman Costume Albums, European Print Culture, and Cross-Cultural Exchange', in *Visual Typologies from the Early Modern to the Contemporary: Local Contexts and Global Practices*, ed. T. Zanardi and L. Klich (London, 2019),

The famous seventeenth-century Ottoman traveller Evliya Çelebi made important observations about colours along the lines of ancient colour correspondences. In his work, skin colours indicated types of personality, dispositions and behaviours; they could also provide insights about one's lifestyle, health and even values. In several instances, he talks about the complexion of people who lived in different locations, which he describes with respect to their environment, climate, food and water, while also commenting on their humoral dispositions. People across the seven climes, according to him, have different skin colours and complexions, some have dark faces, some light. In certain places, because of unhealthy environments, people have a more yellowish complexion, a sign that they are not healthy. He also notes that white skin was aesthetically the most pleasing.[31]

Evliya Çelebi was not alone in observing that people's skin colour and complexion reflected their state of health affected by local environmental and climatic conditions. This idea was informed by humoral theory and long-standing notions of correspondences between health and place.[32] Perhaps even more importantly, this relationship was engrained in well-known theories of physiognomy. According to this, certain physical characteristics – including height, weight, skin colour, hair, eyes, face and body shape – were seen as a reflection of certain character traits. Rooted in the Islamic occult-scientific tradition, physiognomy was especially well received among the Ottoman military and

pp. 45–59; C. Jirousek, *Ottoman Dress and Design in the West: A Visual History of Cultural Exchange* (Bloomington, 2019).

31 B. E. Tekin, 'Evliyâ Çelebi Seyahatnâmesi'nde Renkler' (unpublished MA thesis, Uludağ University, 2018), pp. 92–5.

32 The idea that there was a correspondence between health and place goes back to ancient medicine. See Hippocrates, *Airs, Waters, Places*, trans. W. H. S. Jones (Cambridge MA, 1923). Establishing correspondences of people with places, framed in the context of climate and environment, found a full articulation in the eighteenth century by Montesquieu. For his climate theory, see his famous *The Spirit of the Laws* (*De l'esprit des loix*) of 1748, especially Book XIV, 'On the Laws in Their Relation to the Nature of the Climate', http://montesquieu.ens-lyon.fr/spip.php?rubrique210 (last accessed 28 August 2021). It may be helpful to remember that this environmentalism was used as the intellectual justification for the subjugation and enslavement of African people. For voices opposing the idea of the inferiority of blacks, see, for example, *Dispelling the Darkness on the Merits of the Ethiopians*, a treatise written by the chief judge and member of the Ottoman imperial council Mullah Ali in early seventeenth-century Istanbul. See B. Tezcan, 'Dispelling the Darkness: The Politics of "Race" in the Early Seventeenth-Century Ottoman Empire in the Light of the Life and Work of Mullah Ali', in *Identity and Identity Formation in the Ottoman World: A Volume of Essays in Honor of Norman Itzkowitz*, ed. B. Tezcan and K. K. Barbir (Madison, 2007), pp. 73–95. On the diversity of opinions on this issue in the early modern Ottoman context, also see B. Tezcan, '*Dispelling the Darkness* of the *Halberdier's Treatise*: A Comparative Look at Black Africans in Ottoman Letters in the Early Modern Period', in *Disliking Others: Loathing, Hostility, and Distrust in Premodern Ottoman Lands*, ed. H. T. Karateke, H. E. Çıpa and H. Anetshofer (Boston, 2018), pp. 43–74.

administrative elite, since it facilitated identifying those who possessed talent, intelligence and loyalty – indispensable for climbing the ranks in the Ottoman meritocracy.[33]

To the early modern Ottoman elite, the skin colour of peoples from outside the Ottoman heartlands of Anatolia and the Balkans marked not only their difference but also their perceived inferiority. In this framework, the whiter skin of people in the heartland ('Rumi') was considered to be superior to those who had darker skin. Hence, Arabs and Kurds, as well as such African groups as Nubians, Ethiopians and Sudanese who had darker skin, were judged according to this 'overarching ethno-regional chauvinism'.[34] The sixteenth-century historian Mustafa 'Ali notes that 'the wretched, black-faced Arabs of low descent are of ugly nature and filthy disposition'.[35] Similarly, it was not uncommon to find attacks such as 'that black-faced and most wicked one', raised toward Mullah Ali, the chief judge and member of the Ottoman imperial council in the early seventeenth century, on account of his African origin.[36]

The fair-skinned people of Anatolia and the Balkans were not only held as the moral standard by which everyone of darker skin was to be judged; they also marked the standards of beauty. Classical Ottoman love poetry celebrated the fair skin of the beloved along with large black eyes, arched black eyebrows, eyelashes like arrows and red lips and cheeks, imagined as the highest standards of beauty, worthy of the poet's praise. The beautiful beloved is sometimes 'moon-faced' or described as having skin 'like cotton', so 'delicate and moist'.[37] In poetry, white skin was unambiguously associated with beauty.

Skin colour mattered beyond the diversity represented among Ottoman subjects. Though not unique or exceptional to the Ottoman case, practices of slavery underscored the value attributed to skin colour in that racialised bodies fitted into particular social hierarchies. There was a close association between the function of the slave and his or her

33 E. Lelić, 'Ottoman Physiognomy ('Ilm-i Firâset): A Window into the Soul of an Empire' (unpublished Ph.D. dissertation, University of Chicago, 2017).

34 J. Hathaway, *The Chief Eunuch of the Ottoman Harem: From African Slave to Power-Broker* (Cambridge, 2018), pp. 34–7. Here it may be helpful to note that white skin had different political implications in different historical contexts. For example, the Ottoman imagination of whiteness was different than that of the European. Historical scholarship has shown that colour as racial category gained new political implications especially after the age of explorations, leading to different interpretations through the Spanish and British colonial experiences. See for example P. K. Gilbert, *Victorian Skin: Surface, Self, History* (Ithaca, 2019); S. Seth, *Difference and Disease: Medicine, Race, and the Eighteenth-Century British Empire* (Cambridge, 2018); C. Malcolmson, *Studies of Skin Color in the Early Royal Society: Boyle, Cavendish, Swift* (Farnham, 2013).

35 Mustafa 'Ali, *Mevâ'ıdü'n-Nefâis fî Ḳavâ'ıdi'l-Mecâlis*, ed. M. Şeker (Ankara, 1997), pp. 342, 362: 'Sâyir sevâd-ı vechi ẓâhir olan 'Arablaruñ Nûbîyü'l-aṣl ve Tekrûriyü'n-nesl olanlardan ğayrisinüñ ḥabṣ-i ṭabî'atleri ve kabâḥat ṭıynetleri ve gûn-â-gûn çirkin murdâr sıfatların nice vech ile mükerrerdür'. 'Ve kara yüzlü 'Arablardan ve Hindî nâmındaki bed-aṣl ve bed-neseblerden'.

36 B. Tezcan, '*Dispelling the Darkness*', p. 83.

37 W. G. Andrews and M. Kalpaklı, *The Age of Beloveds: Love and the Beloved in Early-Modern Ottoman and European Culture and Society* (Durham NC, 2005), p. 46.

skin colour. Nuances in skin colour mattered too, as there was a wide spectrum of colour choices in enslavement; it was not only the blacks: white bodies were also enslaved. Black slaves were not a monolithic category, either; a wide spectrum of blackness was at work in Ottoman society. White enslavement was almost exclusively reserved for women sold to elite households, including the imperial household itself, for sexual roles and reproduction.[38] Whether a free Ottoman subject or slave, Muslim or non-Muslim, elite or non-elite, male or female, skin colour was part of a set of meanings and value for all in the Ottoman world. In this vein, the colours of plague embodied medical traditions along with acquired wisdom.

Colours of plague

Ottoman medicine followed the systems of colour concordances described above which can be exemplified in disease names. Turkish words were preferred for disease names, which might also suggest that those were older disease categories that had been long established in their culture. For example, jaundice ('sarılık'), measles ('kızamık'), scarlet fever ('kızıl'), anthrax ('yanıkara') and typhoid fever ('karahumma') were all names diagnosed directly after their colour correspondences using ancient Turkish colour words. Other disease names relied loosely on such associations. For example, night terror ('karabasan', literally black pressure) was experienced as a malicious entity ('mare') exerting pressure on one's chest while they were asleep, bringing on nightmares and making it impossible to get up or wake up. 'Albastı' (literally red pressure) or 'alkarısı' (literally red woman) were used in reference to postpartum fever or childbed infections, because of the ancient belief that an evil spirit targeted women during pregnancy or in childbed (perhaps the association with red was tied to the septicaemia or haemorrhaging that ensued). Not surprisingly, this medical tradition that used colour associations to identify and name diseases also used myriad therapeutic methods that invoked the healing properties of colours and their corresponding herbs, animals and minerals – along with their use in elixirs, charms and talismans – and their planetary correspondences.[39]

These diseases with Turkish colour designations were, however, much older (likely known since at least the Bronze Age). Newer (i.e., late medieval or early modern) diseases typically acquired a name based on loan words from other languages in the medical literature, although they were typically referred to differently in the vernacular. For example, syphilis was named 'frengi' or 'illet-i efrenciye' (literally French disease), likely borrowed from Italian sources that named the disease after the French.[40] Similarly, plague was introduced to Ottoman Turkish as a loan word from Arabic, i.e., 'ta῾un' and 'veba', but

[38] L. P. Peirce, *The Imperial Harem: Women and Sovereignty in the Ottoman Empire* (Oxford, 1993).

[39] For example, a yellow stone is used for jaundice, while a red cloth covers women after childbirth. See F. W. Hasluck, *Christianity and Islam under the Sultans* (London, 1929).

[40] For the term 'frengi', see N. Yıldırım, 'Alaim-i Cerrahin'de (1505) Frengi', *Tıp Fakültesi Mecmuası* 54 (1991), 353–60.

vernacular terms such as 'yumurcak'/'yumrucuk' (bubo), 'ölet' (pestilence or mortality) and 'kıran' (blight) were also used.[41] Interestingly enough, we do not see colour designations in the names of these new(er) diseases.

Islamic medical literature typically used colours as a proxy for diagnosis. As Nahyan Fancy notes, earlier Islamicate medical literature mentioned red, green, black and purple as diagnostic colours for plague buboes. In one of the most well-known moments in the history of medicine, Al-Rāzī's distinguishing between measles and smallpox includes a discussion of colours. Al-Rāzī observed that these diseases were distinguishable not only by where and when their symptoms appear but also by their degree of severity and prognosis, identified on the basis of the colour and location of their respective rashes (if smallpox lesions were black and violet, for example, the prognosis was bad). Ibn Sīnā also stressed the crucial importance of colour in medical diagnosis and treatment. He emphasised the correspondence between colours, temperament and the physical condition of the body. According to Fancy, he also commented on colours as diagnostic help for plague buboes and for the prognosis of the infection. Fancy likewise underscores the important discussion of colours of buboes found in al-Nawawī's work: 'The area surrounding the [swelling] blackens, turns green or reddens into a dingy purple.'[42]

Not unlike other premodern medical traditions, Ottoman medicine also made use of colours in a variety of ways, ranging from diagnosis to treatment and to identifying, naming and classifying diseases. Earlier examples of the Ottoman medical corpus show clear evidence of how colours were used, facilitating the physician's ability to develop a diagnosis in their clinical observations. For example, the fifteenth-century physician and medical writer Hacı Paşa (d. c. 1417) describes the symptoms of plague with great precision and accuracy:

> Plague ['ta'un'] is a feverish swelling or pustules that appear behind the ear, in the armpits, or in the groin area. These painful swellings appear when there is an epidemic and produce a burning feeling. The lesion of the swelling is black or green, or red. It gives nausea, vomiting, thirst, and shortness of breath.[43]

Especially to be noted here are his references to buboes as black, green or red.

Another example comes from an early sixteenth-century plague treatise, titled *Majannah al-ta'un wa al-waba'* (The Refuge from Plague and Pestilence), written by İlyas bin İbrahim (Eliahu ben Avraham) (d. after 1512). The author was an Iberian Jewish physician

41 Varlık, *Plague and Empire*, pp. 11–12.

42 See Nahyan Fancy's chapter 1 in this volume.

43 Hacı Paşa, *Müntahab-ı Şifâ*, ed. Zafer Önler (Ankara, 1990), pp. 172–3: 'ṭā'ūn ıssı veremdür ya sivilcilerdür vebā günlerinde çıḳar zaḥmet verür od gibi göyündürür yarası ḳara ya yeşil ya ḳızıl olur ve ṣayrunuñ göñli döner ḳuṣar ve yüregi oynar ve ögi gider ḳatı ṣuṣar nefes yıyır ve ḳatı ṭarlıġanur ṣolur'.

who came to Istanbul around the turn of the sixteenth century and converted to Islam.[44] In this treatise, he describes plague as follows: 'In the human body, the plague appears like an inflamed boil which gives intense pain and suffering. Its surrounding area is black or green. Its inside is red.'[45] A black bubo, the author added, indicated that the patient was most likely to expire (ṭāʿūn siyāh olursa marīżi bilā-şekk telef ider). This is again an example of a precise reference to a plague bubo, its colour, shape and position, accompanied by information about the patient's prognosis. İlyas's description of the plague bubo is similar to that of Hacı Paşa in that he references the same colours, but he gives a little more detail by noting the colour of the surrounding area of the bubo (black or green) and its inside (red).

We find further interesting observations with respect to colours in the writings of another sixteenth-century Ottoman physician. Writing in the second half of the century, Nidâî comments on colours as a diagnostic and prognostic tool. According to him, when plague buboes were light coloured (white or red), this was a sign that the patient would recover. When buboes were black or green, this meant that the patient would die.[46] Nidâî's observation is important, not only because he also adds white to the mix of colours mentioned by the previous authors, but also because he details the prognosis of the disease on the basis of the various colours of the buboes.

Later writers continued to remark on the diagnostic function of colour. An eighteenth-century physician, Ali Münşi Efendi of Bursa (d. 1733), also commented on the colours of tumours and swellings in his manual for surgery, *Cerrahname*. Though not specific to plague, he comments that malign tumours are darker in colour and, in fact, it is thanks to their colour that they can be distinguished from other kinds of tumours. He also adds that they have no clear shape (amorphous) and are firm to the touch; they cause pain as they grow.[47] A valuable point of comparison comes from Patrick Russell's 1791 *A Treatise of the Plague*, based on his observations of plague patients in Aleppo. Russell, who

44 E. İhsanoğlu, 'Endülüs Menşeli Bazı Bilim Adamlarının Osmanlı Bilimine Katkıları', *Belleten* 58 (1994), pp. 565–605; R. Barkai, 'Between East and West: A Jewish Doctor from Spain', in *Intercultural Contacts in the Medieval Mediterranean*, ed. B. Arbel (Portland, 1996), pp. 49–63.

45 İ. b. İbrahim, *Tevfīkātü'l-hamidiyye fī defʿi'l-emrāzi'l-vebāʾiyye*, trans. A. Ş. Ömeri, ms. Istanbul University Cerrahpaşa History of Medicine Library, 105, pp. 16–17: 'ṭāʿūn vücūd-ı insānda ziyādesiyle mü'ezzī ve mü'ellim iltihāb kesb itmiş bir çıbān olub eṭrāfı siyāh ya da yeşil kendüsi de ḳırmızı bir şeydir'.

46 Nidâî, *Rebîu's-Selâme*, ff. 87b, as cited in E. İstek, 'Osmanlı Hekimlerinin Türkçe Tıp Eserlerinde Veba Hastalığı ve Tedavisi', *Tarih Okulu Dergisi* 11 (2018), 128–52.

47 E. Kâhya, 'Osmanlı İmparatoluğu'ndaki Cerrahi Çalışmalarından Bazı Örnekler', *Türk Kültürü Kongresi Bildirileri (25–29 Eylül 1993, Ankara)* (Ankara, 1999), 2: 345–55: 'Şişin özel bir şekli yoktur; şiş serttir; büyüdükçe ağrılı hale gelir; bu tip şişlerin rengi koyudur; zaten onlar çoğunlukla renkleriyle ayırdedilir'. Also see F. N. Uzluk, 'Bursalı Hekim Ali Münşi Efendi', *Ankara Üniversitesi Dil ve Tarih-Coğrafya Fakültesi Dergisi* 8 (1950); A. Terzioglu, 'Ali Münşi', *Türkiye Diyanet Vakfı İslam Ansiklopedisi* (Istanbul, 1989), 2: 421–2. For manuscript copies of *Cerrahname*, see Istanbul University, TY 4302; Nuruosmaniye 3545; Süleymaniye Library, Halef Efendi 751.

worked as a physician of the Levant Company and was trained in the Western tradition, included in this work 120 case studies of plague patients with detailed observations of the disease. He often includes references to colours when describing the plague buboes and carbuncles. In describing a plague bubo in its early stages, for example, he writes: 'In the incipient state of the bubo, a small, hard, round tumour, was perceived by the finger, more or less deeply seated, but for the most part moveable under the skin, which was yet soft, of its natural colour, and not protuberant'. As the bubo increased in size, it 'took an oblong from, became less movable', but did not have 'outward inflammation' until its advanced stages. 'Its progress to maturity was more or less rapid', but 'once visibly formed', it could follow a different course. In fatal cases, 'it generally retained the natural colour. A few extraordinary cases were met with, in which the bubo itself, or the skin near it, assumed a pale blueish hue'. In other cases, buboes either came to suppuration or gradually dispersed over time. Russell described the size, shape and colour of buboes, carbuncles and other signs of plague on the skin very carefully. He used a range of colours in his descriptions of patients' visible symptoms, with reference to various shades of black, purple, red, blue, yellow and brown, often qualifying them as pale, dusky, dark, deep, bright or livid. It may be interesting to note that, unlike the Ottoman writers, he does not use green in reference to buboes.[48]

As these examples suggest, physicians differed in their use of colours with reference to plague symptoms. The fifteenth- and sixteenth-century Ottoman physicians used a basic colour scheme in their descriptions, primarily using black, green and red. Writing in the late eighteenth century, Russell, trained outside the Ottoman medical tradition, used a much wider range of colours in his clinical descriptions, although significantly omitting green. It is difficult to ascertain exactly how these authors used these colours in a clinical context or whether these colours were meant to be understood exactly the same as in non-clinical contexts. For example, when a text mentioned green in describing a bubo, should this be understood as green in a non-medical context? Probably not, because all these colour designations were used in reference to changes in skin colours. It seems worth noting, however, that green is not a stable category in these clinical descriptions: it was sometimes used almost synonymously with black in reference to plague buboes and generally meant to describe the swelling as being of 'dark colour'. Red (and, in the case of Nidâî, white) is also observed as a colour that is used to describe plague buboes, but often indicated a non-fatal case.

How do we interpret the use of these colours? And what did these colours mean to the writers or their readers? It seems very likely that the authors wrote on the basis of their clinical observations. (In fact, they sometimes boasted that they treated some patients successfully, although it is difficult to comment on their success rate.) Assuming that they observed plague buboes directly – at least some of the times – they chose to use these particular colours to describe plague buboes. The colour descriptions they used are more or

[48] P. Russell, *A Treatise of the Plague* (London, 1791), pp. 113–15.

less in line with the works of earlier authors of the Islamicate medical literature, with the exception of purple. Did the Ottoman physicians describe plague buboes along the same lines as their contemporary European authors? For this, it would be helpful to look at how the European medical literature described the colours of plague buboes.

As they were in the Ottoman context, colours were used to diagnose plague and other infectious diseases in the European medical literature. In the late fifteenth-century death records of Milan, for example, a five-year-old girl was recorded to have died with 'black measles' and a bubo in her left groin. Other examples include cadavers reported to have been 'covered by very black and corrupted "measles"', violet or 'black measles disseminated from the bubo' or 'reddened toward the centre with purplish measles disseminating from it'.[49] Here we find a confirmation that the centre of the plague bubo was noted to be red – an observation also made by İlyas. Black or very black can also be accepted to follow along the general lines that we find in Ottoman authors. What is different in these descriptions is the use of purple or violet to describe lesions as 'measles' – a colour designation that seems to be missing in the Ottoman medical literature. Writing in Venice in the 1570s, Jewish physician Abraham Yagel mentions 'stains' and colours in his plague treatise. Even though he describes the buboes with respect to their locations and how they fill with abscess and pus and suppurate, he does not use colours to describe them. He does, however, refer to colours on a different occasion in his treatise, where he notes: 'they occasionally manifest in the body as stains, as when one sees them as pale green or red, as if arrows pierced there, and this is the illness called "petechiae"'.[50] Writing also in the 1570s, the Genoese surgeon Luchino Boerio described the plague bubo as an elongated tumour that becomes round and pointed; he added 'they were of various colours – yellowish, purple, or black ('citrini, lividi, e negricanti')'. Like other contemporary physicians, Boerio also noted that patients with black buboes had little chance of survival.[51] Another contemporary physician, Girolamo Mercuriale, observed 'scabs, blotches, and spots that were black, purple, or red'.[52]

Here we find an important observation made by Girolamo Mercuriale in his 1577 treatise on pestilence. He writes: 'the reason why it has these various colors is because, since the humor is inflamed and burning, like the nature of fiery things, the fire and flame always seek the upper parts. Hence it comes to be so that it is red at the base; above the base, where there is more fire, it blackens; and at the apex, where the greatest burning comes to be, there is a blister'.[53] This explanation helps us to get a snapshot of a fully inflamed and

[49] See Ann G. Carmichael's chapter 2 in this volume.

[50] See Andrew Berns's chapter 9 in this volume.

[51] S. K. Cohn, *Cultures of Plague: Medical Thinking at the End of the Renaissance* (Oxford, 2010), p. 50.

[52] Cohn, *Cultures of Plague*, p. 51. See also S. K. Cohn, 'Patterns of Plague in Late Medieval and Early Modern Europe', in *The Routledge History of Disease*, ed. M. Jackson (London, 2016), pp. 165–82.

[53] G. Mercuriale, *On Pestilence: A Renaissance Treatise on Plague*, trans. C. Martin (Philadelphia, 2022).

suppurated plague bubo, including its colours. The more fully developed it is, the darker it becomes – whether the author decides to use black, purple or green to refer to it. Considering these different colours used in reference to plague buboes, as well as boils, pustules and carbuncles, it is important to keep in mind that the colour of the bubo changed as it evolved. Since the clinical description we see in the medical literature did not always refer to them at the same stages, we often find them in different colours.

Further evidence for colour designations of plague buboes in the contemporary European medical literature comes from the medical images of 'bubo man' or 'wound man'. These diagrams show plague buboes in the appropriate parts of the body where they appear, namely, in the armpits, behind the ears and in the groin area, but without always labelling them as plague buboes (figure 4.3). They illustrate the glandular swellings as blue-green and sometimes as deep red and vividly weeping.[54] It seems that these drawings also made a reference to the use of colour, not only for diagnosing plague (blue-green buboes), but also for its prognosis (suppurating buboes having a dark red colour). Unlike the textual descriptions of colour, however, here we do not see the colour black for the illustration of plague buboes that we more commonly find in textual accounts. Is it possible that our authors used black (or dark) to describe a blue-green hue? Is it also possible that these clinical colours were not yet well-established or fixed medical categories in the medical literature? To address these questions, it is important to distinguish colours in a medical context from their use in other contexts. In other words, clinical colours did not necessarily have to reflect colours that were understood in everyday life. The use of such colours as red, green or black with respect to plague buboes did not have to correspond to those colours in clothing or other objects. They were the colours visible *on skin*. But a very important distinction to be made here is that those colour designations were made on white skin.

The majority of plague cases seen by both European and Ottoman physicians were likely on white bodies. Hence, the appearance of all sorts of lesions, swellings, boils and pustules, as well as plague buboes, are described as they would have appeared on white bodies. In effect, it was not until the Third Pandemic that the majority of medical writing on plague was to be drawn from non-white bodies. Ironically, that was also the beginning of the microbial identification of plague, which shifted the medical gaze from visible signs of plague on skin (i.e., plague buboes) to ones that could be identified and confirmed only under a microscope. Before the development of medical photography in the nineteenth century and modern medical imaging, those clinical colours were the main tool for the medical community to diagnose, identify, name and classify diseases.

[54] Lori Jones notes that the latter is 'reminiscent of the plague bubo that appears on St Roch's inner thigh, rather than green-blue and fully engorged as they appear in most other instances'. See Jones's chapter 8 in this volume. Also see L. Jones, '"Apostumes, Carbuncles, and Botches": Visualizing the Plague in Late Medieval and Early Modern Medical Treatises', in *Disease and Disability in Medieval and Early Modern Art and Literature*, ed. R. F. Canalis and M. Ciavolella (Turnhout, 2021), pp. 173–200.

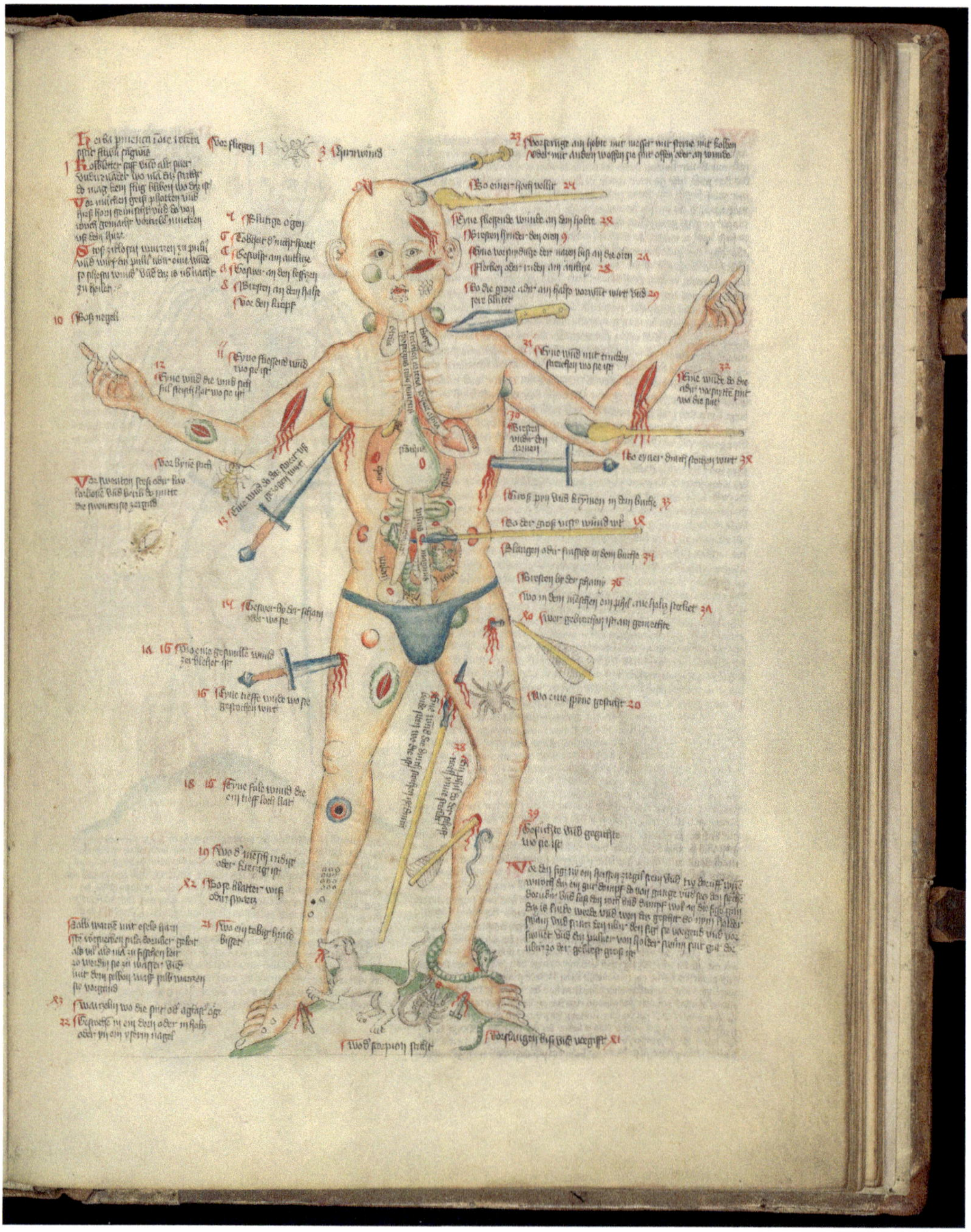

Fig. 4.3. Illustration of a Wound Man in London, Wellcome Collection MS 49, fol. 35r, available under a Public Domain Mark.

Conclusion

The colours of death and disease had many guises throughout history, as the various examples here illustrate. Whether they were used in medical discussions or in religion, literature and art, colours defined, qualified and enhanced the knowledge, experience and imagination of disease and death. Yet colour associations are not timeless or universal. On the contrary, they are very much embedded in culture. Historical context is thus key for interpreting the meaning associated with colours.

Ottoman society, not unlike many others, cultivated its own particular set of colour designations to refer to death and disease, by drawing from earlier traditions to which they added their own cultural experiences. The key components of classical Ottoman culture, both Turkish and Islamic and both separately and in connection with each other, highlighted diverse aspects of colour associations of disease and death: medical and non-medical, traditional and novel, historical and experiential, scientific and emotional.

PART II

Coping, Preventing and Healing

5

The Role of Music in a Franciscan Liturgy for the End of Life, as Evidenced in Manuscript Newberry 24

ELAINE STRATTON HILD[1]

Given the existing, high-quality scholarship on medieval liturgies for end of life preserved in Western European manuscripts, it is not immediately obvious what can be gained from further work with the material. Damien Sicard has examined rituals for the dying in 139 manuscript sources, documenting the transmission patterns of individual prayers and chants and assessing the likelihood of their Roman origins. Frederick Paxton's pivotal publication, *Christianizing Death*, traces the development of deathbed rites from late Antiquity through the Carolingian era, when their overall structures became largely fixed. James Donohue considered several medieval rites as forerunners of the now-current version published by the Roman Catholic Church in the early 1980s. Most recently, Paxton has produced an in-depth discussion and edition of the medieval rites from Cluny Abbey, in France.[2]

Robust as this scholarship is, particularly in terms of source documentation, editorial skill and theological analysis, it neglects one of the deathbed rituals' most integral and formative elements: music. In the Middle Ages, rituals for the dying were largely sung; indeed, Paxton has described them as 'multi-media event[s] of highly choreographed

1 The University of Notre Dame Institute for Advanced Study generously supported the research presented in this chapter. I am also grateful to the staff of the Newberry Library for their assistance.

2 D. Sicard, *La liturgie de la mort dans l'église latine des origines à la réforme carolingienne*, Liturgiewissenschaftliche Quellen und Forschungen 63 (Münster, 1978); F. S. Paxton, *Christianizing Death: The Creation of a Ritual Process in Early Medieval Europe* (Ithaca, 1990); J. M. Donohue, 'The Rite for the Commendation of the Dying in the 1983 *Pastoral Care of the Sick: Rites of Anointing and Viaticum*: A Study Through a Comparison with Its Counterparts in the 1614 *Rituale Romanum* and in the 1972 *editio typica* of *Ordo unctionis infirmorum eorumque pastoralis curae*' (unpublished Ph.D. dissertation, Catholic University of America, 2000). F. S. Paxton, 'Death by Customary at Eleventh-Century Cluny', in *From Dead of Night to End of Day: The Medieval Customs of Cluny*, ed. S. Boynton and I. Cochelin (Turnhout, 2005), pp. 297–318; F. S. Paxton with I. Cochelin, *The Death Ritual at Cluny in the Central Middle Ages* (Turnhout, 2013).

movements, sounds and smells'.[3] Yet scholarship thus far has been limited to texts of the rituals.

Incorporating music into this scholarly discourse integrates a fundamental aspect of the rituals and allows for a more comprehensive understanding. It also provides a different and insightful vantage point. Rather than accessing the rituals through their words – their intellectual content – a focus on the music invites a closer consideration of the rituals' performative aspects and, by extension, of their participants. The following discussion examines both the music and the functions of music in one of the most influential deathbed liturgies of Western Europe, the ritual of the early Franciscan order, as it is preserved in the thirteenth-century Italian manuscript Chicago, Newberry Library, Vault Manuscript 24.

This manuscript is particularly appropriate for a study of this type because among sources that contain medieval rituals for the dying – even among sources of the early Franciscan ritual – Newberry 24 offers some of the most detailed representations of music. In certain positions, the scribal work of Newberry 24 includes pitch-specific music notation, reflecting the melodic pitch content of some of the ritual's chants and making the manuscript an especially informative witness to the ritual's musical aspects. (Indeed, even the surviving manuscript sources from Cluny Abbey, known for their detailed instructions concerning the community's end-of-life liturgy, do not contain musical notation.)

After a brief consideration of the manuscript itself, the context in which it was created and its intended users, the chapter focuses on the ritual for the end of life. More specifically, it examines the five parts of the ritual intended for performance at a dying person's bedside. A close analysis reveals, first, that melody was intended to convey much – if not all – of the material in the bedside liturgy, and second, that this melodic content served several important functions. Far from being an incidental component, or a neutral mechanism for conveying texts, music actually shaped the liturgy in substantial ways. It determined the pacing of the material's delivery; it drew participants into a coordinated community with the demands of shared, precise performance; it shaped specific interpretations of the texts being sung; and it introduced the element of beauty. The two instances at which the scribe provided pitch-specific notation (edited and discussed later) reveal melodies closely intertwined with the texts they convey: melodies that emphasise individual words and images over others and thus suggest particular understandings of the texts. Furthermore, the melodies precisely reflect – and thus, highlight – their texts' syntactic structures.

At first glance, these claims about the functions of music within the ritual might seem improbable. After all, the scribe of Newberry 24 included little music notation and little insight into the specifics of vocal performance in his representation of the liturgy for the dying. The ritual's rubrics use neutral rather than specific verbs. 'Dicantur', for example, could refer to speaking, singing or practically any type of vocal conveyance. How can we know which, if any, portions of the ritual were intended to be sung? A study of the ritual's music begins from this difficult starting point. Newberry 24 does not indicate exactly how

[3] F. S. Paxton, 'Researching Rites for the Dying and the Dead', in *Understanding Medieval Liturgy: Essays in Interpretation*, ed. H. Gittos and S. Hamilton (Aldershot, 2016), pp. 39–56 (p. 54).

– or even if – the ritual was performed. In the liturgy for the dying, the scribe provided a list of items – a litany, prayers, psalms and chants – alongside rubrics to indicate how these items were to be coordinated to the successive stages of the dying process, but he did not provide information about the specific manner in which each item was to be performed. Descriptive accounts of actual performances of this ritual are not preserved, to my knowledge. Moreover, some musical aspects of the ritual could have varied with each performance, depending on the celebrant, the participants who gathered with him and the individual situation in which they sang.

Within these parameters, the scribal work in Newberry 24 must be understood as a prescription, not a description. A consideration of the music in the ritual for the dying is not a consideration of an actual performance. Rather, it is an analysis of a written record – written directions for conducting the liturgy for the end of life – and the scribal work and scribal assumptions that shaped this written record. Thus, an understanding of the ritual's musical component relies on knowledge of scribal practices, particularly of documents containing liturgical material that was performed away from the altar, like the ritual for the dying.[4] A thorough understanding also depends on knowledge of typical performance practices for the specific items that appear in the ritual: litanies, prayers, psalms and responsories. Knowing how these liturgical genres were normally performed allows for informed assumptions about their intended performance within the liturgy for the dying. As will become evident in the following discussion, nearly all of the materials included in Newberry 24 for the deathbed ritual were typically conveyed with melody. In other words, the written words reflect a sung ritual.

The manuscript and its users

Newberry 24 was created during the 1230s, a time when devotion to the recently deceased and canonised Francis was high and friars travelled, established communities and ministered to the sick and dying throughout Europe.[5] The image of Francis lovingly caring for

4 The field of medieval musicology has gained much insight from an extended scholarly discussion on the functions of early music notation and the oral transmission of plainchant. In particular, the scholarship of Leo Treitler challenged musicologists and historians to look beyond the 'expectation that the primary or exclusive function of musical notation is to serve as a non-distorting window on the music with which it is associated'. L. Treitler, *With Voice and Pen* (Oxford, 2003), p. 323. Treitler's most influential publications have been collected in *With Voice and Pen*; see, especially, 'The Early History of Music Writing in the West' and 'Reading and Singing: On the Genesis of Occidental Music Writing', pp. 317–428. A number of responses to Treitler's work have been republished in T. F. Kelly, ed., *Oral and Written Transmission in Chant* (Farnham, 2009).

5 Scholarly dating of the oldest portion of the manuscript that contains the rites for the sick and dying agrees on the decade. Van Dijk suggested that the manuscript was created after 1232, given Saint Dominic's inclusion in the litany: S. J. P. Van Dijk, 'Some Manuscripts of the Earliest Franciscan Liturgy', *Franciscan Studies* 16 (1956), 60–101 (p. 60). Saenger considered Dominic's name to be a later scribal annotation and suggests 'circa 1230': P. Saenger, *A Catalogue of the*

lepers – cleaning their sores with his own hands – became prominent in the saint's hagiography and exemplified the ideal of his order: to willingly live among and serve the sick and needy.[6] Created around the same time as Newberry 24, the image in figure 5.1 reveals a contemporary understanding of Franciscan friars. Francis is pictured in the centre, dressed simply and practically, bending over to wash the legs of a person covered with open sores. Another friar sits to the side, holding a leper on his lap. The image vividly reveals that in the first half of the thirteenth century, Franciscans were understood to be in direct contact with the poorest of the poor: the sick, the dying and the outcast.

Newberry 24 was intended to be a resource for the friars' efforts. The small book measures less than twenty by fifteen centimetres,[7] yet it contains the materials necessary for a friar's daily devotions – the Office liturgy – and three rites for his ministry: visiting the sick ('Ordo ... ad visitandum infirmum'), offering communion to the sick ('Ordo communicandum infirmum') and attending to a person during death ('Ordo commendationis animae' or 'Order for the commendation of the soul'). The inclusion of the rites for the sick and dying in a manuscript that also contains the Office liturgy is unusual. Ordinarily, such rites were part of a book type referred to as a 'rituale', a compilation of liturgies performed by a priest away from the altar. The distinctive combination of materials in Newberry 24, along with its small size, gives strong indications of the book's intended functions: the manuscript was created to assist users in maintaining their liturgical obligations and providing care to the sick and dying while travelling.[8] Van Dijk describes the life of the friars in the

Pre-1500 Western Manuscript Books at the Newberry Library (Chicago, 1989), pp. 43–6. On the basis of Miskuly's dating of the Office of Francis (J. M. Miskuly, 'Julian of Speyer: Life of St. Francis [Vita Sancti Francisci]', *Franciscan Studies* 49 (1989), 93–174), Mitchell considers 1235 to be the earliest possible date: A. W. Mitchell, 'The Chant of the Earliest Franciscan Office' (unpublished Ph.D. dissertation, University of Western Ontario, 2003), p. 85. For the purposes of this chapter, accepting that the manuscript was created between 1230 and 1240 suffices to contextualize it historically. In terms of liturgy, this dating places the manuscript's contents in the earliest layer of distinctively Franciscan liturgical material: after the order's orientation towards the Office liturgy of the papal curia (*Regula bullata*, 1223), yet prior to the liturgical reforms begun by Haymo of Faversham (1241). In terms of the development of the order, the dating of Newberry 24 places its creation after the death and canonization of Francis (1226, 1228) and around the time when papal authority was beginning to loosen the strictest requirements of itinerancy and poverty (*Quo elongati*, issued by Pope Gregory IX in 1230). Robson offers an overview of pivotal dates in Francis's life and the early order in *The Cambridge Companion to Francis of Assisi*, ed. M. J. P. Robson (Cambridge, 2012), pp. xiv–xv. The editorial work evident in Newberry 24 indicates that it was used (or at least updated) throughout the thirteenth century.

6 The first life of Francis, written around 1229 (T. de Celano, *Prima vita*, in *Fontes Franciscani*, ed. E. Menestò, S. Brufani et al. (Assisi, 1995), pp. 275–424), includes encounters between Francis and lepers. Francis's changing attitude towards the sick serves as an indication of his radical conversion.

7 Saenger, *Catalogue*, p. 46.

8 Van Dijk and Donohue also connect the unusual book type – a breviary with rites for the sick and dying – with the itinerant ideals and ministries of the Franciscans. 'The new combination ... is typical of the apostolic and itinerant life of the Order'. S. J. P. Van Dijk, *Sources of the Modern*

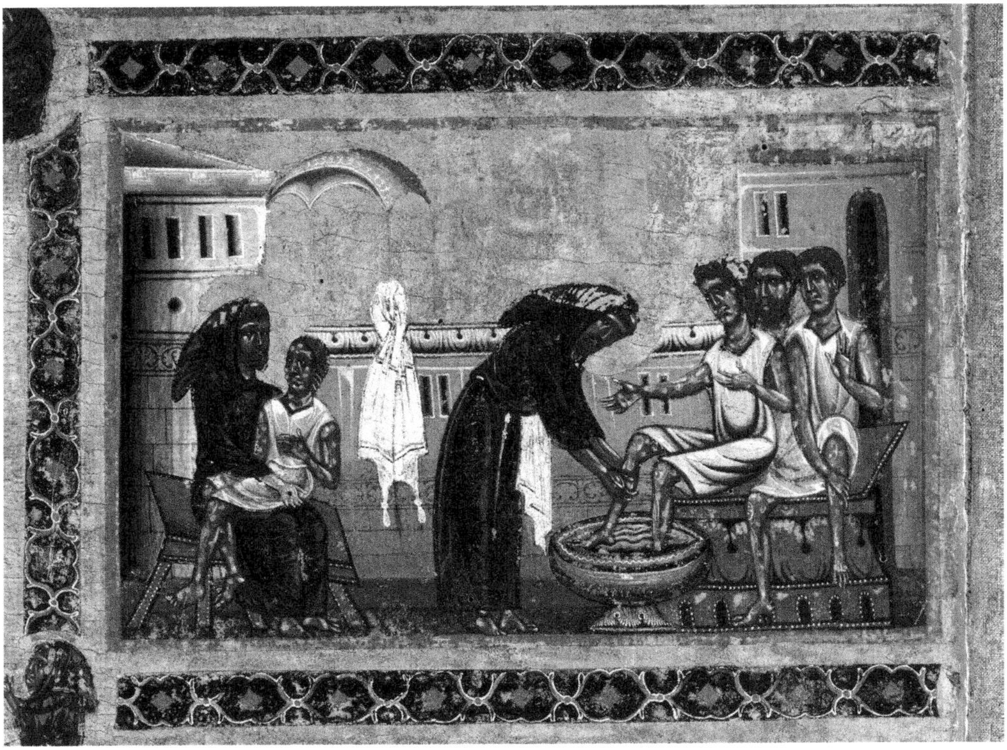

Fig. 5.1. Francis caring for lepers, painting by Coppo di Marcovaldo c. 1245–50, part of *St Francis and Twenty Stories of his Life* ('Bardi Panel') preserved in the Bardi Chapel, Santa Croce, Florence.

Roman Liturgy: The Ordinals by Haymo of Faversham and Related Documents, 2 vols. (Leiden, 1963), p. 138. 'The Franciscans' need for a portable Office book in the thirteenth century was the chief reason why the breviary, rather than the missal, became connected with "going out" and the former became the logical book to contain a ritual for the last sacraments'. Donohue, 'The Rite', p. 201. Van Dijk (*Origins*, p. 225) classifies Newberry 24 as a choir breviary, rather than a portable breviary; the manuscripts he classifies as portable ('portos') have even smaller sizes and most often lack music notation. However, the small size of Newberry 24 contrasts greatly with manuscripts intended only to reside in the choirs of established monasteries. Although not as small as other manuscripts containing the Franciscan liturgies, Newberry 24 would have been easily carried and transported. P. Salmon considers the role of the Franciscans in the development of the breviary as a book type in *L'office divin au moyen âge: histoire de la formation du bréviaire du IXe au XVIe siècle* (Paris, 1967), pp. 152–70. A. Hughes incorporates Newberry 24 into his discussions of notated breviaries in *Medieval Manuscripts for Mass and Office: A Guide to their Organization and Terminology* (Toronto, 2004).

order's early years: 'Travelling in small groups … without chapels, choirs, altars, bells or cemeteries, they preached and prayed, heard confessions and helped the sick wherever they were so allowed'.[9]

The ritual for the dying in Newberry 24

The ritual for the dying in Newberry 24 provides insight beyond a single manuscript version. As the liturgy prescribed for the time of death by the early Franciscan order, this ritual was copied into multiple manuscripts created for the use of friars.[10] Prescribed by a vigorously growing Franciscan order dedicated to serving the sick and dying, the ritual for the end of life within Newberry 24 most likely saw widespread use.[11]

The manuscript's dating to the first half of the thirteenth century suggests that it is one of the oldest documents that preserves the Franciscan liturgy for the dying. As friars established communities throughout Europe, the ritual evidenced in Newberry 24 became widely transmitted, particularly in a slightly revised version from the second half of the century.[12] Elements of the ritual became even more pervasive after they were incorporated into the officially promulgated versions of the Roman Catholic Church.[13]

9 Van Dijk, *Sources*, p. 11. On the Franciscans' itinerant practices and care of the sick, see also L. Silberer, *Klosterbaukunst der konventualen Franziskaner vom 13. Jahrhundert bis zur Reformation* (Petersberg, 2016), p. 30 and O. Schmucki, 'Spiritualität, Askese und Krankheiten nach den Schriften des Franziskus von Assisi', in *Franziskus von Assisi: Das Bild des Heiligen aus neuer Sicht*, ed. D. R. Bauer, H. Feld and U. Köpf (Cologne, 2005), pp. 71–96.

10 Other manuscripts containing early Franciscan liturgies are documented and described by S. J. P. Van Dijk, 'Some Manuscripts' and Mitchell, 'The Chant'.

11 Where Newberry 24 was used for the first decades of its existence has not been precisely determined. The parchment preparation, script and notation indicate conclusively that the manuscript was created in Italy. Following Saenger and Van Dijk, the manuscript was 'in the Franciscan convent of Perugia in the second half of the thirteenth century'. Saenger, *Catalogue*, p. 46; Van Dijk, 'Some Manuscripts', p. 60. The addition of Perugian saints suggests that the manuscript was used outside of Perugia prior to this time.

12 Van Dijk, 'Some Manuscripts' and Mitchell, 'The Chant', investigate the relationships among the earliest Franciscan liturgies, the papal liturgies and the later, revised Franciscan liturgies. Mitchell's study incorporates melodic evidence to do so. Following Van Dijk and Walker, the Franciscan rites for the sick and dying were revised after Haymo's death in 1243 and issued as part of the breviary of 1260: S. J. P. Van Dijk and J. H. Walker, *The Origins of the Modern Roman Liturgy: The Liturgy of the Papal Court and the Franciscan Order in the Thirteenth Century* (London, 1960), pp. 280–91. Donohue offers an analysis – with textual editions and translations of individual items – of the revised Franciscan ritual from 1260, as part of a larger project to better understand the historical underpinnings of the version issued by the Catholic Church in 1980s. Donohue, 'The Rite', particularly pp. 217–37. The Franciscan order's striking expansion in the thirteenth century is documented in map form by R. McKitterick, *Atlas of the Medieval World* (New York, 2004), pp. 150–1.

13 Donohue's study ('The Rite') offers a definitive, detailed analysis of the commonalities between the thirteenth-century Franciscan ritual for the dying and later versions issued by the Roman Catholic Church.

The early Franciscan liturgy for the dying is comprehensive and particularly specific. It provides material for the time when death seems imminent, as well as for the final agony (when the 'soul is struggling to exit'), the precise moment of death and the time at the bedside after death has occurred but before the activities of washing and moving the body have begun. (The ritual's scope extends even further, through the vigil in the church and the burial, but the following discussion considers only the portion of material intended for the bedside.) Multiple, precise rubrics indicate how the material was to be coordinated to these specific stages of the process of dying.

Such detailed rubrics contrast with those of many other medieval deathbed liturgies. As one example, the ritual preserved in the library of Saint Peter's Basilica at the Vatican (in manuscript Arch. Cap. S. Pietro F. 11 pt. A) provides only a single rubric introducing the material for the time of death, with no indication of how the subsequent chants and prayers should be performed or coordinated to the unfolding stages of the end of life. It seems likely that the ritual preserved in the Vatican manuscript was as comprehensive as that of the early Franciscans. It similarly might have accompanied multiple stages in the dying process, yet it is the Franciscan ritual that provides explicit documentation of the intended coordination between the liturgical material and physical events. With its detailed rubrics and pitch-specific music notation, Newberry 24 provides an exceptionally informative perspective on one community's understanding of end-of-life liturgical care.

The context for which the ritual was intended

Giotto's fresco of Francis on his deathbed, shown in figure 5.2, was painted about 100 years after the creation of Newberry 24, yet it depicts a situation similar to the ones for which the manuscript's ritual was intended. A community surrounds the dying person, in order to witness (the man directly behind Francis's head beckons others to come), to bid farewell (the man at the far left of the painting raises his hand as if in acceptance and parting), to mourn (those depicted on the far side of the bed convey emotional responses) and to perform a liturgy (participants at the foot of the bed hold liturgical rods, which perhaps carried flags or banners in the original, undamaged image). Above the people, another community is gathered: angels carry the soul of the dying man heavenwards. Giotto's image visually represents the account of the saint's death from the first life of Francis (written shortly after Francis's death by Thomas of Celano).[14] It also depicts the type of gathering that Newberry 24 assumes for the deathbed liturgy.

The ritual for the dying in Newberry 24 thus presupposes a gathering of people in the presence of the dying person, a gathering with liturgical potential and capability. The ritual's rubrics give no indications of the genders, occupations or religious status (lay, clerical or monastic) of the dying person or other participants. However, we can assume, from the ritual's inclusion in a compilation of Franciscan materials, that at least one friar would have been present and perhaps leading the liturgy when it was performed. Given

[14] De Celano, *Prima vita*, §69–70.

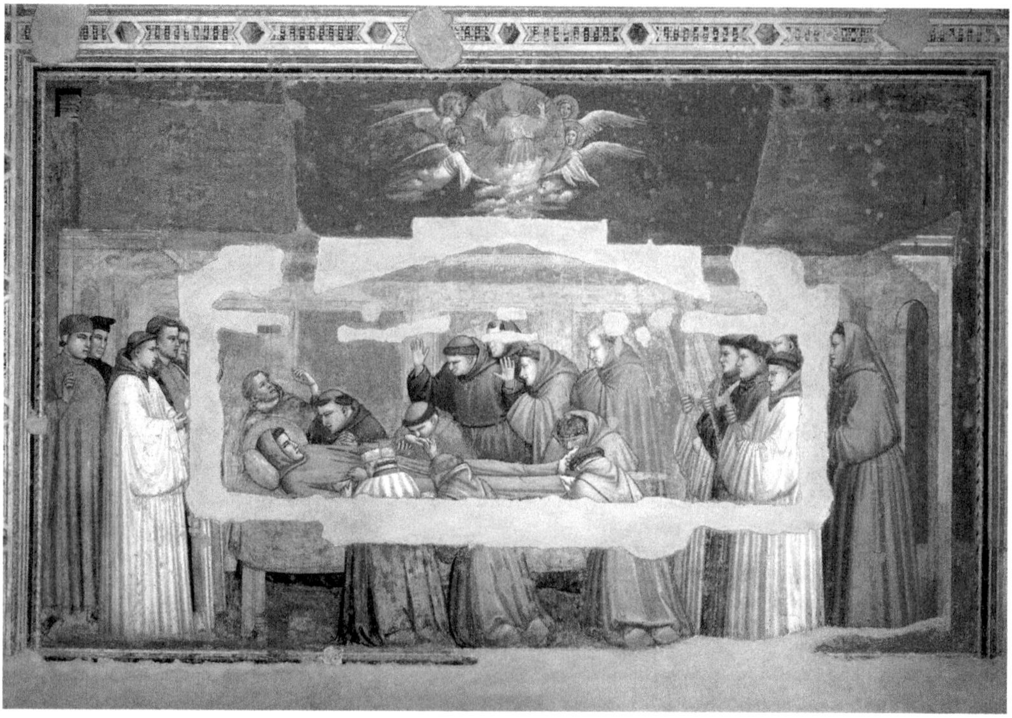

Fig. 5.2. Death of St Francis, painting by Giotto di Bondone c. 1325–28, part of *Stories of St Francis* preserved in the Bardi Chapel, Santa Croce, Florence. © 2021 Photo Scala, Florence.

the Franciscans' outreach, it is likely that the ritual for the dying in Newberry 24 was considered appropriate for use with a broad range of people: men, women and children; lay, clerical and monastic. The gender-specific nouns and pronouns within the liturgy that refer to the dying person appear in the masculine form, yet this is unlikely to indicate that the ritual was performed only for men and boys. The celebrant and participants could well have changed the noun endings and pronouns to the feminine forms as they sang and recited. Alternatively, the masculine forms could well have been considered sufficient, even when the focus of the ritual was a woman or girl.

It also seems reasonable to assume that the ritual could have been used in a variety of settings: the home of a layperson, a monastery or a charitable facility, such as a hospital or hospice. Rather than taking place in a church or chapel – a space dedicated solely to religious acts and rituals – the liturgy for the dying was intended for the intimate space at the bedside. And rather than being designed to unfold with the predictable timing of the Mass and Office liturgies, the ritual for the dying was intended to conform to the individual pacing of a life's ending.

Part 1: The ritual's beginning

Although the scribe of Newberry 24 included notation in only a few positions, music was intended to convey much of the ritual's material, beginning with a litany, a sung chant that involved all gathered participants.

Table 5.1. The Litany

ORDO COMMENDATIONIS ANIME	ORDER OF THE COMMENDATION OF THE SOUL
PRIMUM FIANT LETANIE BREUES AD HUNC MODUM	FIRST LET THE SHORT LITANIES BE PERFORMED IN THIS WAY
Kyrieleison ...	Lord, have mercy ...

The litany in Newberry 24 was not notated, but it was likely intended to be sung.[15] The lack of notation could result from two factors. First, the scribe might have considered music notation to be unnecessary. Medieval litanies that have been preserved with notation reveal that their melodies were often formulaic, consisting of simple, repeating melodic gestures.[16] The scribe might have assumed that the manuscript's users were capable of performing the litany's melody without the aid of written assistance. Second, the scribe might have omitted notation from the litany for the sake of efficiency. With music notation, the litany would have required at least twice as much space on the page as the text alone. Such scribal efficiency is seen in other medieval rituals for the dying, and the manuscript sources tend to present the material in a compact and abbreviated manner. This might have increased the portability of a document carried to the bedside of a dying person.

Performing the litany engaged not only a celebrant but also others gathered at the bedside. The litany names members of the heavenly community in a hierarchical order, beginning with a *Kyrie* entreating the Lord and Christ for mercy.[17] Each name (or collective address) is followed by the imperative request, 'Pray for him' ('ora[te] pro eo'). Litanies were typically performed in a responsorial fashion, with the celebrant or a small group of participants invoking the names of the heavenly personages and the rest of the participants

15 A complete transcription and edition of the ritual's text follows in the Appendix; I have thus not included the original Latin here in the main text. My thanks go to Timothy E. Smith of Loveland Classical Schools for his skilled, generous assistance with the edition and translations.

16 A discussion and examples are provided in D. Hiley, *Western Plainchant* (Oxford, 1993), pp. 51–4.

17 The rubric in Newberry 24 refers to this litany as 'breues' (brief); what makes it relatively short is that it sometimes makes reference to groups, rather than to individual members of the heavenly community. For instance, the apostles Peter, Paul and Andrew are invoked, followed by a plea to 'all of the holy apostles and evangelists'. Francis's name appears fairly high in the list, prior to the holy innocents and Stephen and other martyrs. In the ritual's revised version of 1260, Francis's name appears later in the litany, in the appropriate category of 'monks and hermits' immediately prior to Benedict and Saint Paul the hermit. See Van Dijk, *Sources*, p. 391.

responding with the refrain, 'Pray for him'. This performance practice remained the same in the second half of the litany, which continues as a prayer to Christ and lists each danger from which the dying person should be rescued, followed by the refrain 'Free him' ('libera eum').[18] This format allowed – indeed, invited – those gathered at the bedside to participate in the chant. Significant musical skill was not needed. Refrain melodies were simple and often echoed the melodies of the invocations; participants thus most likely repeated the melody they first heard sung by the celebrant or soloist. The minimal musical demands provided a low barrier to participation for those gathered and the responsorial format provided a simple way for all to join in the prayers of the litany.

The litany's privileged position at the beginning of the ritual suggests a prioritisation: the first task, and the most important way to support the dying person, was to engage the assistance of those in heaven. This first item of the ritual envisions the presence of a community extending beyond the humans, as well as a human community that musically entreats these unseen, yet vital, saints.

Part 2: For the nearness to death

Table 5.2. The Prayer

DEINDE PRO UICINO MORTI	THEN FOR THE NEARNESS TO DEATH
CUM IN AGONE SUI EXITUS	WHEN, IN THE STRUGGLE OF ITS EXIT,
ANIMA UISA FUERIT ANSIARI	THE SOUL IS SEEN TO BE ANXIOUS
FIAT HEC ORATIO	LET THIS BE THE PRAYER
Proficiscere anima christiana …	Go forth, Christian soul …

For the final moments of life – the time that the rubric refers to as 'uicino morti' – the ritual prescribes a prayer that was probably recited with a simple melody. The typical performance practice for liturgical prayers in the Middle Ages involved one person reciting the text with formulaic melodic gestures.[19] These recitation melodies were neither complicated nor elaborate, yet they strictly controlled the conveyance of the texts. The melodies consisted of repeating gestures that were applied to the texts' syntactic units – clauses and sentences. A rising melodic gesture conveyed the first syllables of each syntactic unit, then the majority of the unit was conveyed with a single repeating pitch (the reciting tone). Its

18 The named threats include '[God's] wrath … the dangers of death … a bad death … base lusts … the powers of the devil … every evil'. The litany then names the means – provided by Christ – through which the dying person can be saved: 'through your birth … through your holy cross … through your death and grave … through your glorious resurrection … through your miraculous ascension … through the favor of the holy spirit'. The litany ends, as it began, with a repetition of the *Kyrie*'s three-fold plea for mercy.

19 Hiley's discussion of the melodies used for reciting liturgical prayers appears in *Western Plainchant*, pp. 49–51.

final syllables were conveyed with a descending gesture. The musical contours signalled the beginnings and endings of clauses and sentences, thereby facilitating the intelligibility of the text in performance.

The metaphor of death as a journey permeates this part of the ritual. The prayers offer detailed, vibrant images of the soul's successful passage, in which dangers are conquered through the help of the saints and the mercy of God, and the soul is finally received into the heavenly community. As with the litany, the prayers populate the experience of dying with heavenly companions and advocates. Far from being isolated, the dying person is portrayed as being in good company. These ideas would have been made more accessible in performance by the melodic articulation of the beginnings and endings of the prayers' syntactic units. Even in this text-heavy, idea-rich portion of the ritual, in which the intellectual contents of the texts seem to be paramount and prioritised, music incorporated an aspect of audible appeal. Although the recitation melodies were simple, they created patterns of repetition and symmetry and presented theological understandings with the beauty of organised sound.

Part 3: If the soul is uneasy …

Table 5.3. The Psalms

SI ANSIATUR ADHUC ANIMA	IF THE SOUL IS STILL UNEASY
DICANTUR HII PSALMI	THESE PSALMS OUGHT TO BE UTTERED
PSALMUS Confitemini …	PSALM Acclaim … [117]

The following material addresses – and integrates – the dying person's anxiety into the ritual.[20] In cases of continuing unease, the ritual prescribes the performance of two psalms depicting God as a merciful figure, able and willing to relieve human suffering. The first of these two psalms (Psalm 117) calls on Israel, the house of Aaron and finally those who fear the Lord to proclaim 'Forever is His kindness'.[21] Recited within the context of the ritual, those gathered at the bedside joined the community of the psalm in proclaiming God's love.

The psalm also portrays God relieving anguish and offering powerful assistance: 'From the straits I called to Yah. Yah answered me in a wide-open place. The Lord is for me, I shall not fear … The Lord is for me among my helpers, and I shall see the defeat of my foes … My strength and my might is Yah, and He has become my rescue'. Additionally, the psalm evokes the image of a gate, which could have been understood, in the context of the ritual, as a metaphor for a successful death: 'Open for me the gates of justice – I

20 ANSIATUR] *read as* ANXIATUR.

21 Translations follow R. Alter, trans., *The Hebrew Bible*, III, 276–91, in which the psalms are numbered as 118 and 119.

would enter them, I would acclaim Yah. This is the gate of the Lord – the just will enter it'. The psalm orients the dying person towards God – and away from people – as a source of assistance: 'Better to shelter in the Lord than to trust in humankind. Better to shelter in the Lord than to trust in princes'. The God portrayed in Psalm 117 is a source of rest and assurance, one who offers comfort to a suffering person and whose unwavering love provides help against any obstacle.

The subsequent psalm prescribed by the ritual (Psalm 118) continues the articulation of God's steadfast, reliable characteristics. The narrative voice of this psalm praises and adheres to the law and rules of God, even while suffering: 'My being longs for Your rescue, for Your word I hope ... Though I was like a skin-flask in smoke, Your statutes I did not forget'. God is portrayed as a dependable source of wisdom and guidance: 'Forever, O Lord, Your word stands high in the heavens. For all generations Your faithfulness. You made the earth firm and it stood'. Thus, in the face of continuing anxiety, the ritual prescribes a large dose of theological reassurance: a depiction of God as willing and able to help a suffering person.

Reassurance most likely came not only from the intellectual content of the psalms, but also from the manner in which they were performed. Psalms were typically sung, with participants divided into two groups that performed verses in alternation. Psalm melodies (often referred to as 'tones') were simple, but they nonetheless provided the organisation of sound and time common to all music.[22] Like the melodies for prayers, psalm tones prescribed the conveyance of texts in a way that clearly delineated the beginnings and endings of syntactic units. Collectively reciting a psalm required participants to attend to one another carefully, in order to match pitch and pacing. To begin performing a verse simultaneously, singers also needed to breathe together. The deliberate, disciplined use of time might well have added an element of calm and reassurance for both the attending community and the dying person. At the moment of highest anxiety, the ritual prescribes texts depicting a loving, powerful God, conveyed with beautiful sound.

Part 4: At the departure of the soul

Table 5.4. The Responsory and Verses

EGRESSA ANIMA AUTEM	AT THE DEPARTURE OF THE SOUL HOWEVER
DICATUR HOC RESPONSORIUM RECITANDO	THIS RESPONSORY OUGHT TO BE UTTERED, RECITING
Subuenite	Come help...
VERSUS Suscipiat	VERSE May Christ ...
VERSUS Requiem eternam	VERSE Rest eternal ...

22 Hiley's discussion of psalm tones appears in *Western Plainchant*, pp. 58–64.

	(fol. 253)
RESPONSORIUM Svbuenite sancti dei occurrite angeli domini suscipientes animam eius offerentes eam in conspectu altissimi	RESPONSORY Come help, saints of God Hurry, angels of the Lord taking up his soul offering it in the sight of the most high
VERSUS Svscipiat te Christus qui uocauit te et in sinu Habrae angeli deducant te	VERSE May Christ, who has called you, receive you and to the bosom of Abraham may the angels lead you
Susci<pientes>	Taking <up his soul offering it in the sight of the most high>
VERSUS Requiem <eternam dona eis domine et lux perpetua luceat eis>	VERSE Rest <eternal give them, Lord and let perpetual light shine on them>
Offerentes	Offering <it in the sight of the most high>

The ritual prescribes song to accompany the moment of death: the responsory *Subvenite*, along with the verses *Suscipiat* and *Requiem eternam*.[23] The chants appear in this portion of the ritual in abbreviated form and the scribe references them only by their first words. More comprehensive versions of the chants, with music notation, appear on folio 253 in a later part of the ritual meant for the time immediately prior to burial. It is highly likely, but not possible to prove definitively, that the melodic settings written on fol. 253 were also intended for use at the deathbed. This scribal practice – of notating a chant fully only in one position and using cues to refer to it in other positions – was typical and made efficient use of a manuscript's space.

23 The manuscript shows evidence that a second scribe made changes to the rubrics. These changes bring the rubrics into conformity with those of the revised version of the ritual from 1260. EGRESSA ANIMA] *corrected from* EGRESSA ANIMA DE CORPORE. RESPONSORIUM RECITANDO] *corrected from* RESPONSORIUM. The genre designations of RESPONSORIUM and VERSUS suggest that the chants were used in the Office liturgy and that they were interwoven in performance: portions of the responsory were repeated after each verse. The texts of the responsory *Subvenite* and its verse *Suscipiat* are evident in one of the oldest extant documents containing a deathbed ritual (the late eighth-century manuscript Berlin Öffentliche Wissenschaftliche Bibliothek MS lat. 105 Phillipps 1667). In *Christianizing Death*, Paxton traces the historical development of the rites for the dying, including the use of individual chants; see especially pp. 108 and 115–16. *Subvenite* and *Suscipiat* are discussed in Sicard, *La liturgie*, pp. 66–8 and edited by R. J. Hesbert, *Corpus antiphonalium officii* (Rome, 1963–79), IV, 421, no. 7716. The Cantus database allows for an investigation of their transmission patterns in notated Office manuscripts: University of Waterloo, 'CANTUS: A Database for Latin Ecclesiastical Chant', http://cantusdatabase.org/ (accessed 24 August 2019). VERSUS Requiem eternam] VERSUS Requiem eternam CUM Req<uiem> e<ternam>.

The texts of these chants present an understanding that, at the time of death, the soul was beginning a journey. The chants simultaneously describe and accompany a moment of transfer, when the dying person moves from the care of the earthly community into the care of the heavenly. The text of *Subvenite* calls upon angels and saints to come and carry the dying person's soul 'into the sight of the most high'. These helpers are told to 'hurry': the soul's journey is beginning and the urgent time for their assistance has arrived. The text of the verse *Suscipiat* addresses the dying person's soul directly, offering a blessing and a hope for the journey: 'May Christ, who has called you, receive you'. The scribe of Newberry 24 indicated that after the performance of this verse, the final words of the responsory should be repeated: 'Taking up his soul, offering it in the sight of the most high'. With this return to the responsory, the perspective – and the text's addressee – again shifts: the singers no longer address the dying person directly, but, rather, refer to him with third-person pronouns. The text of the second verse, *Requiem eternam*, also uses third-person pronouns as it asks God to grant eternal peace and perpetual light.

This shift from second-person to third-person pronouns is far from trivial. The verse *Suscipiat* marks the final time at the deathbed when the dying person is addressed directly. In this way, the chants mark the poignant transition: the dying person changes from someone who resides in the community – and is able to be spoken to – to someone who is in another place and can only be spoken about. The chants thus address and bridge the vital moment of change and also provide a structure of acceptance. The words of the chants transfer the soul, in the listeners' imaginations, from its residence in the human body to a residence in the heavenly realm – in the 'sight of the most high'.

A close examination of the manuscript's music notation (figures 5.3 and 5.4) reveals that the chants' melodies reinforce – and even expand upon – the understandings offered in the texts. For example, the melody conveying the words 'Hurry, angels of the Lord' reflects the text's urgency. The music with these words contains multiple, rapid expansions: with the first two syllables of the word 'occurrite' (hurry, figure 3.3, line 2), the melody ascends a fifth (from 'e' to 'b-flat' or 'b', marked with the first arrow of line 2). The melody conveying the word 'angeli' (angels) repeats and intensifies this gesture, with an ascent of a fifth with higher pitch content ('f' to 'c', marked with second arrow of line 2). For the final word of the statement, 'domini' (of the Lord), the melody echoes these previous gestures with an ascent of a fourth with lower pitch content (from 'e' to 'a', marked with the third arrow of line 2). These quick ascents lend an energy and impetus to the melody that was not present in the chant's beginning (seen in line 1). Examining the melody's ambitus reveals a similar situation. In the chant's beginning, the melody stays within a narrow range (spanning only a fourth, from 'd' to 'g'), but in line 2, it rises into a new range (reaching the pitches 'b' and 'c') and increases its ambitus to an interval of a sixth while conveying the words 'Hurry, angels of the Lord'. The repeated, swift ascents and the upward expansion of the ambitus contribute to the musical depiction of urgency, reflecting the text's image of haste.

The melody also offers an aural image of the dying person's soul being brought into God's presence. The words referring to the soul ('animam eius' and 'eam') are conveyed with

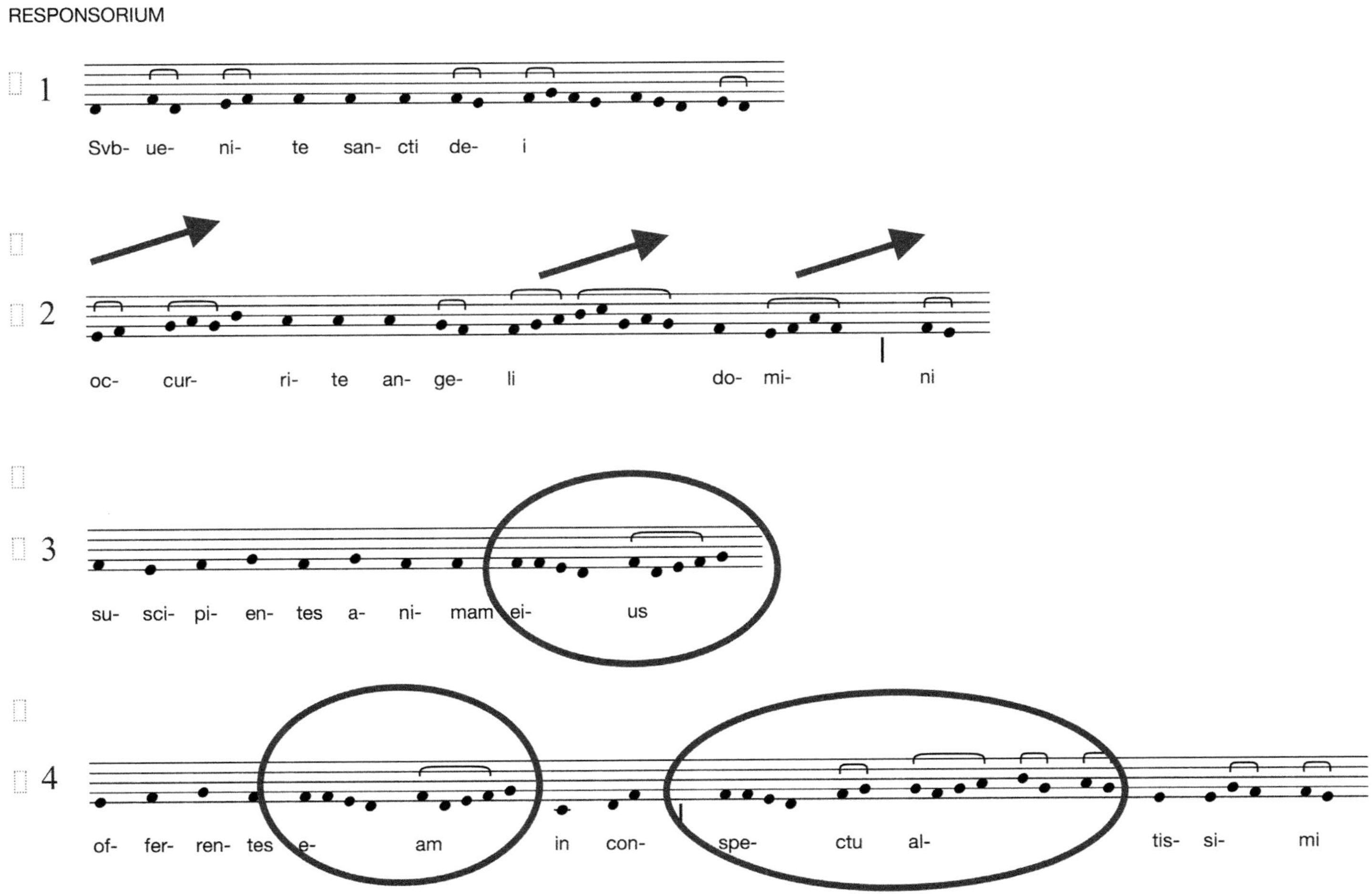

Fig. 5.3. Chant for the moment of death: Subvenite, edited from Newberry 24, fol. 253 by Elaine Stratton Hild.

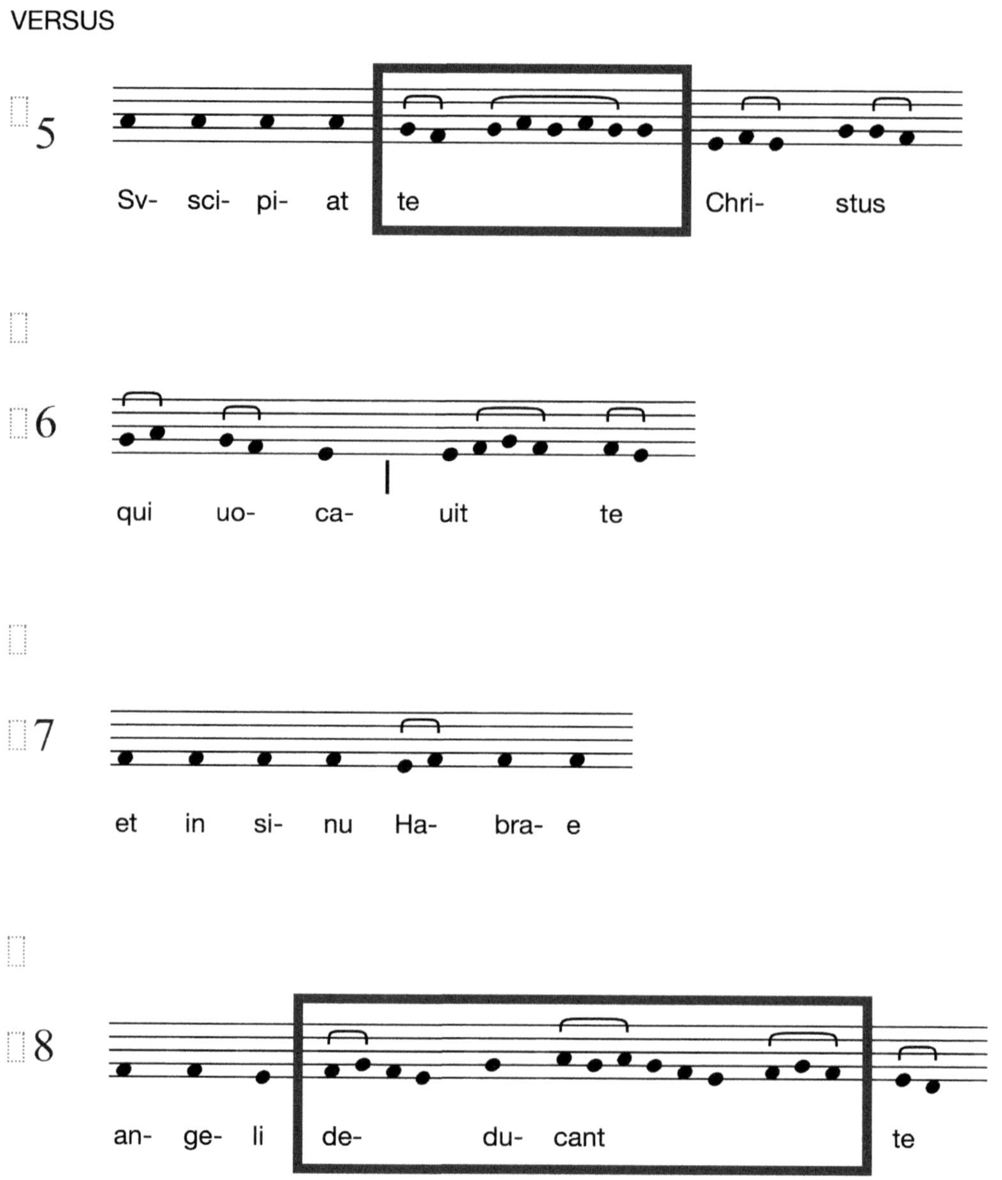
VERSUS
5
Sv- sci- pi- at te Chri- stus
6
qui uo- ca- uit te
7
et in si- nu Ha- bra- e
8
an- ge- li de- du- cant te

Fig. 5.4. Chant for the moment of death: Suscipiat, edited from Newberry 24, fol. 253 by Elaine Stratton Hild.

a repeated musical gesture (circled in lines 3 and 4). This gesture is striking: it contains leaps, changes in direction and multiple pitches conveying each syllable. It becomes associated with the dying person's soul through musical repetition. After the distinctive gesture conveys the two mentions of 'soul', it then returns once more, in a position that gives it much poignancy, while articulating the word 'conspectu' (in the sight [of the most high], circled in bold in line 4). By using the musical gesture to convey the word 'conspectu', after it has become associated with 'soul', the musical setting creates an audible encounter between the soul and the 'most high'. But instead of continuing with an exact repetition of the previous instances (which finished on the pitch 'g') the gesture now unfolds with a greater ascent, climbing to the highest notes of the phrase ('b-flat') with the word 'altissimi' (highest). In this way, the melodic gesture associated with 'soul' transforms and melds into the melody conveying the words referring to God. What is prayed for in the text – that the soul be brought into the presence of the most high – becomes the reality of the melody. The text speaks of the soul being offered in the sight of God and the melody depicts it.

In doing so, the melody offers its own image of the soul's destination. The words 'in the sight of the most high' ('in conspectu altissimi', line 4) are conveyed with the chant's longest melodic ascent, creating an audible sense of spaciousness. The melody articulates the word *in* with the lowest pitch of the chant ('c'). It then rises while conveying the word 'conspectu', and by the first syllable of 'altissimi' it has climbed the interval of a seventh (to 'b-flat'). This extended, sweeping ascent articulates the words 'in conspectu altissimi' in a manner unlike any other words in the chant. According to the melody, when the soul is in the presence of God, it has risen to an extraordinary, expansive place.

The melody of the following verse, *Suscipiat* (figure 5.4, lines 5–8), gives prominence to the most vital words of the chant's text, those that offer the dying person the reassurance of companionship. As mentioned above, this chant is the final time at the deathbed that the attending community addresses the dying person directly. The melody emphasises this direct address in its articulation of the first instance of the word 'te' (you, indicated with a rectangle in line 5). While previous syllables of the verse were conveyed with only one pitch, and thus received little emphasis in performance, the syllable 'te' is conveyed with six pitches, giving it a strong articulation. The pitches conveying this word are also the highest in the verse's ambitus, providing even more prominence in performance. Only one other word in this verse is conveyed with such melodic emphasis: the word 'deducant' (lead, marked with a rectangle on line 8) is articulated with extended melismatic gestures and pitch content in the upper reaches of the chant's range. With these marked conveyances of the words 'you' and 'lead', the melody emphasises the companionship prayed for in the text – the understanding that the dying person will be accompanied and guided. The melodic content of the chant thus gives prominence to the text's most reassuring expressions.

The chants focus on the dying person, yet it is also appropriate to consider their impact on the ritual's other participants. Through their melodic content and requirements for performance, the chants controlled the use of time and prescribed meaningful activity – singing – for those surrounding the deathbed and witnessing the end of a life. In this most poignant of moments, music provided structure. The singers of the chants were required to breathe and perform in a controlled, disciplined and precise manner. Even those who simply listened would have experienced music structuring the moments and leading the community through the extraordinary transition of loss.

Part 5: Afterwards

Table 5.5. Afterwards

POSTEA	AFTERWARDS
Kyrieleison Christeleison Kyrieleison	Lord have mercy; Christ have mercy; Lord have mercy
Pater noster PRIUATE Et ne nos …	Our Father … SILENTLY And lead us not …

Even after the moment of death, the ritual continued to provide those gathered at the bedside with liturgical, musical material, designated with a rubric of one word: 'afterwards'. Before the activity of cleaning and moving the body, the ritual directs those gathered to perform a chant, prayers and verses with responses.

The first item in this part of the ritual is the three-fold prayer for mercy: *Kyrie eleison, Christe eleison, Kyrie eleison.* This chant, like the litany, probably involved the gathered participants rather than only a celebrant or soloist. Customary performance practices with the *Kyrie* included a three-fold repetition of each invocation, often performed in alternation, either with a single person leading and the rest of the participants responding or with two groups alternating.[24] In this position in Newberry 24, the first letters of each invocation (K, C and K) are written in red ink, a colour the scribe used in other places to designate rubrics and the beginnings of chants. This scribal use of coloured ink gives prominence to the beginning of each invocation of the *Kyrie* and suggests that in performance, each invocation contained more substance and complexity than the two words written on the page.

Were the chant to have been sung through by one person, the scribe likely would have used red ink on only the first initial (to mark the chant's beginning) and black ink for the remainder. Instead, the *Kyrie* was likely intended to be performed with repetitions of invocations and alternation of participants. The melody recorded on fol. 253 (with the *Kyrie* performed prior to the burial) was most likely also intended for the moments after death. As seen in other parts in the ritual for the dying in Newberry 24, the scribe chose to reference chants by their first words and to write them in full in only one later position, most likely as a space-saving mechanism. The Breviary of Saint Claire (held in Assisi, San Damiano), which contains a similar version of the ritual, also supports this understanding. The breviary has musical notation in this position in the ritual, offering further indications

24 On the melodic traditions of the *Kyrie*, including the three-fold repetition of each invocation, see Hiley, *Western Plainchant*, pp. 150–6.

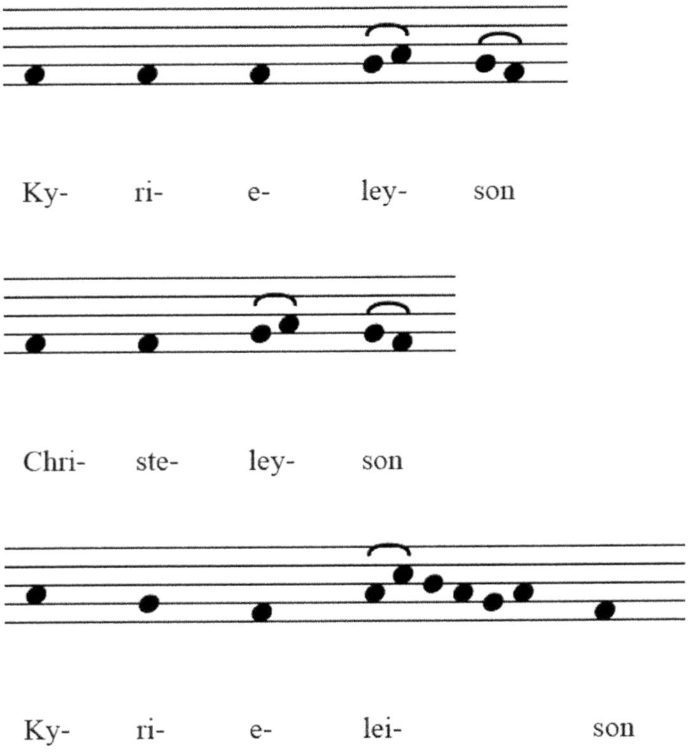

Fig. 5.5. Chant for the time immediately following death: Kyrie eleison, transcribed from Newberry 24, fol. 253 by Elaine Stratton Hild.

that in the early Franciscan liturgy the intention was for the *Kyrie* to be sung in the moments after death.[25]

As figure 5.5 shows, the melody recorded for the *Kyrie* closely conforms to the text's syntactic structures. The first invocation, 'Kyrieleyson', is conveyed with an arch-shaped melodic gesture. That the gesture begins and ends on the same pitch ('f') lends a sense of completion to its ending. The second invocation, 'Christeleyson', is conveyed with a repetition of this melodic gesture. In this way, the second invocation is also presented as a distinct and complete melodic unit and the two invocations sound as recognisably distinct iterations. The melodic conveyance of the third invocation introduces variation with a higher range, beginning a third higher with the pitch 'a' and rising to the highest pitch of the chant, 'c'. Yet even with this melodic distinction and intensification, the third musical gesture ends with the pitch 'f', creating a coherence with the previous invocations. The

[25] See L. Bracaloni, *Il primo rituale Francescano nel breviario di S. Chiara* (Quaracchi, 1923), p. 78.

chant conveys the three invocations as distinct melodic entities and the beginnings and endings of the melodic gestures are coordinated with the beginnings and endings of the syntactic units.

The next item prescribed by the ritual – the prayer *Pater noster* – would have been familiar to those gathered. While the rubric directs participants to say the first portion of the prayer 'priuate' (most likely, silently), the final statements, beginning with the words 'et ne nos' (and lead us not), were probably recited with two groups alternating verses. Following the *Pater noster*, the scribe recorded an additional series of statements and responses. The scribal inclusion of coloured initials suggests that these were also performed in alternation between a celebrant and other participants. Those gathered thus prayed on behalf of the dying person collectively.

Why these specific items, immediately following death? The *Pater noster* and the *Kyrie* were two of the most common and frequently performed items in the Franciscan liturgy. Those reciting these items at the deathbed would most likely have already recited them multiple times during the day. The familiarity itself might have offered comfort; bringing these well-known items into the deathbed liturgy might well have grounded the monumental experience of witnessing a life's ending in daily religious practices.

The final prayer at the bedside, *Tibi domine commendamus animam famuli tui*, succinctly expresses the religious function of the ritual: 'To you, Lord, we commend the soul of your servant'.[26] Those gathered entrusted their companion to the care of God. The prayer also articulates the deceased person's new status: 'dead to the world … alive to you'. With this prayer, the ritual provides an explicit confirmation of two levels of change: the person is now deceased and the earthly community has transferred one of its members to the care of the heavenly community. By assigning this prayer to the bedside, prior to the activities of washing, transporting and burying the body, the ritual indicates that the explicit articulation of this religious understanding took momentary precedence over more practical matters. As with the ritual's earlier prayer, a simple melody most likely conveyed this final material at the bedside.

Conclusion

Unlike the liturgies of the Mass and Office, the liturgy for the dying was intended to accompany events with unpredictable timing. Possible positions of flexibility in the pacing of performance are evident throughout the ritual. The specific rubrics provide points of orientation during the process of dying. Their division of material into five parts, each corresponding to a stage in the process, suggests that time could have been allowed in between sections, in order to accommodate the variable progress of an individual's passage through the stages.

[26] The translation follows Paxton, *Christianizing Death*, p. 147 n. 71. See also Sicard, *La liturgie*, pp. 355–8.

For example, the material in the second section of the ritual, indicated for *uicino morti* (proximity to death), might not have been sung until the celebrant judged that death was truly imminent. This particular section of the ritual reveals another position of flexibility. The rubric refers to only one prayer, yet the scribe included six. It is quite likely that a celebrant or soloist could have used as many prayers as seemed appropriate, given the timing of the individual's situation. The rubric 'Si anxiatur adhuc anima' (if the soul is still uneasy), which precedes the third portion of the ritual, suggests yet another point of flexibility. The wording implies that the material in the section was to be used only if the dying person seemed to be struggling extensively. This section thus seems to have been conceived of as optional; in some circumstances, it might not have been used at all. Similarly, the psalms prescribed in this section consist of large portions of text, requiring many minutes to sing. If death occurred during the performance of the psalms, it is quite conceivable that, rather than continuing with subsequent psalm verses, the celebrant simply might have shifted to the following section of the ritual and the material indicated for the moment of death. Through the rubrics' points of orientation and the material designated for each stage in the process of dying, the ritual offered structure to a variable and unpredictable progression.

The use of melody would have provided even more structure, particularly to the delivery of the texts. Much of the material at the bedside seems to have been intended for performance with simple melodies, unrecorded in the manuscript. Indeed, assuming typical performance practices, almost the entirety of the material at the bedside would have been conveyed with melody. The minimal music notation included in the ritual most likely reflects the efficiency of the scribe's work and his understanding of what the manuscript's users would have needed in order to perform the ritual appropriately. The litany, psalms and prayers would have been conveyed with formulaic melodies articulating the beginnings and endings of syntactic units. With these items, as well as the *Kyrie* following death, the melodies would have controlled the delivery, pacing and pitch content of the texts.

For chants with recorded melodies – particularly the responsory *Subvenite* and the verse *Suscipiat* – the notation reveals how music shaped the conveyance of the texts. The melodic settings emphasise individual words (through the use of higher pitch content and gestures with multiple pitches) and draw connections between words (by the use of melodic repetition). With these musical means, the sung performances would have guided listeners towards specific understandings: reassurances that the hopes expressed in the chants' words – the hopes for assistance, companionship and a heavenly destination for the dying person's soul – would be realised.

Because the performance involved not just a single celebrant, but also others gathered at the bedside, the musical component of the ritual controlled both the delivery of the texts and the interactions among those in the attending community. A collective performance required coordination of breath, as well as matching of pitch and pacing. In short, those gathered were drawn together into a coordinated, precise effort to realise the liturgy.

In these ways – in the specific, detailed rubrics providing points of orientation, in the prescription of material for each stage in the dying process, in the music that controlled the delivery of texts and the interactions among participants – the ritual offered meaningful structure and actions for the attending community. The prescription for the time of death was a gathering of witness, liturgical support and – in the music that conveyed the texts – beauty. The experience of death was to be accompanied with song.

Appendix

Table 5.6. Order of the Commendation of the Soul

ORDO COMMENDATIONIS ANIME		ORDER OF THE COMMENDATION OF THE SOUL	
fol. 252-b			
PRIMUM FIANT LETANIE BREUES AD HUNC MODUM		FIRST LET THE SHORT LITANIES BE PERFORMED IN THIS WAY	
Kyrieleison		Lord, have mercy	
Christeleison		Christ, have mercy	
Kyrieleison		Lord, have mercy	
cum Maria ora pro eo		with Mary pray for him	
Omnes sancti angeli	orate	all holy angels	pray <for him>
Sancte Abel	ora	Saint Abel	pray …
Omnes chorus iustorum	orate	all the chorus of the just	pray …
Sancte Abraham	ora	Saint Abraham	pray …
Sancte Johannis baptista	ora	Saint John the Baptist	pray …
Omnes sancti patriarche et prophete	orate	all holy patriarchs and prophets	pray …
Sancte Petre	ora	Saint Peter	pray …
Sancte Paule	ora	Saint Paul	pray …
Sancte Andrea	ora	Saint Andrew	pray …
Omnes sancti apostoli et euangeliste	orate	all holy apostles and evangelists	pray …
Sancte Francisce	ora	Saint Francis	pray …
Omnes sancti innocentes	orate	all holy innocents	pray …
Sancte Stephane[27]		Saint Stephen	
Omnes sancti martires orate pro eo[28]		all holy martyrs	pray for him
Sancte Siluester	ora	Saint Silvester	pray …

27 later addition, interlinear

28 later addition, lower margin

Omnes sancti pontifices et confessores	orate	all holy pontiffs and confessors	pray …
Sancte Paule hermite	ora	Saint Paul the hermit	pray …
Sancte Benedicte	ora	Saint Benedict	pray …
Omnes sancti monachi et heremite	orate	all holy monks and hermits	pray …
Sancta Lucia	ora	Saint Lucy	pray …
Omnes sancte uirgines	orate	all holy virgins	pray …
Omnes sancti et sancte dei	orate	all saints of God	pray …
Propitius esto	parce ei domine	be merciful	spare him, Lord
Propitius esto	libera eum domine	be merciful	free him, Lord
Ab ira tua	libera	from your wrath	free …
A periculo mortis	libera	from the dangers of death	free …
A ma<la> morte[29]	libera	from a bad death	free …
A penis inferni	libera	from punishments of hell	free …
A potestate diaboli	libera	from the powers of the devil	free …
Ab omni malo	libera	from every evil	free …
Per natiuitatem tuam	libera	through your birth	free …
Per sanctam crucem tuam	libera	through your holy cross	free …
Per mortem et sepulturam tuam	libera	through your death and burial	free …
Per gloriosam resurrectionem tuam	libera	through your glorious resurrection	free …
Per ammirabilem ascensionem tuam	libera	through your miraculous ascension	free …
Per gratiam spiritus sancti paracliti	libera	through the favour of the holy spirit advocate	free …
In die iudicii	libera	in the day of judgment	free …
Peccatores te rogamus		transgressors, we ask you,	
audi nos		hear us	
Vt parcas ei rogamus audi nos		to spare him, we ask you, hear us	
Kyrieleison		Lord, have mercy	
Christeleison		Christ, have mercy	
Kyrieleison		Lord, have mercy	

[29] Illegible note in margin

DEINDE PRO UICINO MORTI	THEN FOR THE NEARNESS TO DEATH
CUM IN AGONE SUI EXITUS	WHEN, IN THE STRUGGLE OF ITS EXIT,
ANIMA UISA FUERIT ANSIARI[30]	THE SOUL IS SEEN TO BE ANXIOUS
FIAT HEC ORATIO	LET THIS BE THE PRAYER
Proficiscere anima christiana <…>	Go forth, Christian soul …
ORATIO	PRAYER
Deus misericors deus clemens <…>	Merciful God, gentle God …
fol. 252v	
ORATIO	PRAYER
Commendo te omnipotenti deo karissime frater <…>	I commend you to almighty God, beloved brother …
ORATIO	PRAYER
Svscipe domine seruum tuum <…>	Receive, Lord, your servant …
ORATIO	PRAYER
Commendamus tibi domine animam famuli tui <…>	We commend to you, Lord, the soul of your servant…
fol. 252v–b	
ORATIO	PRAYER
Delicta iuuentutis et ignorantias eius <…>	The transgressions of his youth and his ignorances…
SI ANSIATUR[31] ADHUC ANIMA	IF THE SOUL IS STILL UNEASY
DICANTUR HII PSALMI	THESE PSALMS OUGHT TO BE UTTERED
PSALMUS	PSALM
Confitemini	Acclaim… [117]
PSALMUS	PSALM
Beati immaculati USQUE Ad dominum cum tribularer	Happy whose way is blameless… [118] UNTIL To the Lord when I was in straits… [119][32]

30 ANSIARI] *read as* ANXIARI

31 ANSIATUR] *read* ANXIATUR

32 Translations of the psalms follow R. Alter, trans., *The Hebrew Bible,* III: 276–91.

EGRESSA ANIMA[33] AUTEM	AT THE DEPARTURE OF THE SOUL HOWEVER
DICATUR HOC RESPONSORIUM RECITANDO[34]	THIS RESPONSORY OUGHT TO BE UTTERED, RECITING
Subuenite	Come help…
VERSUS Suscipiat	VERSE May Christ receive…
VERSUS Requiem eternam[35]	VERSE Rest eternal…
POSTEA	AFTERWARDS
Kyrieleison	Lord, have mercy
Christeleison	Christ, have mercy
Kyrieleison	Lord, have mercy
Pater noster PRIUATE	Our Father… SILENTLY
Et ne nos	And lead us not…
VERSUS Requiem eternam	VERSE Rest eternal <grant him, Lord>
R Et lux perpetua	RESPONSE And let light perpetual <shine upon him>
VERSUS A porta inferi	VERSE From the gate of hell
R Erue domine animam	RESPONSE Save his soul, Lord
VERSUS Requiescat	VERSE May he rest <in peace>
R Amen	RESPONSE Amen
VERSUS Domine exaudi	VERSE Lord, hear <my prayer>
R Et clamor	RESPONSE And let my cry <come before you>
VERSUS Dominus uobiscum	VERSE The Lord be with you
R Et cum spiritu tuo	RESPONSE And with your spirit
ORATIO Tibi domine commendamus <…>	PRAYER To you, Lord, we commend…

33 The manuscript shows evidence that a second scribe made changes to the rubrics. These changes bring the rubrics into conformity with those of the revised version of the ritual from 1260. EGRESSA ANIMA] *corrected from* EGRESSA ANIMA DE CORPORE.

34 RESPONSORIUM RECITANDO] *corrected from* RESPONSORIUM

35 VERSUS Requiem eternam] VERSUS Requiem eternam CUM Req<uiem> e<ternam>

TUNC FRATRES QUIBUS PRECEPTUM FUERIT LAUENT CORPUS <...>	THEN THE BROTHERS WHO HAD BEEN DIRECTED OUGHT TO WASH THE BODY...

6

Medical and Spiritual Healing of Death and Disease in Medieval Miracle Stories

JENNIFER C. EDWARDS[1]

Introduction

Visitors to saints' shrines during the European Middle Ages (c. 500–1500) believed that miraculous healings would cure worthy petitioners, something secular healers could not offer with their skills. Indeed, miracle tale collections promulgated by saints' cults argued that their patrons' spiritual healing was superior to that of secular practitioners. According to saints' lives, ill or injured people needing medical assistance typically sought care from secular practitioners first, before seeking it from saints. It was perhaps only in the direst cases that people turned to saints; few diseases or conditions, it seemed, were beyond the miraculous healing abilities of saints, who, according to large numbers of miracle reports, reversed even death.

A saint's life offered propaganda for his or her cult, as well as justification for the holy person's admission into the Church's litany of saints. The primary purpose of miracle stories was thus to demonstrate the power of God and the sanctity of the intercessor. Descriptions of secular healers in such texts typically demonstrated the failure of their interventions, thereby proving the superiority of the saint's curative power. At times, such narratives even claimed secular medical expertise for the saints, such as calling Luke the great healer, depicting Saints Cosmas and Damian in surgery and describing in detail the medical attention that Saint Elizabeth provided to sick men and women. In fact, this hagiographical approach actually shows great respect for medical workers, since it is only when the best possible secular care has failed that the saint's cure is deemed remarkable. Similarly, it is only when the saint demonstrates better medical talent than a secular expert that her charity is considered holy. Rather than attacking the medical profession, such

1 I thank Nükhet Varlık and Lori Jones for their generosity, patience and encouragement and Janine Larmon Peterson for her thoughtful and generous comments. This chapter began as conference presentations for 'The Healing Arts Across the Mediterranean: Communities, Knowledge, and Practices' at Rutgers University, following a kind invitation from Nahyan Fancy, the 2014 'Berkshire Conference for Women's Historians' and the American Association for the History of Medicine in 2017. I am grateful to the warm and receptive audiences for all three papers, especially Monica Green, Dyan Elliot, Mickey Moran, Sara Ritchey, Winston Black, Nicole Archambeau and Ann Carmichael.

texts make reference to secular practitioners in order to demonstrate both that the patient's issue had no mortal solution and that the miracle or holy treatment was truly glorious.

Scholars have consulted documents related to the cult of the saints since at least the 1970s for information about medieval medicine, patients, disease and disability.[2] Texts such as saints' lives, miracle tales and canonisation proceedings document the medieval experience of illness, injury and disability as well as the search for treatment and cure. While there are many reasons for scepticism when reading hagiographical literature – adherence to formulae, repetition of topoi and emphasis on miracle and faith – it is necessary to recognise that the hagiographer had an obligation to accuracy and credibility in discussing medical interventions. In fact, hagiography's

> very purpose, that of focusing convinced, secure (and financially rewarding) devotion upon the saint, ensures that its authors cannot afford to be inaccurate in matters of detail, for were they to be so, their treatises would lose their credibility before they had gained even a part of their point ... Thus, the picture they give us ... of the 'medicus', on call with his diagnostic and drugging and cupping and surgical skills, and sharp and varied iron instruments, can legitimately be used to fill out the others we have.[3]

Since these documents are so numerous, their examination has much to yield for the histories of disease and disability.

Medical practitioners in medieval Europe included literate, educated physicians, as well as surgeons, barbers, herbalists, apothecaries, midwives, monastic infirmarians, astrologers and so-called wise or cunning persons. Women served in all of these positions and ministered to the physical needs of their community, but they were increasingly pushed into marginal, low-status and less respected positions over the course of the central and later Middle Ages. This was especially the case in areas where and at times when licensing became more common.[4] The sick accorded female and male saints equal healing authority,

2 H. J. Magoulias, 'The Lives of the Saints as Sources of Data for the History of Byzantine Medicine in the Sixth and Seventh Centuries', *Byzantinische Zeitschrift* 57 (1964), 127–50; E. F. Frey, 'Saints in Medical History', *Clio Med* 14 (1979), 35–70; J. Jansen, ed. and trans., *Medizinische Kasuistik in den 'Miracula Sanctae Elyzabet:' Medizenhistorische Analyse und Übersetzung der Wunderprotokolle am Grab der Elisabeth von Thüringen (1207-31)* (Frankfurt, 1985); V. J. Flint, 'The Early Medieval "Medicus", the Saint – and the Enchanter', *The Society for the Social History of Medicine* 2 (1989), 127–45; J. Ziegler, *Medicine and Religion, c. 1300: The Case of Arnau de Villanova* (Oxford, 2005); I. McCleery, '*Multos ex medicinae arte curaverat, multos verbo et oratione*: Curing in Medieval Portuguese Saints' Lives', *Studies in Church History* 41 (2006), 192–202; J. Duffin, *Medical Miracles: Doctors, Saints, and Healing in the Modern World* (Oxford, 2009); M. Johnson, 'In the Bursting of an Eye: Blinding and Blindness in Medieval Ireland's Hagiography', in *Wounds and Wound Repair in Medieval Culture*, ed. K. DeVries and L. Tracy (Leiden, 2015), pp. 448–70. See also Jenni Kuuliala's chapter 7 in this volume for a discussion of infirmity and death wishes in medieval French and Italian canonisation processes.

3 Flint, 'Early Medieval "Medicus"', pp. 135–6.

4 Salerno was the centre of medical learning in Europe by the late twelfth century, while Bologna, Paris and Montpellier followed during the thirteenth century: N. G. Siraisi, *Medieval and*

however, and sought their healing power with confidence. Increasingly after the twelfth century, classically trained male physicians attempted to code medical authority as male, further marginalising even those female healers who were expert in gynaecology. Saints' cults, however, continued to depict female ability to heal the sick through spiritual devotion, arguing that this holy power was greater than that of the most skilled (male) physicians.

In this chapter, I first examine evidence for women's roles in medieval medical practice that reveals not only their presence but also their marginal, low-status positions. Second, I examine the medical interventions that female saints offered as part of the high-status community of holy healers. Third, I discuss the treatment of medical experts in hagiographical texts, especially examining Jacobus de Voragine's thirteenth-century *Legenda aurea*, or *The Golden Legend*. The chapter demonstrates that medieval European Christians considered saints important medical workers whose spiritual healing power was superior to that of earthly physicians and that female saints enjoyed a status as healers that more earthly female medical workers did not have. Yet, while hagiographers celebrated female saints' thaumaturgic healing power and the more mundane healing interventions that they offered as charity to the sick, such as bathing, feeding, bandaging and applying ointment, there nevertheless was a gendered difference in the *Golden Legend*'s presentation of male and female saints' relationship with secular healing. This is likely due to institutionalising trends that, by the thirteenth century, placed greater emphasis on the university training that limited and marginalised women's roles in the professional medical fields. It also reflects the formalisation of the canonisation process that limited the creation of new female saints. Together, these two contemporary trends shaped the portrayal of saints' relationship with healing, especially via the presentation of the Dominican Jacobus de Voragine.[5]

Early Renaissance Medicine: An Introduction to Knowledge and Practice (Chicago, 2009), p. 188. Licensing started as early as the mid-twelfth century and was common but not omnipresent by the fourteenth century. In all places, it involved a demonstration of literacy: J. Shatzmiller, *Jews, Medicine, and Medieval Society* (Berkeley, 1994), p. 14; L. García-Ballester, M. R. McVaugh and A. Rubio-Vela, 'Medical Licensing and Learning in Fourteenth-Century Valencia', *Transactions of the American Philosophical Society* 79 (1989); M. R. McVaugh, *Medicine before the Plague: Practitioners and Their Patients in the Crown of Aragon, 1285–1345* (Cambridge, 1993), p. 69, 78. The impact of licensing and an emphasis on education and literacy are examined by M. H. Green, *Making Women's Medicine Masculine: The Rise of Male Authority in Pre-Modern Gynaecology* (Oxford, 2008).

5 Canonisation procedures became increasingly formal and controlled by the papacy over the course of the thirteenth century: A. Vauchez, *Sainthood in the Later Middle Ages* (Cambridge, 1997), pp. 22–57 (p. 27); this process had a 'detrimental effect on the promotion and ultimate selection of female saints': J. T. Schulenburg, *Forgetful of Their Sex: Female Sanctity and Society, ca. 500–1100* (Chicago, 1998), p. 5.

Women as medical practitioners

Over the course of the twelfth century, an increased emphasis on literacy and on university training limited high-status medical practice almost completely to male physicians, although this was not a systematic or comprehensive shift. Cities with larger numbers of university-trained physicians witnessed stronger control of healing professions and greater marginalisation of women.[6] In places without such a strong presence of educated male physicians, women and less formally educated men were better able to continue practising medicine.

Yet medieval women continued to practise medicine in most fields: they were physicians, surgeons, barbers, apothecaries and midwives. They had male and female patients and worked alongside their male colleagues. Learning much more than this about female medical practitioners in the Middle Ages remains a challenge, however, since evidence of such women is elusive. The sorts of documents traditionally used to extract biographical information about medieval medical workers (such as legal, notarial and guild records) do not record women and, since they lacked university training, female medical workers were likely of the 'middling or lower artisanal classes' who did not appear in most archival records.[7] Married women likely appeared in records under their husbands' names, making married female practitioners 'invisible in the documents' of activities that they may have engaged in alone.[8] Since women often engaged in multiple occupations in the Middle Ages, had careers that fluctuated over the course of the life cycle and participated in 'low-status, marginal positions within the trades', women's work in the medical fields was often transitory and fluid, again less likely to leave a record.[9]

Without a university education, medieval women were not able to practise at the highest levels of the medical fields, nor were they able to gain full access to the medical guilds. Here, too, the improvement in record keeping over the course of the Middle Ages actually works against our ability to study women: as understanding of Arabic, Hebrew and ancient medical texts improved, those with university educations and training in theoretical medicine were seen as the only experts, especially in legal contexts. This excluded women, who had difficulty accessing that training.[10] Licensing regulations imposed between the twelfth and sixteenth centuries in European kingdoms likely exacerbated these problems, as both

6 Green, *Making Women's Medicine Masculine.*

7 M. H. Green, 'Documenting Medieval Women's Medical Practice', in *Practical Medicine from Salerno to the Black Death*, ed. L. García-Ballester, R. French, J. Arrizabalaga and A. Cunningham (Cambridge, 1994), pp. 322–52 (p. 327).

8 Ibid., p. 327. Green suggested that even our 'criteria … for identifying practitioners themselves preclude documentation of women's medical practice' because we look for explicit labels that were not attached to women; ibid., p. 328.

9 Ibid., p. 332. Women's '"careers" … show greater fluctuation than men's, depending on their position in the life cycle or their marital status' which leads to difficulty in occupational labelling. Ibid., p. 324.

10 Ibid., p. 350.

men and women who practised on the margins without official regulation are less likely to appear in documentary sources.[11]

Female practitioners are not completely invisible in the available records, however. A trial of six unlicensed practitioners in fourteenth-century Paris included the healer Jacoba Felicie and three female colleagues.[12] Female practitioners in various occupations have also been identified in Venice, Paris, Manosque, Florence and across Iberia, although often at times when licensing was not strict or in numbers that declined over time.[13] And, at the very least, most medical theorists accorded women a role in the 'medical care of other women, if only in the role of manual assistant to the male physician … and in the rarely challenged role of birth attendant', since men observed the taboo of manually examining a woman.[14] As was true in other medieval guilds, husbands might have trained their wives and fathers their daughters, particularly apothecaries, surgeons and barbers, who did not normally require university education to practise. For example, Juan de Luna taught his daughter, who in turn taught her son. Women may also have occupied positions that required less start-up capital or that charged less money to patients.[15] In Marseilles, the Jewish midwife Floreta d'Ays might have attracted business because she charged less money than a Christian midwife.[16]

The female healer known as Trota, to whom the famous Trotula is often credited, was known to diagnose and cure 'as a master'; authors describing her respected her expertise.[17] Monastic women in medieval England also demonstrated medical abilities, mostly

[11] M. H. Green, 'Women's Medical Practice and Health Care in Medieval Europe', *Signs* 14 (1989), 434–73 (p. 452); and Green, 'Documenting', p. 335. See Margaret Pelling's suggestion that women in early modern England were usually unlicensed, involved in multiple occupations and used family networks to gain training: 'Medical Practice in Early Modern England: Trade or Profession?' in *The Professions in Early Modern England*, ed. W. Prest (London, 1987), pp. 90–128.

[12] Green, 'Women's Medical Practice', p. 452.

[13] L. Münster, 'Women Doctors in Medieval Italy', *Ciba Symposium* 10 (1962), 136–40; D. Jacquart, *Le milieu médical en France du XIIe au XVe siècle: en annexe 2e supplément au 'Dictionnaire' d'Ernest Wickersheimer* (Geneva, 1981); K. Park, *Doctors and Medicine in Early Renaissance Florence* (Princeton, 1985); D. Herlihy, *Opera Muliebra: Women and Work in Medieval Europe* (Philadelphia, 1990); B. Coury, 'Contributions à l'histoire sociale des praticiens parisiens à la fin du Moyen Âge: aspects méthodologiques', *Sources, travaux historiques* 5 (1986), 13–28; G. Dumas, 'Les femmes et les pratiques de la santé dans le Registre des plaidoires du Parlement de Paris, 1364–1427', *Canadian Bulletin of Medical History* 13 (1996), 3–28 (p. 10–12); McVaugh, *Medicine before the Plague*, pp. 103–7.

[14] Green, 'Women's Medical Practice', p. 473; and also M. H. Green, 'From "Diseases of Women" to "Secrets of Women": The Transformation of Gynaecological Literature in the Later Middle Ages', *Journal of Medieval and Early Modern Studies* 30 (2000), 5–39.

[15] Green, 'Documenting', pp. 333–34.

[16] M. H. Green and D. L. Smail, 'The Trial of Floreta d'Ays (1403): Jews, Christians, and Obstetrics in Later Medieval Marseille', *Journal of Medieval History* 34 (2008), 185–211 (p. 198 n. 53).

[17] M. H. Green, ed. and trans., *The Trotula: An English Translation of the Medieval Compendium of Women's Medicine* (Philadelphia, 2002), pp. 48–50.

on a low-status and practical level, with the 'infirmaress' following directions given by a consulting physician.[18] At least two women in medieval England also tended men, by dispensing medicine and performing surgery for the monks at Westminster abbey.[19] Women in Salerno, the 'mulieres Salernitane', appear as experts in twelfth-century medical texts discussing folk medicine and ritual. Authors discussing these women did not attribute to them any facility with medical theory, however, and women were routinely disconnected from the abstract, theoretical, university-educated medical thinking of the Middle Ages. While women owned medical books, they do not appear to have engaged strongly with medical literature.[20]

Part of the problem of seeing women in the documents might lie in how we define medical practitioners. One possibility is the inclusive notion of 'any individual whose occupation is basically concerned with the care of the sick'.[21] Alternatively, one could limit the definition to only those women who identified explicitly with medical work, either by charging for labour or by receiving community recognition for their work. The largest category of female practitioner that fits this definition was the midwife, but even midwives are elusive in the sources, since they had no guilds and were not licensed until the late Middle Ages. No special training was expected of them beyond that gained in their own childbearing. In the later Middle Ages, men sought greater control over women's health that may have displaced female medical workers from gynaecological practice.[22] The problem of identification extends into the early modern period.[23]

Women's healing activities were also important at home. While women were called as expert medical witnesses in court, held licences to practise medicine and were hired to practise in Iberia, however, they were not labelled in ways that explicitly identified them as medical practitioners. Focusing on the 'wide range of expert activities both to maintain health and to cure or relieve sickness that were conducted in households' increases the spectrum of healers who fit the broader definition noted above. We must remember that

18 F. Getz, 'Women Medical Practitioners in England (act. c. 1200–1475)', in *Oxford Dictionary of National Biography* (Oxford, 2004); many thanks to Monica Green for sharing this reference with me.

19 Getz, 'Women Medical Practitioners in England'. According to Getz, since the surgeon was called in 'after others had failed', her expertise might have been particularly respected.

20 M. H. Green, 'The Possibilities of Literacy and the Limits of Reading: Women and the Gendering of Medical Literacy', in *Women's Healthcare in the Medieval West: Texts and Contexts* (Aldershot, 2000), pp. 4–5. 'We have, then, a situation where both women's literacy and the quantity of medical literature … were simultaneously increasing, yet where women's access to the literate culture of medicine seems not to have been growing at a comparable pace'.

21 M. Pelling and C. Webster, 'Medical Practitioners', in *Health, Medicine, and Mortality in the Sixteenth Century*, ed. C. Webster (Cambridge, 1979), pp. 165–235 (p. 166); Green, 'Documenting', pp. 335–36.

22 Green, 'Documenting', pp. 337–39; Green, *Making Women's Medicine Masculine.*

23 M. Pelling, *The Common Lot: Sickness, Medical Occupations, and the Urban Poor in Early Modern England* (New York, 1998).

there is a 'continuum of women's practice whose original focus is the everyday experience of care within the household'.[24] Women's healing in the domestic sphere was more common than – and often preferred to – the services of more formally trained professionals.

Women's medical care thus was a central component of the medieval household economy. Medieval Europeans turned to female medical practitioners when ill or hurt and relied on women's medical care as surgeons, apothecaries, midwives and physicians, even if women's work in these fields was temporary, occasional or informal. Women did not gain high-status positions or receive significant authority within the medical field, instead losing ever more ground over time. Women dominated the position of midwife, but this position also became masculinised, de-professionalised and thus marginalised.[25] Women working on the margins of the medical field may have offered lower fees and been more available, however, and so they continued to practise.

Women as saints

Women were also a minority within the community of saints, making up only 17.5 per cent of the more than 800 saints examined in a 1982 study.[26] While women did not become saints in the same numbers as men and their access to sanctity shifted through conventions such as canonisation procedures, female saints nevertheless were a constant presence in the lives of medieval Christians. The cults of so-called universal saints – such as the Virgin Mary, Mary Magdalene, Saint Anne, Thecla and Helena – filled the church calendar and focused the devotional lives of Christians across Europe. Local saints symbolised popular devotion, being women recognised for a holy life and power. Women became saints as martyrs, nuns, mothers, virgins, queens and ascetics. *Vitae* (*Lives*) depicting their holy biographies repeat themes of virginity, charity, self-sacrifice, asceticism, care of the sick and miraculous healing. These holy women offered charity during their lives, giving money and food to the needy and nursing care to the sick. Saints offered medical treatments as part of their charity and worked miracles, both during their lives and posthumously. Many saints' *vitae* depict holy women washing wounds, applying ointments, bandaging cuts or broken limbs and nursing the ill and disabled. For example, the sixth-century queen Saint Radegund tended the bodies of sick people at Athies: 'she washed them herself in warm baths and cared for the putrefaction of their sickness ... Before she washed them she prepared by her own hand a potion that would restore those exhausted from sweating'.[27] Not only

24 M. Cabré, 'Women or Healers? Household Practices and the Categories of Health Care in Late Medieval Iberia', *Bulletin of the History of Medicine* 82 (2008), 18–51 (p. 50); I thank the author for sharing her work with me.

25 Green, 'Women's Medical Practice', pp. 446–52; Green, *Making Women's Medicine Masculine*.

26 D. Weinstein and R. M. Bell, *Saints and Society: The Two Worlds of Western Christendom, 1000–1700* (Chicago, 1982).

27 Venantius Fortunatus, 'De Vita Sanctae Radegundis Libri Duo: Liber I', in *Monumenta Germaniae Historica: Scriptores Rerum Merovingicarum 2*, ed. Bruno Krusch (Hanover, 1888), pp.

did she nurse their diseased bodies, but she also created her own tonic, as an apothecary would, to restore their strength. At Poitiers, Radegund

> washed the heads of the poor, scrubbing away each scab, mange and worm, not squeamish about any rotten flesh and now and then removing worms, purging putrid skin, combing one by one the heads she had washed herself. In the manner of the Gospel, she even covered in oil the sores and wounds revealed by softening the skin or irritated by nails, soothing spread of disease.[28]

She tended people with leprosy and 'washed their faces and hands, she applied oil to their ulcers, and fed each one'.[29] Thus Radegund cleaned dirty wounds, treated them with ointments and created her own medications to care for the sick.

The thirteenth-century Beguines are particularly well known for devoting their lives to nursing the sick members of their communities, whom they bathed, kissed, fed and tended.[30] According to the *Life of St Marie d'Oignies*, the saint even suffered the diseases of her friends: 'she was sick with the sick … sometimes she even felt their afflictions in her own limbs'.[31] Marie then called a priest who blessed the area of the pain 'and in a miraculous manner the pain fled to another place, as if dreading the power of the Holy Cross'. Repeating this blessing eventually removed all the pain. Saint Douceline de Digne, who established the Beguines in Marseille, offered healing charity to several people. Among them was a young Beguine whose limbs were so swollen that she could not walk until Douceline washed her on Holy Thursday, leaving no trace of the illness 'even though the doctors had abandoned her as lost'.[32] By nursing the sick and taking on lives of charity,

---

364–77 (p. 366): 'ipsa eas lavans in termis morborumque curans putredines … quos ante lavarat, eisdem sua manu miscebat, ut fessos de sudore sumpta potio recentaret'. The translation here and elsewhere is mine unless noted otherwise. A full English translation is also available in Venantius Fortunatus, 'The Life of the Holy Radegund', in *Sainted Women of the Dark Ages*, ed. and trans. J. A. McNamara and J. E. Halbourg (Durham NC, 1992), pp. 70–105.

28 Fortunatus, 'Vita', p. 370: 'capita lavans egenorum, defricans, quidquid erat, crustam, scabiem, tineam, nec purulenta fastidiens, interdum et vermes extrahens, purgans cutis putredines, singillatim capita pectebat ipsa, quae laverat. Ulcera vero cicatricum, quae cutis laxa detexerat, aut ungues exasperaverant, more euangelico oleo superfuso, mulcebat morbi contagium'.

29 Ibid., p. 371: 'facies lavabat, manus, ungues et ulcera et rursus administrabat, ipsa pascens per singula'.

30 C. W. Bynum, *Holy Feast and Holy Fast: The Religious Significance of Food to Medieval Women* (Berkeley, 1988).

31 'The Middle English Version of Jacques de Vitry's *Life of St. Marie d'Oignies*', trans. Sarah McNamer, in *Medieval Hagiography: An Anthology*, ed. T. Head (New York, 1999), pp. 709–27 (p. 726).

32 P. de Porcellet, *La vie de sainte Douceline: fondatrice des Béguines de Marseille*, ed. J. H. Albanés (Marseille, 1879), pp. 169–71 (p. 170): 'la quall li meje avian per mort dezamparada, aissi cant dezesperat de sa salut e de son gariment'.

these saints became family caregivers to the needy rather than for their own children, parents or husbands.

Beyond this charitable care for the bodies of the sick, saints also worked healing miracles – sometimes during their lives but more commonly after their deaths. As saints, these holy women became intercessors, conduits for the mighty power of God and focal points for the prayers of those in need. Sick people, disabled people and their loved ones petitioned saints to heal them and, according to numerous recorded miracles, the saints responded.

There was little beyond the healing power worked through the saints. In addition to her nursing care, Radegund also miraculously cured:

> In fact, if anyone despaired of a wound or pustule, the saint's attendant offered a vine leaf, pretending this to be her work. Then, reluctantly the saint made the sign of the cross secretly over the leaf, which was carried to the desperate one and placed on the wound. A cure soon healed the wound.[33]

Indeed, Venantius Fortunatus, Radegund's biographer, credited her with great skill: 'A nun who spent a whole year freezing cold in day and burning hot at night, not able to move a step for six months while lying lifeless' came to Radegund's attention. After bathing her, the saint

> remain[ed] alone together with the sick woman for two hours as a doctor (*medica*). She assessed the diseased limbs, to what extent the illness affected the shape of her body from head to heel. Then wherever her hands touched, sickness fled from the listless patient and she who had been placed in the warm water by two persons left it healthy; she for whom wine had no flavour accepted it, drank, and was restored. What more? The following day, when she was supposed to migrate from the world, she processed in public, healed.[34]

Fortunatus depicted her as a doctor in treatment, patience and bedside manner. Radegund's treatment resulted in a complete cure.

Saints' shrines memorialised the holy women, maintained their relics and became destinations for pilgrims, penitents and petitioners. Clergy or other caretakers at the shrines recorded reports of miracles credited to the saints' posthumous power. These records became especially important in advertising the shrine. Even if miraculous cures were

[33] Fortunatus, 'Vita', p. 371: 'Denique, si quis pustulae desperaret de vulnere, offerebat ministra sanctae folium pampani, mentiens sibi opus hoc esse. Sic vix obtento signaculo, portans ad desperatum, vulneri superposito, mox occurrrebat remedium'.

[34] Fortunatus, 'Vita', pp. 373–4: 'Monacha quaedam toto anno in die gelata frigore, per noctem cremate igne, sex mensibus nec gressum movens, cum iaceret exanimis.... Remanente tantum sola simul aegrota cum medica fere per horas duas. Quantum est corporis forma, a capite usque ad plantam infirma membra conbaiulat. Dehinc, quo manus attingebat, fugiebat dolor de languida, et, quam duae deposuerant, exit salubris de tepida; quae vinum nec odorabat, accepit, bibit, et refecta est. Quid plura? Sequenti die; cum iam speraretur migrare de saeculo salva processit in publicum'.

worked in a dream or at the patient's home, it was necessary to travel to the shrine to give thanks for the miracle where it could be recorded. While early records of saints' miracles included stories of protection for the saint's possessions, 'personnel' and institutions, over time healing cures became the main focus of miracle collections.[35] Female saints thus healed and their healing miracles were promoted by the faithful, who saw their shrines as a source of medical care.

In Oxford, Saint Frideswide cured pilgrims who drank holy water from her shrine, and she healed a girl whose father measured her with a thread, coated the thread with wax and offered the candle as a votive at her shrine.[36] In over one hundred recorded miracles, the saint cured blindness, deafness, fever, madness, epilepsy, paralysis, skin disease, tumours, ulcers and general 'illness' suffered by those who visited her shrine. According to the *Liber Eliensis*, Saint Æthelthryth healed a man suffering from swelling in his limbs that was 'meant to test his patience, so that the glory of God and the merit of the dear virgin might be made manifest in him'.[37] Æthelthryth appeared to him in a dream and told him that 'relief from [his] wretched infirmity and the restoration of [his] health lie in Ely' and if he travelled there he would 'quickly rejoice in … health'. He followed these directions and was cured through the holy water at the saint's spring. The shrine provided a destination where the ill could request a cure or thank the saint for a miracle.

Some saints made promises to care for a specific group under their protection, such as Saint Margaret of Antioch's promise to protect pregnant women:

> if any woman calls to me in the labor of childbirth,/ or better, reads my life, Lord be merciful to her./ Nor let her die, but bring forth that child to view/ All safely from his mother's womb with all his limbs in place./ Save both mother and child, Lord, for love of me./ Lord, for our mother's love, may this prayer be granted.[38]

Miracle tales and saints' lives thus established that these holy women had power over blindness, deafness, troubled limbs, paralysis and all manner of illness, which they routinely cured. While they were not included among the medical practitioners in a standard definition, Christians saw their healing care as valid and important a route to health as the treatment offered by a physician, surgeon or apothecary. They thus offered female saints respect and status not accorded to mundane women healers.

35 Ward, *Miracles*, p. 67.

36 Ward, *Miracles*, p. 85. Radegund healed Goda in a similar miracle with a candle made to the same length as Goda's height. Fortunatus, 'Vita', p. 374; see McNamara, ed., 'Life', p. 84.

37 'The Book of Ely', trans. J. Paxton, in *Medieval Hagiography*, ed. Head, pp. 459–94 (pp. 481–2).

38 'Life of St. Margaret from the *South English Legendary*', ed. and trans. W. R. Larson, in *Medieval Hagiography*, ed. Head, pp. 683–91 (p. 690).

Miracles over medicine

Some holy biographies or miracle tales describing saints' power to heal claimed that miraculous healing was *superior* to the medical abilities of secular healers. In these stories, a patient suffering disease or some disability first exhausted secular medical expertise and, finding the result unsatisfactory, then sought the care of a saint.[39] In his thirteenth-century compilation of holy stories, the *Golden Legend*, Jacobus de Voragine repeatedly depicted saints curing, both posthumously and during life, people who had first sought the care of a secular healer. Jacobus took pains to portray secular medical workers as experts and competent in their field.[40] A Dominican from Genoa, Jacobus (1228–98) began compiling his 'readings on the saints' c. 1260.[41] The collection became enormously popular, with more than one thousand manuscripts and hundreds of incunabula surviving.[42] This collection reflects a popular understanding of the ways in which medieval Christians perceived relationships between medical and spiritual healers. While the focus of Jacobus's stories is, of course, on the holy deeds of the saints, his discussion of medical workers reveals more respect for their abilities than one might have expected. Given the popularity of the *Golden Legend*, its discussion of secular healers also indicates a broader sense of the relationship between medicine and spirituality in medieval Christian European communities in the thirteenth century.

The *Golden Legend* contains 182 chapters, 156 of which focus on saints; another ten focus on Christ and three on the Virgin Mary. Of the saints earning a chapter, 82 per cent are male and 18 per cent female.[43] Twelve per cent of the entire book, or 14 per cent of the chapters on saints, contain some reference to secular medicine. Some of these references, as discussed below, demonstrate quite sophisticated understanding of contemporary medical theory. Forty-seven per cent of the stories depict the saint having superior medical expertise. Another 19 per cent include references to Christ or Luke the Evangelist as great

39 R. Finucane, *Miracles and Pilgrims: Popular Beliefs in Medieval England* (Aldershot, 1977), p. 59 notes that at least 10 per cent of medieval English pilgrims seeking a miraculous cure had previously sought secular help.

40 R. Koopmans, *Wonderful to Relate: Miracle Stories and Miracle Collecting in High Medieval England* (Philadelphia, 2011), p. 193; Finucane, *Miracles and Pilgrims*, p. 64. Finucane also reminds us that the canons of the Fourth Lateran Council in 1215 stated a preference for the priest and spiritual welfare over physician and physical welfare.

41 On Jacobus, see A. Boureau, *La Légende Dorée: Le système narratif de Jacques de Voragine (†1298)* (Paris, 1984); E. Cushing Richardson, *Materials for a Life of Jacopo da Varagine* (New York, 1935).

42 The standard modern edition is Iacopo da Varazze, *Legenda aurea*, ed. G. P. Maggioni, 2 vols., 2nd edn (Tavarnuzze, 1998). The edition used in J. de Voragine, *The Golden Legend: Readings on the Saints*, 2 vols, trans. W. G. Ryan (Princeton, 1993), hereafter *GL*, was *Legenda aurea vulgo Historia Lombadica dicta*, ed. T. Graesse (Leipzig, 1845). Ryan claims that it was the only book more widely read than the Bible (I, xiii).

43 This mirrors the findings in Weinstein and Bell, *Saints and Society*. Four of the *GL* chapters contain both male and female saints. I am counting here by chapter, rather than by number of saints referenced in the *GL*, since the 10,000 Virgins might complicate the analysis.

healers. The final third make reference to medical work – such as doctors diagnosing the man that Agnes had rejected with lovesickness, a successful healer being frightened on the cusp of his martyrdom but receiving counsel from Saint Vitalis and Saint James the Dismembered being advised by onlookers that doctors could reassemble him.[44] Jacobus used the words 'medicus' (healer) and 'physicus' (physician) to describe medical practitioners in most of these cases. He made no reference to 'medica', or secular female healers. There are, in fact, no clear examples of female medical practitioners of any kind in the text, except for saints, who are described in healing roles during their lives and working miracles after their deaths.

Where they mention medical healing, miracle stories typically seek to demonstrate that contemporary medicine is not up to the task of healing a challenging case; the miracle thus can demonstrate the superiority of faith and God. Some hagiographers actively depicted medical healers as charlatans giving bad advice, but the *Golden Legend* avoided this.[45] Instead, Jacobus respected the methods of the healers he described and demonstrated a deep understanding of medical theory. Jacobus tells of a widow named Galla who

> was a very hot-blooded woman, and her doctors told her that unless she gave herself again to the embraces of a husband, the excessive internal heat would cause her to grow a beard, unnatural as that would be. This actually happened, but she felt no concern about the external deformity because she loved inner beauty more.[46]

Jacobus makes reference to humoral theory, the idea that balance between the four humours – blood, phlegm, black bile and yellow bile – determined health and personality. Because Galla was not fulfilling her wifely duty to her husband, she had grown too hot from an excess of yellow bile that would cause her to grow a beard. By not following medical advice, Galla showed that chaste inner beauty was superior to outer appearance.[47]

Similarly, in his chapter on the Purification of the Virgin, Jacobus drew a contrast between spiritual and medical understanding of embryo development: 'One is that the child is brought into the Temple building on the fortieth day, just as the soul most frequently enters the body, as into its temple, on the fortieth day: this we learn from the

44 Most of these were physical issues, but we might consider St Vitalis offering some mental healthcare as well.

45 Gregory of Tours, for example, practically 'gloats' over the 'medical shortcomings' of doctors who exacerbated the sufferings of an epileptic, failed to heal Gregory's dysentery and were unable to cure cataracts. All of these were healed by holy miracles due to the intercession of saints. Flint, 'Early Medieval "Medicus"', p. 134.

46 *GL*, I, 349. *Legenda aurea*, lxxxiv, ed. Maggioni, I, 573–4: 'ualde ignea conspersio corporis inesset, ceperunt medici dicere quia nisi ad amplexus uiri rediret, calore nimio contra naturam barbam habitura esset. Quod ita post factum est. Sed illa nihil exterius deformitatis timuit, quia interiorem speciem amauit'.

47 This is similar to the life of Saint Wilgefortis, who grew a beard to avoid marriage. My thanks to the readers for these comments on the significance of Galla in showing Jacobus's medical knowledge and similarity to Wilgefortis.

Scholastic History. (The physicians, however, say that the male body is completely formed in forty-six days)'.[48] This explanation was entirely Christian, as forty-six days is thought to be the time between Christ's conception and birth. Nevertheless, Jacobus demonstrated that secular medical treatments had not succeeded in order to glorify the saint. This respect is commonplace in hagiography: people went to saints only 'as a last resort when conventional methods had failed'.[49]

In several of Jacobus's stories, the petitioner had exhausted all the available remedies without success before seeking out a saint. He told a story about a 'lady named Petronia, who had suffered for a long time from a very serious illness and had tried many remedies without the slightest success'.[50] In the life of Saint Peter Martyr, a nun from a monastery in the diocese of Constance had 'suffered [for a year or more] from painful gout in her knee, and no remedy had been found to cure it'.[51] In the same life, 'A man, named Rufinus, from Canapicio of the Villa Mazzati, fell seriously ill. A vein had ruptured in the lower part of his body and blood flowed out continually; and no doctor was able to find a remedy.'[52] In these cases, Jacobus demonstrated that the healer was an expert in his craft and had offered the best possible care. The patient was not healed, however, and thus turned to God and the saints for healing.

Indeed, the *Golden Legend* reveals a great deal of respect for medical workers, even ascribing their methods to the saints. Some saints embraced the language and culture of medical knowledge so thoroughly that they acted as doctors themselves. In a well-known example of holy medicine, a man whose leg was 'totally consumed by a cancer' slept while Saints Cosmas and Damian appeared to him (figure 6.1),

> bringing salves and surgical instruments. One of them said to the other: 'Where can we get flesh to fill in where we cut away the rotted leg?' The other said: 'Just today an Ethiopian was buried in the cemetery of Saint Peter in Chains. Go and take his leg, and we'll put it in place of the bad one'. So he sped to the cemetery and brought back the Moor's leg, and the two saints cut off the sick man's leg and inserted the Moor's in its

48 *GL*, I, 143–4; *Legenda aurea*, xxxvii, ed. Maggioni, I, 238–9: 'Vna, ut per hoc intelligitur quod sicut puer XL die in materiale templum inducitur sic XL die a conceptione ut sepius anima in corpus tamquam in suum templum infunditur, sicut dicitur in scholastic hystoria licet physici dicunt quod in XLVI diebus corpus perficiatur'.

49 J. Ziegler, 'Practitioners and Saints: Medical Men in Canonization Processes in the Thirteenth to Fifteenth Centuries', *Social History of Medicine* 12 (1999), 191–225 (p. 194).

50 *GL*, I, 48. *Legenda aurea*, xxxvii, ed. Maggioni, I, 84: 'quedam matron nomine Patronia ... diu infirmitate grauissima torqueretur et multa adhibens remedia nullum sentiret liberationis uestigium'.

51 Ibid., 264. *Legenda aurea*, lxi, ed. Maggioni, I, 434: 'per annum et amplius grauem guttam in genu perpessa est ita quod nullo remedio poterat liberari'.

52 Ibid. *Legenda aurea*, lxi, ed. Maggioni, I, 435: 'Vir quidam de Canapicio de uilla Mazati nomine Rufus ualde infirmitatem incurrit; nam uena fracta in inferioribus partibus anterius sine cessatione sanguinem emittebat ita quod a nullo medicorum aliquid sibi remedium poterat adhiberi'.

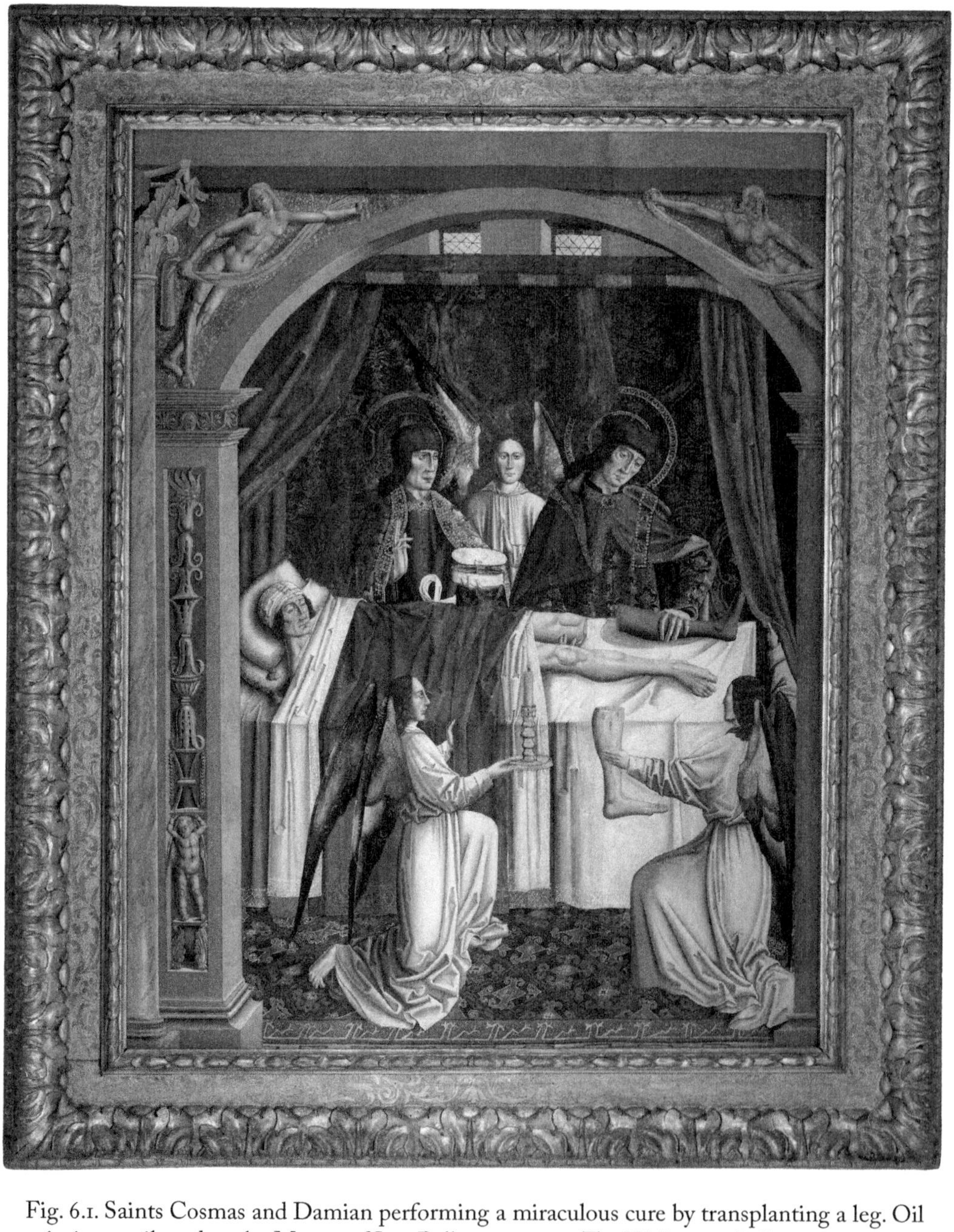

Fig. 6.1. Saints Cosmas and Damian performing a miraculous cure by transplanting a leg. Oil painting attributed to the Master of Los Balbases, c. 1495. The Wellcome Collection, available under a Public Domain Mark.

place, carefully anointing the wound. Finally they took the amputated leg and attached it to the body of the dead Moor.[53]

Saints do not normally require surgical instruments to be able to work their posthumous cures, nor do they typically require a cadaver from whom to take healthy tissue. The story is a fascinating example of surgery using holy power over dead bodies not just for resurrection miracles, but also to restore health to an injured man's limb, not something secular surgeons could offer. The story's conclusion that Cosmas and Damian also restored the dead man's leg by attaching the amputated one to him, an unnecessary step for a man who had already died, might lead us to expect a resurrection miracle for the dead man, yet none is forthcoming.[54] The saints employed surgical methods, with results completely out of reach to secular surgeons, and performed in a dream with real-world effects. The *Golden Legend* flags gendered differences within the miraculous work of the saints, however: there is no similarly surgical work performed by a saintly woman.

Jacobus made it clear that faith healings worked by saints had no limitations. When Saint Basil was 'seriously ill with the malady of which he was to die, he called for a Jew named Joseph, a man highly skilled in the art of medicine'.[55] Although Basil's doctor was an expert, Basil was not interested in his medical expertise and did not ask him for any medical assistance; instead he intended to convert the healer by demonstrating the power of God. In this example, Jacobus had no criticism for Joseph's expertise, since he does not treat Basil. Instead, Basil prayed to God to delay the time of his death so as to convince Joseph of the power of Christ. Similarly, during the martyrdom of Saint James the Dismembered, the bystanders begged James to perform the required sacrifice to the pagan god so that he might live, despite the loss of his hands, since 'there are expert physicians who will be able to ease your pain!'[56] Although he acknowledged the expertise of the physicians who might be able to comfort him, James rejected the deception required to gain their

53 *GL*, II, 198. *Legenda aurea*, cxxxix, ed. Maggioni, II, 980: 'unguenta ac ferramenta secum portantes. Quorum unus alteri dixit: "Vbi carnes accipiemus ut abscissa carne putrida locum uacuum repleamus?" Tunc ait alter: "In cimiterio Sanci Petri ad uincula hodie Ethiops recens sepultus est. De illo ergo affer ut huic suppleamus". Et ecce, ad cimiterium properauit et coxam Mauri attulit. Precidentesque coxam infirmi coxam Mauri eius loco inseruerunt et plagam diligenter ungentes coxam infirmi ad corpus Mauri mortui detulerunt'.

54 The man's black skin may offer one explanation for the neglect of a miracle for him, but, this seems a missed opportunity. Laura Ingallinella is exploring a French version of the narrative that does not contain any reference to race or faith; see 'Il "miracolo della gamba nera" dei santi Cosma e Damiano: fonti e rimaneggiamenti nell'agiografia latina, greca e romanza', in *'Que ben devetz conoisser la plus fina': Per Margherita Spampinato*, ed. M. Pagano (Avellino, 2018), pp. 345–67 and the forthcoming 'Making the "Miracle of the Black Leg": Racialized Bodies in Late Medieval Hagiography'.

55 *GL*, I, 112. *Legenda aurea*, xxvi, ed. Maggioni, I, 186: 'positus in infirmitate qua et mortuus est, quendam Iudeum nomine Ioseph medicinali arte ualde peritum ... uocavit'.

56 *GL*, II, 345. *Legenda aurea*, clxx, ed. Maggioni, II, 1221: 'sint tamen peritissimi medici qui tuis doloribus ualenant subuenire'.

assistance. The martyrdom continues. While Jacobus's emphasis was on the superiority of faith, he described secular practitioners as capable and competent.

In the *Golden Legend*, saints also deny medical expertise that has been ascribed to them by others, insisting that their ability to heal does not come from human learning but, rather, from faith. In the life of Saints Barlaam and Josaphat, Jacobus clearly drew the contrast between secular and miraculous medicine. Barlaam observed that the prince's tutor had trouble with his eyes, knowledge he had 'though I'm no expert in medical matters'.[57] And in the story of the Apostle Saint James, the Emperor Vespasian insisted that Albanus must be a physician because he came from Jerusalem:

> Vespasian: 'You come from the land of the wise men, you know the art of medicine, you are a physician! You must cure me!' ... he had had some kind of worms in his nose....
>
> Albanus: 'My lord, I know nothing of medicine and therefore am unable to cure you.'
>
> Vespasian: 'Cure me or die!'
>
> Albanus: 'He who gave sight to the blind, drove out demons, and raised the dead, he knows that I have no knowledge of the art of healing.'[58]

While Albanus went on to cure Vespasian of these worms, he insisted that he did so as a believer and not as a medical expert.

The success of the saint's healing miracle would be undermined if the practitioner were unskilled or inexpert in his field; indeed, 'respect for the *medicus* in the community must have been high to make him a suitable foil for the saint'.[59] The presence of medical workers in these stories establishes, first, that the person really suffered from some malady; second, that proper medical care had been offered; and third, that the malady persisted despite the doctors' best efforts. Only in these cases could the saint's miraculous healing be recognised. Of course, Jacobus was not alone in demonstrating respect for the medical profession while also arguing for the power of the saints: in the early medieval period, Caesarius of Arles, Isidore of Seville and Cassiodorus Senator all respected the expertise and care of the secular healer and even encouraged their communities to seek such expert assistance.[60]

57 *GL*, II, 358. *Legenda aurea*, cxxxix, ed. Maggioni, II, 1242: 'Ego autem medicinalis artis non expers'.

58 *GL*, I, 273. *Legenda aurea*, lxiii, ed. Maggioni, I, 453–4: 'Cui Vespasianus: "De terra sapientum uenis, artem nosti medicaminis, medicus es, curare me debes". Vespasianus enim qoddam genus uermium naribus insitum ... gerebat ... Cui uir ille [Albanus] respondit: "Artem medicaminis domine, nescio, et ideo te curare non ualeo". Cui Vespasianus: "Nisi me curaueris, morte morieris". Cui ait ille: "Ille qui cecos illuminauit, demones effugauit, mortuos suscitauit, ille nouit quia medendi artem ignoro"'.

59 Flint, 'Early Medieval "Medicus"', p. 136.

60 Ibid., p. 132.

This tendency to contrast saints' efforts with secular healing, in order to demonstrate the power of spiritual healing, continued into the thirteenth century. By this point, canonisation inquests were emphasising testimony from medical workers who had made their failure explicit, pushing them to acknowledge that 'what had happened could not have been caused by any kind of medical intervention ... [that] the cure was made by divine power and not by medical means'.[61] The expertise of secular medical workers, who acknowledged that the person had been ill, that the best remedies had been attempted and that the only cure was miraculous, were all essential for demonstrating the saint's holy power.

Secular healers occasionally recognised that a wound was beyond their best care, as happened in the story of Francisca that was told during the canonisation proceedings of Celestine V. Francisca developed a fistula after being hit in the foot by a stone and Magister Riccardo of Sulmona refused to treat her, recognising her injury as a lost cause. Later Riccardo testified that Peter of Morrone (the future Celestine V) had healed her despite the desperation of her case.[62] Within the same proceedings, a medical doctor named Benedetto of Sulmona testified to Peter's miracles. He had reason to respect Peter's skills as a healer, since he had sought the latter's help for the blindness of his own daughter, Catania. After doctors had previously been unable to 'help her in any way', Benedetto had personally witnessed the healing miracle. Several doctors testified regarding Catania's story, confirming her blindness, their inability to heal it and the completeness of the cure that Peter of Morrone worked.[63]

The same pattern appears in unsuccessful canonisation inquests for Italian saints, whereby 'the recipients of the miracles stressed that they had first gone to a succession of doctors'.[64] Documents for Anthony Peregrinus and Facio of Cremona claimed several miracles after secular medical care had failed. Anthony healed a boy three days after an injury when 'human remedies were worth nothing', an abbot with an untreatable abscess and a man with a nerve problem.[65] Facio also cured an abscess that had plagued a woman for fourteen years. This demonstration of thaumaturgical healing was essential to arguments for sanctity.

Testimony at Delphine de Puimichel's canonisation inquest also demonstrated her holiness, superior to any healing a physician could offer. Master Laurence 'believed that

[61] Ziegler, 'Practitioners and Saints', p. 198.

[62] Ibid., p. 197. As Ziegler suggests (p. 206): 'When a medical man recognized the superiority of celestial medicine through the saint's mediation, the saint's curative omnipotence could not easily be contested by potential critics or sceptics'. See also R. Brentano, 'Sulmona Society and the Miracles of Peter of Morrone', in *Monks, Nuns, Saints and Outcasts: Religion in Medieval Society*, ed. S. Farmer and B. H. Rosenwein (Ithaca NY, 2000), pp. 79–96.

[63] Brentano, 'Sulmona Society', p. 91.

[64] J. L. Peterson, *Suspect Saints and Holy Heretics: Disputed Sanctity and Communal Identity in Late Medieval Italy* (Ithaca, 2019), pp. 25–7.

[65] Sicco Polenton, 'Vita Beati Antonii Peregrini', *Analecta Bollandiana* 13 (1894): 417–25 (p. 423): 'nihil remedia humana valebant'.

he had the epidemic illness [plague] and he knew that those who contracted the illness soon died. He also knew that against this illness no remedy had efficacy'.[66] Following a neighbour's suggestion, Laurence vowed that if he were healed he would visit the tomb of Delphine with a gift. He survived. Alazays Mesellano, for whom the 'doctors had no hope that she should be freed of the illness', similarly vowed to gift Delphine's tomb and recovered; she clearly did not share the doctors' loss of hope.[67]

As in the *vitae* and miracle tales, the canonisation testimony demonstrates that Christians faced with disease consulted doctors, but in the most hopeless cases that threatened permanent disability and death and in which the doctors could do no more, the ill turned to holy people. With them, they found their faith rewarded. Rather than competing with saints, the physicians' testimony demonstrated that the holy community solved the direst cases that went beyond the possible interventions of the medical experts. The canonisation testimony reveals this drive to demonstrate superiority over secular medicine, even in the case of a holy woman who would not otherwise enjoy medical superiority over physicians. It is worth observing, however, that the same institutionalising trend that limited women from the elite echelons of medicine also affected saints. As canonisation became a formal and papacy-controlled process with inquests and intense documentation requirements in the thirteenth century, women had a more difficult time meeting the requirement for sanctity. Delphine's case, for example, did not succeed.

Miracle stories spotlighting medical workers

Returning to the *Golden Legend*, dynamic stories about healing medicine in the text demonstrate the superiority of the saints to other practitioners. Two patients in the *Golden Legend* suffering from 'the stone' feared undergoing surgery to relieve their suffering.[68] Jacobus tells of a girl in Sicily whose

> mother, in this dangerous situation, commended her to God and Saint Dominic. The following night the saint appeared to the girl, placed in her hand the stone that had caused her so much pain, and departed. When she awoke and found herself cured … The

66 N. Archambeau, 'God Helps Those Who Help Themselves: Negotiating a Miracle in the Fourteenth-Century Canonization of Delphine de Puimichel', *Anuario de Estudios Medievales* 43 (2013), 7–25 (pp. 7–8): 'fuit febre gravatus, et nichilominus afflictus morbo vocato in vulgari *lo cat*, quo cum quis tactus erat tunc temporis, moriebatur communiter, adversus morbum illum nullo remedio prevalente'. Ultimately Delphine was not canonised, but the witness testimony follows typical patterns for such inquests.

67 J. Cambell, *Enquête pour le procès de canonisation de Dauphine de Puimichel, Comtesse d'Ariano* (Turin, 1978), p. 436: 'medici non sperarent quod deberet liberari a dicta infirmitate'; N. Archambeau, *Souls under Siege: Stories of War, Plague and Confession in Fourteenth-Century Provence* (Ithaca NY, 2021), p. 119.

68 Such fears about surgery were fair, as even the Persian physician Rhazes refused to undergo surgery for cataracts when he went blind late in life: McVaugh, *Medicine before the Plague*, p. 35.

> mother took the stone to the friars' house and, to commemorate this great miracle, [they] hung it in front of an image of Saint Dominic.[69]

Similarly, in the story of Saint Augustine, healers

> recommended that the stone [in a boy] be cut out, but the boy's mother, fearing that her son would die, invoked Augustine's aid. No sooner had she finished her prayer than the boy passed the stone with his urine and was completely cured.[70]

In both cases, the saints intervened to save the faithful from the pains and dangers of surgery, not by performing the procedure like Cosmas and Damian, but by removing the need to do so.[71] In these stories, there is no accusation that the surgeons were unskilled; the fear was all on the part of the patient or the patient's mother. Jacobus simply acknowledged that surgery was frightening and dangerous. In each of these stories, the saint demonstrates the superiority of faith over medicine. The patient is saved from having to undergo the risks of surgery, with not just the stone removed but also fear and anxiety.

One further story also suggests that there were other risks involved with surgery. Jacobus tells of a knight who was so grievously wounded in battle that his hand hung loose from his wrist. Doctors and friends advised him to have the hand amputated, but the knight, embarrassed of being maimed, instead had the hand tied in place with bandages and medicaments. He then invoked Saint Mark's aid and the injury was immediately righted, save for a scar: evidence of the miracle and a monument to the great blessing granted to the knight.[72] Here, faith saved the knight from both the dangers of surgery and the apparent shame of living as an amputee.

While miracle tales were intended to focus devotion on the saint's holy deeds, some collections also conveyed medical knowledge, such as William of Canterbury's twelfth-century collection of Thomas Becket's miracles that used a lot of medical terminology. In describing the saint's miraculous healing of kidney stones, leprosy, epilepsy, diabetes or an ulcer, William explained the nature of these problems so that his readers might both understand the medical issues involved and fully appreciate Becket's healing powers and his ability to treat 'the "causes" of disease'.[73] Rather than seeing the saint and healer as

69 *GL*, II, 56. *Legenda aurea*, cix, ed. Maggioni, II, 740: 'mater eius pro instanti periculo filiam suo Deo et beato Dominico commendauit. Sequento ergo nocte dormienti puelle beatus Dominicus astitit et in manu eius quo torquebatur lapidem posuit et abscessit; quem puella euigilans et se liberatam inueniens … Mater uero lapidem ad domum fratrum attulit et ipsum in memoriam tanti miraculi coram ymagine Dominici suspenderunt'.

70 *GL*, II, 129. *Legenda aurea*, cxxxix, ed. Maggioni, II, 861: 'incidi deberet, mater pueri mortis sibi timens periculum beatum Augustinum deuote in sui filii subsidium inuovauit. Statimque fusa oratione puer lapidem cum urina emisit et plenam sanitatem recipit'.

71 There are similar cases in *GL*, II, 126–7.

72 *GL*, I, 247.

73 Koopmans, *Wonderful to Relate*, p. 184.

opposed or competing, William connected the two roles and used one to better establish the other.

Female saints as holy healers

Female saints were also thaumaturgical healers, often outperforming their male counterparts in miracle working.[74] Many female saints' lives and miracles focused on treating injury and illness, including thaumaturgic healings, even resurrection. The holy stories of female saints such as Umiltà of Faenza also included medical knowledge superior to that offered by secular healers. In the *Golden Legend*, female saints cured, tended and treated in healing ways, but not in reference to mundane medicine. With one exception, Jacobus contrasted miraculous and secular healing only in chapters for male saints.

Chapters on female saints in the *Golden Legend* account for 19 per cent of those that discuss secular medicine in some way. Yet, in these stories on female saints, Jacobus did not contrast holy women's medical interventions with those of secular healers as he had done for the male saints. None of the *Golden Legend*'s healing miracles that were worked through the intercession of a holy woman included a reference to the medical establishment. Recipients of miracles in Jacobus's stories of holy women do not mention first seeking aid from a physician or surgeon. Only one chapter on a female saint even comes close to contrasting secular healers directly with the saint's ability: doctors advised Saint Paula to drink wine and avoid water, but she refused and nearly convinced an admonishing bishop to avoid wine as well. In the other cases, Saint Peter disguised as a physician comforted Saint Agatha, physicians diagnosed Agnes's spurned lover with lovesickness and, in the chapter on the Purification of the Virgin, physicians have different views on embryology. The *Golden Legend* describes thaumaturgical healings in the chapters on female saints and discusses charity to the poor and ill, but Jacobus avoids describing women secular healers or demonstrating female saints' healing in comparison with secular medicine. There is a similar lack of secular female healers in the canonisation proceedings.[75]

While Jacobus does not contrast female saints' miraculous power or charity with the medical work of secular practitioners, he does display similar medical interventions of these saints' significant intercessory power. Jacobus tells us that Saint Martha cured King Clovis's kidneys, Mary Magdalene helped a woman conceive and cured blindness, Savinia cured a girl of illness, Agnes cured Constance of leprosy and Elizabeth cured blindness, restored a hand and cured illness. Mary Magdalene, Christina and Elizabeth each resurrected the dead. Mary Magdalene brought a dead woman back to life after two years, which is especially impressive, and brought another a man back just long enough to make his confession. Elizabeth displayed extensive charity to the poor and sick: she bathed ill

74 See Weinstein and Bell, *Saints and Society*: while 17.5 per cent of their sample were female, 22.3 per cent of miracle-workers were female, and women comprised 27.2 per cent of those with wonder-working relics.

75 Ziegler, 'Practitioners and Saints'.

people, established a hospital for the poor and tended a woman 'with a horrible leprosy whom she bathed and put to bed, cleansing and bandaging her sores, applying remedies, trimming her fingernails, and kneeling at her feet to loosen her shoes'. Elizabeth was also severe when her advice was rejected: 'She prevailed upon the sick to confess their sins and to receive holy communion, and when one old woman flatly refused, she had her whipped to change her mind.'[76] Jacobus included these stories of holy women healing and treating the sick; he just did not reference medical workers in establishing their healing powers as he had done with male saints. This is all the more surprising, since he took seriously Saint Catherine's capacity to dispute, noting that experts in logic and rhetoric were sent to dispute with her and praised her preaching. To find such narratives for holy women, we need to go beyond the *Golden Legend*.

The story of a miraculous healing bestowed upon a petitioner only after s/he had sought the care of an earthly healer does appear in other collections of miracles worked by female saints written both before and after the *Golden Legend*. In the sixth-century life of Saint Radegund, for example, the saint healed a young girl who received medical treatment but still did not recover. A woman named Goda was ill and did not respond to medicine; much like the woman that Frideswide healed, however, Goda was miraculously cured when a candle was made to the length of her own height and lit.[77]

Saint Umiltà of Faenza's (d. 1310) life repeatedly demonstrates the saint's superior healing power over secular medical care (figure 6.2). She even healed her own body through prayer:

> One time, when she was afflicted with a tumor in her kidneys, having been assigned a nurse by the abbess (who thought that Umiltà did not want a doctor), and fearing that the stink of her wound would be disturbing to the convent, she gave herself to prayer. At once, as soon as she arose from prayer, she was cured. When the sister who had been assigned to her as a nurse, intending to treat her in the usual way, discovered that she was cured and that there was no sign of there having been any wound.[78]

Umiltà also healed her fellow nuns after all hope of success from the doctors had been lost. A sister began to bleed from her nose and all remedies proposed by physicians proved unsuccessful.

[76] *GL*, II, 311. *Legenda aurea*, clxiv, ed. Maggioni, II, 1169: 'Ipsos autem infirmos ad confessionem et communicationem inducens uetulam quandam penitus renuentem uerbere castigatam induxit'.

[77] Fortunatus, 'Vita', p. 374; see McNamara, ed., 'Life', p. 84.

[78] M-A. Stouck, ed., *Medieval Saints: A Reader* (Toronto, 1998), p. 456; 'De S. Humilitate Abbatissa Ordinis Vallumbrosani Florentiae', *Acta sanctorum quotquot toto orbe coluntur vel a catholicis scriptoribus celebrantur*, 68 vols. (Brussels, 1863–87) [hereafter *AASS*], May V, 206: 'Dum quodam tempore cancro quodam graviter in renibus esset laesa, tenendo (ut aestimabat) quia medicum nolebat, curatricem deputatam ab Abbatissa; ne foetore gravaretur Conventus, orationi se dedit: a qua surgens confestim sanata fuit. Et tum Soror, quae sibi ab Abbatissa in curatricem data fuerat, more solito curare eam volens, ipsam sic sanatam reperit, ac si nulla ibi laesio unquam fuerit'.

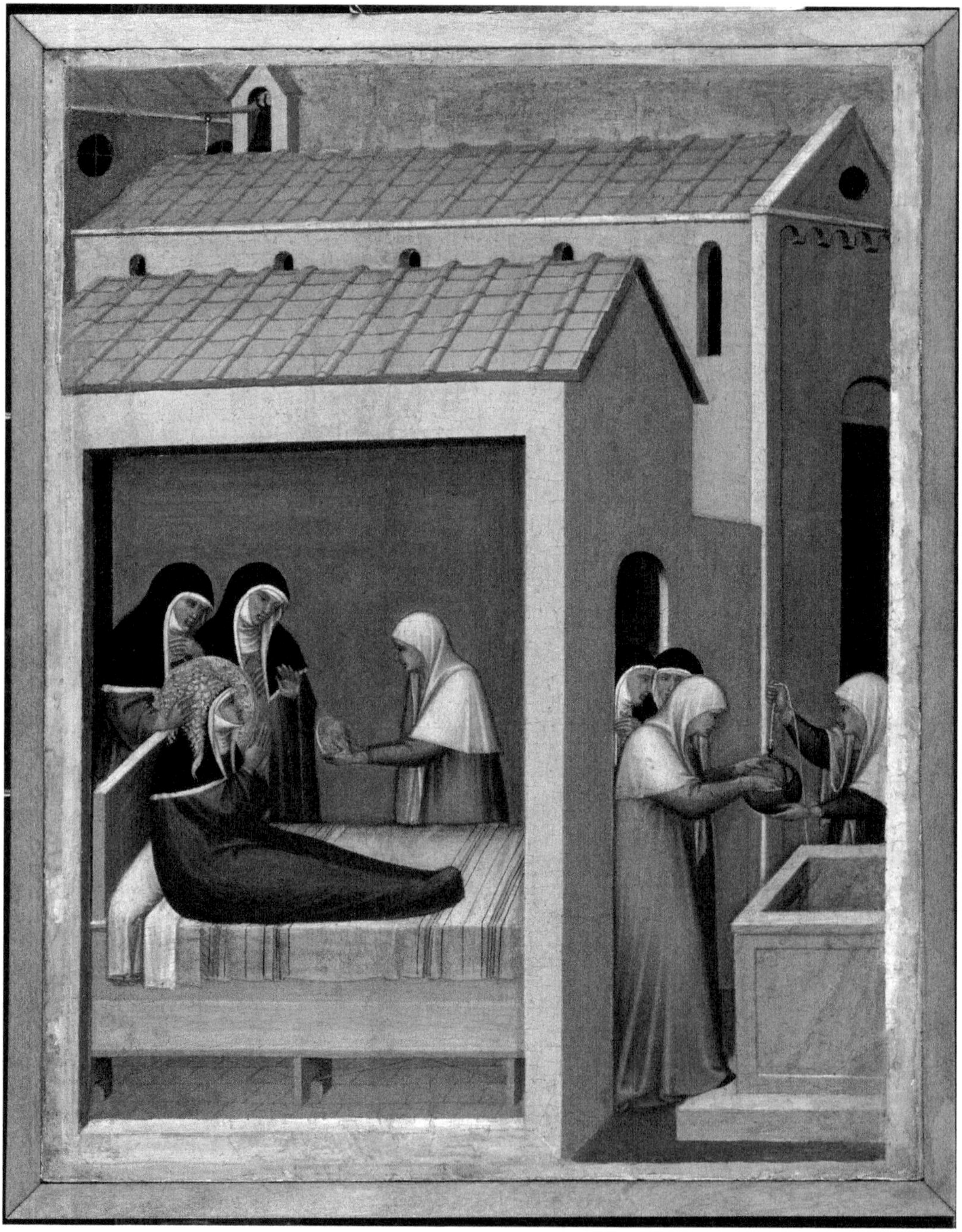

Fig. 6.2. The ice miracle of Saint Humilitas, panel by Pietro Lorenzetti, c. 1341 Gemäldegalerie der Staatlichen Museen zu Berlin, Creative Commons Attribution–NonCommercial–ShareAlike 3.0 Germany (CC BY-NC-SA 3.0 DE).

> When the pious nurse Umiltà heard this, as was her custom, she sweetly invoked the supreme physician, made the sign of the cross over her, and at once the sister was completely cured, with all her strength restored.[79]

She likewise offered treatment to pilgrims who had been given grave sentences from the surgeon. A man who was supposed to have his foot amputated was healed by her touch.

Similarly, Saint Christina the Astonishing (d. 1224) demonstrated her holy power by resisting the ministrations of a secular healer. After a man broke Christina's leg, her sisters hired a healer who bound her broken shinbone with medicated bandages. 'After the physician had left, she drew off the bandages since she thought it shameful to have any doctor for her wounds but Jesus Christ'. According to Christina's *vita*, Jesus indeed healed her and 'healed from all hurt, she walked … and danced … and praised and blessed him for whom alone she had chose to live or die'.[80] These saints not only healed, they provided cures that were beyond the means of even the most competent medical workers, male or female.[81]

Female saints thus were not only healers: their superior healing explicitly contrasted with secular treatments. The fact that Jacobus did not use the same topos of the superior healer for women, despite the appearance of that theme elsewhere in female saints' narratives, likely results from his role as a thirteenth-century elite male cleric, a Dominican and an archbishop of Genoa. His stories of female saints demonstrate great respect for them, including their healing powers, but he wrote at a time of transition where medical expertise and high-status sainthood were both becoming entrenched as male prerogatives. He rested women's authority as saints in their virginity and suffering, while emphasising the superior expertise of holy men.

Conclusion

References to healers in miracle stories like those included in the *Golden Legend* took a variety of forms, but Jacobus's stories portrayed physicians respectfully. The failure of secular healers' very best efforts left the saint room to demonstrate the superior healing ability of Christ and his intercessors – not because the medicine had failed, but because

79 Stouck, *Medieval Saints*, 460–61; 'De S. Humilitate Abbatissa Ordinis Vallumbrosani Florentiae', p. 209: 'Quod dum nutrix pia persensit, summum medicum dulciter ex more advocans, super eam signum Crucis indidit, et confestim resumptis viribus plenissime curate fuit'.

80 Stouck, *Medieval Saints*, 441; Thomas of Cantimpré, 'De S. Christina Mirabili Virg. Apud Trudonopolim in Belgio', *AASS* July V, 653: 'medico recedente, apposita detrahebat, indignum ducens alium suis plagis medicum adhiberi praeter Salvatorem nostrum Jesum Christum … sanata ab omni incommodo, per aream cellarii deambulabat ac tripudians, laudans et benedicens illum, cui soli mori et vivere delegisset'.

81 In some cases, though, people who threatened the saint's shrine or ignored her orders could find themselves ill, paralysed or worse. Saint Æthelthryth (d. 679) specialized in this sort of healing/cursing punishment. See Paxton, 'Book of Ely'.

no earthly medicine could help. Jacobus was writing at the same time that medical licensing and expectations for university educations were limiting women's access to medical fields *and* as canonisation inquests formalised that process, making it harder for women to become saints. This context may explain why Jacobus's text used medicine to emphasise male holy power but did not do the same for female saints, despite that topos appearing in other female saints' narratives written both before and after the *Golden Legend*. These investigations increasingly valued the testimony of medical practitioners to support claims for miraculous cures. By depicting physicians positively and respecting their expertise, Jacobus's readings also supported the testimony of physicians in such trials.

Moreover, since the *Golden Legend* circulated broadly around the Mediterranean world, Jacobus's positive valuation of medical workers – who were bested at their best only by the power of God – might influence much of the Christian population to respect not only the holy power of saints but also the medical expertise of physicians. Thus, rather than competing with medical healing, Jacobus's discussion of holy miracles uses both medical healing and spiritual healing to demonstrate the possible treatments available to the sick and wounded in medieval communities.

Holy women devoted themselves to the care of the sick without regard for their own safety or health, and their charitable sacrifice demonstrated sanctity in an age without the martyrdom of persecution. Saints nursed the ill by washing their wounds, applying ointments, preparing healing potions and bandaging their limbs. As conduits of holy power, these women performed holy miracles, healing petitioners who sought their care in life or after death. Saints worked such cures at their shrine or in dreams and without the limitations of secular healing. Although women were also earthly medical practitioners engaged as physicians, surgeons, apothecaries and midwives, such women did not receive the respect given their male peers, nor were they able to attain the heights of their fields. Female saints received great respect as healers, however, even if their authority was not always represented in the same ways as that of their holy male colleagues. Including saints who healed within our definition of 'medical workers' better fits the practice of medieval Christians and demonstrates the respect accorded to women treating disease, disability and even death in medieval Europe, while attending to these distinctions reveals the operation of patriarchy even in holy communities.

7

Infirmity and Death Wishes in Medieval French and Italian Canonisation Processes

JENNI KUULIALA[1]

A vast majority of miracles recorded in late medieval Europe were cures. There was a culturally established pattern for a proper miracle narrative, and various emotions were used to highlight its central aspects. A core element of a miracle was the presence of a severe situation that no human remedy or assistance could resolve. Other important features were the idea to ask the saint for assistance, the actual petition, the miracle and, finally, its joyous aftermath. In terms of healing miracles, the dire situation was typically a fatal illness, accident or chronic/long-term infirmity that caused the patient significant functional hindrances, pain and/or other discomfort. The narratives often point to the severity of the situation by referring to the emotions it caused for the future 'miraculé' (miraculously cured person) and/or for his or her family members. At the same time, hope and trust in the saint's ability to help were inherent in the narratives. Personal devotion, including a firm belief in the saint's powers, was crucial for obtaining a miraculous cure. Eventually, proper devotion resulted in the hoped-for situation – the miracle and its aftermath – followed by great joy and gratitude.[2]

By nature, miracle narratives are therefore emotional scripts. In her book on medieval affective meditation, Sarah McNamer defines such scripts as 'quite literally scripts for the performance of feeling'.[3] Miracle narratives are a different type of source than affective literature, but some clearly were meant for public or private reading. They are also known

1 The writing of this chapter has been funded by the Academy of Finland Centre of Excellence in the History of Experiences, Faculty of Social Sciences, Tampere University. I wish to thank Ville Vuolanto and the editors of this volume for their insightful comments.

2 The narrative pattern of a miracle has been analysed in S. Andrić, *Miracles of St. John Capistran* (Budapest, 2000), pp. 228–38; M. Goodich, *Miracles and Wonders: The Development of the Concept of Miracle, 1150–1350* (Aldershot, 2007), pp. 93–9; G. Klaniczay, 'Miracoli di punizione e *malefi- cia*', in *Miracoli: Dai segni alla storia*, ed. S. B. Gajano and M. Modica (Rome, 2000), pp. 109–36. See also J. Kuuliala, 'Proving Misfortune, Proving Sanctity. Reconstructing Physical Impairment in Fourteenth-Century Miracle Testimonies', in *Miracles in Canonization Processes: Structures, Functions, and Methodologies*, ed. C. Krötzl and S. Katajala-Peltomaa (Turnhout, 2018), pp. 197–226.

3 S. McNamer, *Affective Meditation and the Invention of Medieval Compassion* (Philadelphia, 2010), p. 12. See also J. Hillmann, 'Internal Theater and Emotional Scripts in French Jesuit Meditative Literature', in *Affective and Emotional Economies in Medieval and Early Modern Europe*, Palgrave

to have been popular topics for dinner-table conversations and other social situations.[4] The circulating stories guided people in their emotional practices and in the ways they later reported their experiences.

In this chapter, I discuss one rare but striking way that the need for a healing miracle was presented: a wish that the infirm person would die. Most often these wishes appeared in descriptions that emphasised the severity of the 'miraculé's' medical condition. There is also a small group of cases in which the petitioner asked the saint to liberate them or their children from their infirmity to either a healthy state or death. These narratives put the emotions of the persons involved in focus in an unconcealed, obvious manner. In what kinds of situations were such expectations and sentiments recorded? Whose emotions and sentiments were central for the miraculous? What might have prompted the death wishes? I also address here the connection between these wishes and communal devotional practices.

The source material consists of canonisation inquest documents recorded between the thirteenth and fifteenth centuries, in the areas of present-day France and Italy. Canonisation processes were conducted by the papacy from the early thirteenth century in order to investigate a putative saint's life, merits and deeds.[5] During the inquests, dozens or even hundreds of people, clerics, nuns and laypeople alike were interrogated under oath about the holy man or woman's life and miracles. The witnesses were not allowed to recite their memories freely, but were, rather, interrogated by the papal commissioners, usually following a ready-made list of questions.[6] These lists contained the elements included in the cultural pattern of a miracle, enhancing its significance and giving space for the expression of emotions. Often an interpreter was needed to translate between the interrogator and the witness, while a notary translated the depositions from vernacular languages into Latin.[7] The resulting documents thus reflect the views of the witnesses and cultural ideas

Studies in the History of Emotions, ed. A. Marculescu and C.-L. Morand Métivier (Cham, 2018), pp. 143–66, for the usage of this concept.

4 See S. Yarrow, 'Narrative, Audience and the Negotiation of Community in Twelfth-Century English Miracle Collections', in *Elite and Popular Religion*, ed. K. Cooper and J. Gregory, Studies in Church History (Woodbridge, 2006), pp. 65–77 (pp. 74–5).

5 The practicalities and legal developments of canonisation processes have been most comprehensively studied in G. Klaniczay, ed., *Procès de canonisation au Moyen Âge. Aspects juridiques et religieux* (Rome, 2004); R. Paciocco, *Canonizzazioni e culto dei santi nella* christianitas *(1198–1302)* (Assisi, 2006); A. Vauchez, *La sainteté en Occident aux derniers siècles du Moyen Âge. D'après les procès de canonisation et les documents hagiographiques* (Rome, 1988 [1981]); T. Wetzstein, *Heilige vor Gericht. Das Kanonisationserfahren im europäischen Spätmittelalter* (Cologne, 2004).

6 The practicalities of testifying about miracles have recently been analysed in C. Krötzl and S. Katajala-Peltomaa, ed., *Miracles in Canonization Processes: Structures, Functions, and Methodologies* (Turnhout, 2018).

7 C. Krötzl, 'Prokuratoren, Notare und Dolmetscher. Zu Gestaltung und Ablauf der Zeugeneinvernahmen bei spätmittelalterlichen Kanonisationsprozessen', *Hagiographica* 5 (1998), 119–40.

about the miraculous,[8] but these aspects are available to us only through the juridical and theological requirements of the process. Any analysis must focus on the interpretations, memories and retellings of the events as they were formed in the interaction between the various parties involved in the inquest.

In canonisation testimonies, illness and disability[9] intermingle with lived religion, which sees religion as a communal space in which people participated and performed their social roles.[10] These social roles include the performance not only of various religious rituals but also of appropriate emotions, sentiments and reactions, which were, as noted above, important aspects in the veneration of saints. Research on medieval disability has shown that people with various impairments were not automatically excluded from societal activities; rather, they were often productive members of their communities.[11] However, as the following analysis demonstrates, conditions that we would label as chronic illnesses or disabilities today could also be associated with sentiments such as grief and anguish, occasionally even abhorrence or shame. These sentiments are not just negative, but they helped with obtaining the miracle, an important event for the whole community, and particularly for strengthening the social importance of the person invoking the saint.[12]

In the testimonies, death wishes intermingle with caretaking of the severely infirm. They also overlap with the role medical practitioners played in forming emotions related to the miraculous. As Barbara H. Rosenwein concludes in her seminal work *Emotional Communities in the Early Middle Ages*, no equivalent term for emotion existed in medieval writing. Furthermore, although many medieval terms for various emotions are basically

8 See M. Goodich, '*Mirabilis Deus in sanctis suis*. Social History and Medieval Miracles', in *Signs, Wonders, Miracles: Representations of Divine Power in the Life of Church*, ed. K. Cooper and J. Gregory (Woodbridge, 2005), pp. 135–56, for finding witnesses' voices in the testimonies.

9 The term 'disability', especially in its modern, political and cultural sense, did not exist in the Middle Ages. Various health issues were labelled as *infirmitates*, infirmities. J. Kuuliala, *Childhood Disability and Social Integration in the Middle Ages: Constructions of Impairments in Thirteenth- and Fourteenth-Century Canonization Processes* (Turnhout, 2016), pp. 32–43; I. Metzler, *Disability in Medieval Europe: Thinking about Physical Impairment during the High Middle Ages, c.1100–1400*, (London, 2006), pp. 4–5; H.-W. Goetz, 'Vorstellungen von menschlicher Gebrechlichkeit in frühen Mittelalter', in *Homo debilis. Behinderte – Kranke – Versehrte in der Gesellschaft des Mittelalters*, ed. C. Nolte (Affalterbach, 2009), pp. 21–55.

10 S. Katajala-Peltomaa and R. M. Toivo, 'Religion as an Experience', in *Lived Religion and the Long Reformation in Northern Europe c. 1300–1700* (Leiden, 2016), pp. 1–19.

11 On medieval disability, see, for example, J. R. Eyler, ed., *Disability in the Middle Ages. Reconsiderations and Reverberations* (Aldershot, 2010); Kuuliala, *Childhood Disability*; Metzler, *Disability in Medieval Europe*; I. Metzler, *A Social History of Disability: Cultural Considerations of Physical Impairment* (London, 2013); C. Nolte, ed., *Homo debilis. Behinderte – Kranke – Versehrte in der Gesellschaft des Mittelalters* (Affalterbach, 2009); W. J. Turner and T. Vandeventer Pearman, ed., *The Treatment of Disabled Persons in Medieval Europe: Examining Disability in the Historical, Legal, Literary, Medical, and Religious Discourses* (Lewiston, 2010).

12 See L. A. Smoller, 'Miracle, Memory, and Meaning in the Canonization of Vincent Ferrer, 1453–54', *Speculum* 73 (1998), 429–54.

translatable, they had a variety of meanings and connotations that only partly overlap with modern concepts.[13] In terms of the expressions of grief and desperation that are at the core of the death wishes examined in this chapter, it is important to focus on socially sanctioned ways of expressing emotions and reactions. Following Monique Scheer's conceptualisation in 'Are Emotions a Kind of Practice',[14] I primarily approach the witnesses' sentiments as ritual practices and devotional expressions.

The sentiments and wishes analysed in this chapter pertain to medieval ideas about curability and incurability.[15] In order to receive and prove a healing miracle, physicians (or other healers) had to be unable to help. In other words, the condition had to be incurable. At the same time, there was always the possibility that divine help existed and could be received; yet the petitioner also had to believe that the saint was able to heal the condition (recognising, of course, that in the end it depended on God).[16] As Mary Lindemann has pointed out, the various practices of healthcare and healing must be taken seriously in research and 'on their own terms';[17] for the people being discussed here, a miracle cure was indeed a possibility. Although the lived reality was most likely more diverse and people simultaneously sought help from various healing agents (physicians, apothecaries, folk healers, saints, etc.), the narrative structure of a miracle required proof that earthly healing attempts had proven futile and were no longer used after a petition to the saint had been made.[18]

Expecting death, hoping for cure

In any analysis of canonisation documents, language and translation are crucial issues that must be taken into account. It is possible that translations were closer to the witnesses' words when they spoke a Romance language, but we have no evidence of this. Therefore, it

13 B. H. Rosenwein, *Emotional Communities in the Early Middle Ages* (Ithaca, 2007), pp. 3–4. See also N. Archambeau, 'Tempted to Kill: Miraculous Consolation for a Mother after the Death of Her Infant Daughter', in *Emotions and Health, 1200–1700*, ed. E. Carrera (Leiden, 2013), pp. 47–66 (pp. 48–9), for the problem of terminology when studying emotions in hagiographic texts.

14 M. Scheer, 'Are Emotions a Kind of Practice (And Is That What Makes Them Have a History)? A Bourdieuian Approach to Understanding Emotion', *History and Theory*, 51 (2012), 193–220.

15 See Metzler, *Social History of Disability*, p. 6; Metzler, *Disability in Medieval Europe*, p. 71, on the problem of the concept, especially in its medical sense.

16 See, for example, N. Siraisi, *Medieval and Early Renaissance Medicine. An Introduction to Knowledge and Practice* (Chicago, 2009), p. 42.

17 M. Lindemann, *Medicine and Society in Early Modern Europe* (Cambridge, 2010), p. 86.

18 The versatility of treatments available has been called medical pluralism; see especially D. Gentilcore, *Healers and Healing in Early Modern Italy* (Manchester, 1998). For the requirement that no medical help was used after a petition to the saint, see L. Ackerman Smoller, 'Defining the Boundaries of the Natural in Fifteenth-Century Brittany: The Inquest into the Miracles of Saint Vincent Ferrer (d. 1419)', *Viator* 28 (1997), 333–60 (pp. 345–7); C. Krötzl, 'Saints, Healing and Communities in the Later Middle Ages: On Roles and Perceptions', in *Infirmity in Antiquity and the Middle Ages: Social and Cultural Approaches to Health, Weakness and Care*, ed. C. Krötzl, K. Mustakallio and J. Kuuliala (Aldershot, 2015), pp. 255–64.

is impossible to know exactly what words the witnesses used as they described their sentiments, or even whether the interpreters and notaries had fully understood the witnesses' innermost meanings.

The issue of vocabulary and language is concretised in the depositions that used the Latin word 'sperare' (to expect). In the 1377 Breton canonisation inquest of Duke Charles of Blois, the word is frequently used to denote difficult situations in which the saint's assistance was gravely needed. The nobleman Gaufridus Budes testified about the cure of an 'armiger' (armour-bearer) who was badly hurt in a battle against the English: a spear broke a vein in his neck. Gaufridus paraphrased the words of a surgeon who gave a poor prognosis (figure 7.1). The expression the testimony records is 'ac magis sperabatur de morte ipsius, quam de vita'. This, like other similar statements, could be translated as 'expecting his death rather than him staying alive'.[19] Here, as in other similar cases in Charles's canonisation process, the word 'sperare' was used in situations in which the illness or injury was so severe that the consensus was that the patient could not survive – at least not without divine intervention. Similarly, in the mid-fifteenth-century Breton hearing of St Vincent Ferrer, a woman was expected/feared to die of plague ('sperabatur ipsam mori') because everyone else in the village with similar symptoms had died. In the same hearing, a pregnant woman was reportedly expected ('sperabat') to die of her infirmity without a doubt ('sine dubio').[20]

Such examples and expressions are repeated throughout the documents. They had a clear purpose: to demonstrate that death was the expected outcome and that while all hope for *human* remedy was lost,[21] that of divine help was omnipresent. In medieval thinking, despair was considered to be a sin when it denoted denying God's mercy. It therefore directly opposed confession. Yet the word itself had different connotations. According to Alexander Murray, the type of 'desperatio' (despair) that appeared in miracle narratives was the despair of the present, the 'failure of some perfectly concrete and carnal hope'.[22] While the verb 'sperare' denoted an expected or feared outcome and was used when the patient's condition was considered to be fatal, 'desperatio' – or rather the verb 'desperare' (to despair) – was associated both with fatal illnesses and with situations that could be labelled as (feared) permanent disability.

As an example of the former, a physician named Amadasius testified in St Nicholas of Tolentino's inquest, held in Tolentino and Marches in 1325, about the attempted but failed cure of a nobleman suffering from fever. He stated that the three doctors who had

19 Vatican City, Biblioteca Apostolica Vaticana, MS Vat. lat. 4025, fol. 122r–v. See also MS Vat. lat. 4025, fols. 131v, 142r, 142v, 159r, 174v, 175r, 177r for the usage of similar expressions.

20 P.-H. Fages, ed., *Procès de la canonisation de saint Vincent Ferrier pour faire suite à l'histoire du même saint* (Paris, 1904), pp. 73, 78, 83, 221.

21 The verb 'sperare' was not the only one used in such situations, as 'dubitare' (to suspect) and 'credere' (to believe) were also used. See, for example, N. Occhioni, ed., *Il processo per la canonizzazione di S. Nicola da Tolentino* (Rome, 1984), p. 595, where a man testified that it was suspected he would much more probably die than live ('quasi dubitabatur potius de morte quam de vita').

22 A. Murray, *Suicide in the Middle Ages; Volume 2: The Curse on Self-Murder* (Oxford, 2010), p. 374.

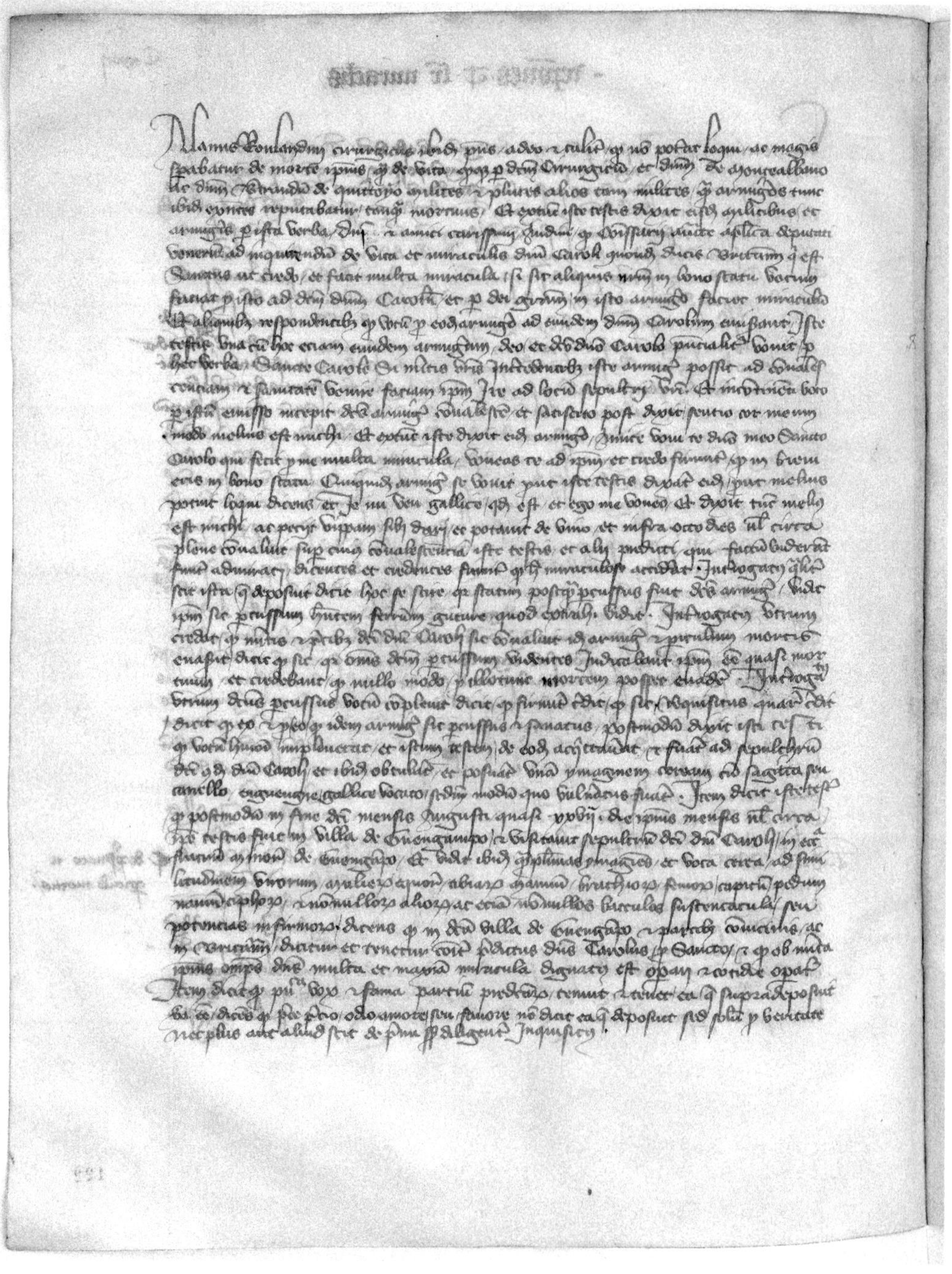

Fig. 7.1. Page from the Breton canonisation inquest of Duke Charles of Blois in 1377, including the testimony of Gaufridus Budes. Vatican City, Biblioteca Apostolica Vaticana, MS Vat. lat. 4025, fol. 122v.

tried to cure him had given up on him ('de eo desperaverant').[23] A similar expression related to physicians' verdict was recorded in the canonisation process of St Louis of Toulouse (Marseille, 1308). Micholana de Rocaforti, a Cistercian nun eventually cured of spasms that had prevented her from taking care of herself, stated that she 'did not expect to receive her health because physicians said that there was no hope of her recovery' ('immo erat desperata de sanitate sua, pro eo quia medici dicebant quod nulla spes erat de sua convalescentia').[24] The word 'desperata' again relates to the prognosis. The question was not about despair in the sense that Micholana had given up hope that God and the saints had the ability to help, but, rather, that humans had any ability to cure her.

Regardless of their wording, such statements by physicians, as well as the references to their verdicts by other witnesses, had the purpose of underscoring the saint's power. Physicians' scientific expertise helped to prove that the miraculously cured condition was incurable by their methods.[25] This does not mean that they were considered incompetent, but quite the opposite – they had done their best and a physician was not even supposed to promise too much.[26] The fact that they had given up – and the sentiments that their verdict of incurability caused – therefore proved and prompted a miracle. Witnesses tended to place the invocation and the miracle at the most difficult moment:[27] the patient or their family members had ceased to believe or expect that a mundane cure could be found and, as their last resort, had decided to invoke a heavenly healer.

For severe illnesses that were considered fatal, it is of course possible that in some cases 'sperare' included an expectation or a wish for the patient's death, but this is usually impossible to deduce.[28] The pregnant Breton woman mentioned above is an exception, since her death would have doomed her unborn child to perdition. Illnesses such as plague or a

23 Occhioni, *Il processo*, p. 579.

24 'Processus canonizationis S. Ludovici ep. Tolosani', in *Analecta Franciscana sive chronica aliaque varia documenta, Tomus VII. Processus Canonizationis et Legendae variae Sancti Ludovici O. F. M. Episcopi Tolosani*, ed. Collegio S. Bonaventura (Quaracchi, 1951), pp. 1–269 (p. 210). Another witness to the same miracle, a 'beguina devota' (Beguine) Stephania de Rotgerio, used a similar expression when referring to her own sentiment, saying that she herself did not expect that Micholana would regain her health and considered her illness incurable. 'Processus canonizationis S. Ludovici ep. Tolosani', p. 213.

25 Vauchez, *La sainteté*, p. 549.

26 See D. Lett, '*Judicium Medicine* and *Judicium Sanctitatis*. Medical Doctors in the Canonization Process of Nicholas of Tolentino (1325): Experts Subject to the Inquisitorial Logic', in *Church and Belief in the Middle Ages: Popes, Saints, and Crusaders*, ed. S. Katajala-Peltomaa and K. Salonen (Amsterdam, 2016), pp. 153–70; J. Ziegler, 'Practitioners and Saints: Medical Men in Canonization Processes in the Thirteenth to Fifteenth Centuries', *Social History of Medicine* 12 (1999), 191–225 (especially p. 217).

27 Smoller, 'Defining the Boundaries', p. 345.

28 One list of translations for the word has been provided in C. du Cange et al., *Glossarium mediae et infimae latinitatis*, 10 vols. (Niort, 1883–87), VII, 552a–b; the translations in du Cange's *Glossarium* are not, however, based on the same documents analysed in this chapter.

severe wound were known to be mostly fatal. If the expectation that the patient would die included a wish that it would happen soon, it was undoubtedly caused by the community's wish that the suffering be shortened. However, as these narratives are about miracles, there was always an element of hope that the person would be healed and survive once a petition was made to the saint. Retrospectively, the hope was also realistic, since it had resulted in the miracle. We can only guess how many people invoked saints in vain, with no response to their lingering hope for a miraculous cure.[29]

Wishing for a child's death

Occasionally the death wish was explicitly stated and the reasons specified. In these testimonies, the witness quite clearly stated that death was a better option than a situation in which the chronically ill or disabled patient would continue to suffer. The anxieties and worries of the witness, who was always a family member, were the primary grounds for their sentiments. As an example, in Cesena in 1253 or 1254, a man named Ugolinus gave testimony in the canonisation inquest of Italian hermit John Buoni. Ugolinus recounted that his son, Dalborgus, had suffered for eight years from a very large hump on his neck. The hump caused the boy a great deal of 'anxiety and tribulations' ('ansietatem et tribulationem'), preventing him from working or taking care of most tasks. Due to the 'ansietas' (anxiety) that he suffered, Dalborgus made so much noise while in bed that no one in the house could sleep.[30]

Ugolinus took his son to various physicians in Cesena and Rimini, but that was futile. Given all this, Ugolinus 'desired more the death of his son Dalborgus than him being afflicted in such a way' ('Unde cum dictus testis potius affectaret dictum filium suum Dalborgum mortuum, quam sic tribulatum'). Furthermore, he testified that he did not know what to do, except that he wanted to die because of his pain ('dolor'). Eventually, Ugolinus told Dalborgus to go to John Buoni, who was still alive at the time, stating that if that did not help, he would send his son to a monastery because he was unable to live in the world. Dalborgus met John Buoni, was given some bread by the brothers of his order and thus was healed. Dalborgus himself gave a more specific description of his symptoms: the hump made his breathing laborious and also caused the noise he made while sleeping. His narration is otherwise quite similar to that of his father, but it lacks the emphasis on anxiety and pain and does not refer to any death wishes.

More testimonies with similar wishes appear in John Buoni's process than in any other. A man named Bartholomaeus, whose two-year-old son suffered from an epilepsy-like

[29] On the undoubtedly large number of petitioners who were left without a miraculous cure and whose stories were never recorded, see J. Arnold, *Belief and Unbelief in Medieval Europe* (New York, 2005), pp. 86, 94, 222; R. C. Finucane, *Miracles and Pilgrims. Popular Beliefs in Medieval England* (New York, 1995 [1977]), pp. 81–3; Vauchez, *La sainteté*, pp. 530–1.

[30] *Acta sanctorum quotquot toto orbe coluntur vel a catholicis scriptoribus celebrantur*, 68 vols. (Brussels, 1863–87) [hereafter *AASS*] Oct, IX, 823–4.

paralysis, stated in the same hearing that during the seizures he (the son) emitted foam and looked like a monster ('emittebat spumam et erat tunc quoddam monstrum ad videndum'). Bartholomaeus preferred his son's death to his staying alive ('ipse testis potius dilexisset illum filium suum mortuum quam vivum'). A neighbour further testified that the father had said that the child was not worth a denar and therefore he preferred the boy's death ('quod non habebat carum dictum filium suum, quasi in valorem unius denarii, immo potius eum mortuum affectabat').[31] Here the father's reported sentiment is mainly one of repulsion, perhaps even a failure of an offspring who did not fulfil expectations. The boy's mother, Honesta, testified that she could not stand to watch her son during his seizures because of the great pain it caused ('pro nimio dolore non poterat sustinere videre eum'). She further added that she did not know what to do with her son, since medical means did not help; she too rather wished to see him dead than vexed in such a manner ('dicta testis nesciret, quid faceret de dicto filio suo, imo potius voluisset eum vidisse mortuum quam sic tribulatum'). Eventually the couple decided to make a 'votum' (vow) to John Buoni and the boy was healed.[32] The mother's deposition clearly states that the reason for her wish was precisely the suffering of the child and her own helplessness. At the same time, the narration shows that the couple decided to act together at the moment they both had reached their ultimate state of helplessness.

A sense of helplessness is evident also in the testimony of a woman named Benvenuta. She described the miraculous cure of her stepdaughter Cancellaria, who had suffered from severe fistulas between the ages of three and eighteen. After several physicians had pronounced the girl withered and ruined and her condition impossible to cure ('medici dicebant eam marcidam et adeo corruptam quod numquam poterat liberari'), Benvenuta did not expect Cancellaria to recover and preferred her death ('desperata de convalescentia ejus, imo potius affectabat eam mori').[33] In her own testimony, Cancellaria, who had become a nun, did not refer to such wishes, nor did the other women who had travelled with the two women to John Buoni's shrine.[34] That a verdict of incurability could prompt such wishes is also stated in the testimony of Guilia, the mother of a severely disabled three-year-old child. She testified that after hearing that the girl would remain 'contracta' (crippled), she 'wanted to die and said that she wished her daughter were dead' ('dicta testis cum audiebat hoc, volebat mori, et dicebat: Utinam mortua esses, filia mi').[35] She did not specify who had convinced her of the girl's incurability by earthly means. Her

31 *AASS* Oct, IX, 879. A neighbour woman Bellavicina testified about her own reactions to the child's infirmity in quite a different manner. She said it was a 'mirabilis compassio' (wonderful compassion) to see the small child's body with so much tribulation and suffering. Ibid., p. 880.

32 Ibid.

33 *AASS* Oct IX, 870.

34 During their pilgrimage to Cesena, they travelled by boat to Ravenna and then walked from there. They had a neighbour woman Bona, who was blind, with them and Benvenuta paid for her journey. Bona was also cured at the shrine. Ibid. pp. 870–1.

35 Ibid., p. 827.

son testified that everyone in the house wished the girl would die because she looked like a monster on the ground ('potius affectarent eam mortuam quam sic vivam, imo mors ejus fuisset gaudium omnibus de domo, quia videbatur dicta Agnese quoddam monstrum super terram').[36] The mother and son's statements appear to reflect somewhat different connotations and causes, but the notarial process may be the reason for this. Overall, the testimonies highlight the importance of communal and medical consensus regarding curability. Relatives and neighbours played a crucial role in defining an infirm bodily state and in making the decision to ask for the help of a saint.[37] Similarly, in addition to individual experience, communal opinion also defined health.[38]

It was usually the parents or other family members of severely disabled children who made statements about death wishes. In only one case that I have found is their reason directly stated to have been only about the child's suffering. A thirty-year-old man named Guilliermus di Colle Alto testified in Peter of Morrone's (Celestine V) inquest (Sulmona, 1306) about his own cure more than a decade earlier. He had a severe inflammation in his right knee, which made the whole leg 'lost and powerless' ('perditum et impotens'). The 'medici' (physicians) were of the opinion that surgeons should cauterise the leg. Guilliermus's parents, however, preferred that he would remain ill and die rather than having to bear him going through the operation ('magis volebant eum quasi derelictum longo tempore ipsam infirmitatem pati et mori ex ea quam sustinere possent quod ferro abscideretur').[39] Cauterisation was one of the most feared and painful medical procedures in the Middle Ages,[40] but here too we also witness the view that parents were responsible for finding a cure for their infirm children.[41]

In all other examples, like in those from John Buoni's inquest discussed earlier, death wishes can be interpreted as the ultimate epitome of the parents' (or other family members')

36 Ibid., p. 828.

37 For example, S. Katajala-Peltomaa, 'Gender, Networks, and Collaboration: Pilgrimages in Fourteenth-Century Canonization Processes', in *De Amicitia. Friendship and Social Networks in Antiquity and the Middle Ages*, ed. K. Mustakallio and C. Krötzl (Rome, 2011), pp. 231–43.

38 Finucane, *Miracles and Pilgrims*, p. 73.

39 *Il Processo di canonizzazione di Celestino V*, ed. A. Marini, 2 vols. (Florence, 2015–16), II, 36–9.

40 For cauterisation, see, for example, Finucane, *Miracles and Pilgrims*, p. 61; Siraisi, *Medieval and Early Renaissance Medicine*, pp. 116–18, 161–2. Medical professionals seem often to have been reluctant to perform such drastic operations. Ziegler, 'Practitioners and Saints', p. 223.

41 L. Haas, *Renaissance Man and His Children: Childbirth and Early Childhood in Florence, 1300–1600* (New York, 1998), p. 162. In hagiographic material, however, the primary nurturing role was more often the mother's. R. C. Finucane, *The Rescue of the Innocents: Endangered Children in Medieval Miracles* (New York, 2000), pp. 99–100; S. Katajala-Peltomaa, *Gender, Miracles and Daily Life: The Evidence of Fourteenth-Century Canonization Processes* (Turnhout, 2009), especially pp. 115–20; D. Lett, *L'enfant des miracles: Enfance et société au Moyen Âge (XIIe–XIIIe siècle)* (Paris, 1997), p. 141. In Scandinavian miracles, the father's role appears more active than in the southern European ones: S. Katajala-Peltomaa, 'Masculinity and Lived Religion in Late Medieval Sweden', *Scandinavian Journal of History* 38 (2013), 223–44.

pain over the child's condition, caused by a mixture of the child's suffering and their own weariness or even shame. Benedictus Thomasii de Sulmona testified in Peter of Morrone's hearing held in Sulmona in 1306 that he had wished for his 'crippled' ('contractus') son's death because he found him abominable ('ipsi testi dictus filius suus abhominabilis adeo, quod pocius mortem quam uitam eius desiderabat').[42] Blacacius, the eldest son of a 'miles' (soldier) and therefore the future guardian of his sister Rixenda, a girl eventually cured of deafness, stated in Louis of Toulouse's hearing that it was believed her deafness could not be cured ('credebat quod nullo modo posset a dicta surditate curari') and that everybody in the house had wished for the girl's death because they were ashamed of her deafness ('verecundabantur quod ita erat surda, ita quod magis vellent mortem quam vitam eius').[43] These accounts appear rather gruesome to modern sensibilities. Psychological studies on modern Western societies, however, have shown a variety of parental emotions and thoughts upon hearing about their child's serious disability; these include grief, guilt and frustration.[44] I have argued elsewhere that reports of such sentiments in miracle testimonies usually derive from parents' or other caretakers' troubles in fulfilling their social roles as guardians, which was the primary reason for their shame; otherwise, it is a rare emotion in canonisation testimonies.[45] Miracles that healed children also healed their parents' pain, helplessness and confusion:[46] the parent was usually the one who prayed to the saint and therefore the saint, while curing the child, gave their specific grace to the mourning guardian.[47]

Wishing for one's own death

The death wishes of ill and disabled children's parents can be explained in terms of their responsibilities and the significance that those responsibilities played in making a miracle necessary. What about the even more sporadic cases in which an infirm adult expressed the wish to die?

A woman named Bonaventura who was suffering from a condition she called 'ismania' (phrenesis, according to the Bollandists who edited the text) testified that it made her hold

42 *Il Processo di canonizzazione di Celestino V*, ed. Marini, pp. 140–1.

43 'Processus canonizationis', ed. Collegio S. Bonaventura, p. 154.

44 See, for example, N. M. Glover-Graf, 'Family Adaptation Across Cultures towards a Loved One Who Is Disabled', in *Psychosocial Aspects of Disability: Insider Perspectives and Strategies for Counselors*, ed. I. Marini, N. M. Graf and M. J. Millington (New York, 2011), pp. 169–94; E. J. Bruce, C. L. Schultz and K. X. Smyrnios, 'A Longitudinal Study of the Grief of Mothers and Fathers of Children with Intellectual Disability', *British Journal of Medical Psychology* 69 (1996), 33–45.

45 Kuuliala, *Childhood Disability*, pp. 114–25, 146–8.

46 This was expressed by one father in John Buoni's inquest, whose small daughter was severely disabled. He 'mourned greatly' ('doleret multum') for the child's condition, because the girl 'did not live or die' ('nec moriebatur nec vivebat'). *AASS* Oct IX, 864.

47 See also D. Webb, 'Friends of the Family: Some Miracles for Children by Italian Friars', in *The Church and Childhood*, ed. D. Wood (Oxford, 1994), pp. 183–95.

her head, eyelids and eyes 'like a fool' ('tamquam fatua'); this made her feel very ashamed ('verecundabatur multum'). She did not know what to do, since medical treatment was useless, and so she wished for death much more than to continue living like that ('potius affectaret mortem quam sic viveret'). She made a vow to John Buoni and God and in return received a miraculous cure.[48] In the process of St Louis of Toulouse, a man named Ferrarius Salvanis from Carpentras testified about his cure from a 'horrible infirmity' ('horribilem morbum') in his thighs, which were full of fistulas and worms. The illness made him unable to stand on his feet and to work. Physicians could not cure him. Ferrarius reported that both he and his wife expected that he could not be cured in any manner. Wishing for his death much more than staying alive (like that), at the suggestion of his wife, Ferrarius made a vow to St Louis ('optans magis mori quam vivere, ad persuasionem uxoris sue devovit se beato Ludovico').[49]

These two conditions were considered severe, the first primarily socially and the latter physically, and both also prevented the patients from performing their social roles. A bad leg with less drastic symptoms and consequences typically did not evoke such sentiments, but Ferrarius' condition was extremely serious. Especially, the worms can be read as an epitome of the danger and fear that long-lasting wounds could cause.[50] In a manner similar to those of the children discussed above, Ferrarius Salvani's testimony directly connects failed medical treatments and no expectation of a mundane cure with the idea of asking for a saint's help. Bonaventura's testimony presents the issue in a similar manner: the wish to die rather than living with such a condition led to the invocation. Like the parents who wished for their children's death, these two adults were, besides their physical suffering, unable to take care of their social roles. This added further to their distress. Especially if their illness had the danger of becoming fatal, these people were lingering in a state that could even be defined as liminal: being neither fully alive in spirit nor yet dying.[51] Although not directly stated, this connection implies that losing one's zest for life because

48 *AASS* Oct IX, 821.

49 'Processus canonizationis', ed. Collegio S. Bonaventura, p. 227.

50 There are occasional narratives about fistulas that cause social problems because of stench. The early fourteenth-century miracle collection of St Louis IX of France, based on the now largely lost canonisation testimonies, records the cure of a young apprentice, Guillot. After working for a Parisian cloth-fuller for a couple of years he acquired an illness in his leg that caused fistulas. Eventually, the stench coming from his leg became so bad that the other workers did not want to be in the same room with Guillot. This prompted the master to suggest that he should have his leg amputated so that he could again earn his bread among other people. Guillot refused and was finally cured at Louis IX's shrine. G. de Saint-Pathus, *Les Miracles de Saint Louis*, ed. P. B. Fay (Paris, 1931), pp. 21–3.

51 Irina Metzler has discussed the liminal status of disabled people in *Disability in Medieval Europe*, pp. 155–6. In some of the sources used in this chapter, the same idea can be seen, but it should not be seen as describing the status of the disabled in general. The severity of the condition played a crucial role, as did the possibility of death. For further discussion, see Kuuliala, *Childhood Disability*, pp. 194–5.

of a severe infirmity was not only the final straw that required saintly assistance, but also was part of the problem that the saint was being asked to address.

In his study of suicide in the Middle Ages, Alexander Murray writes about miracle narratives from high medieval England, analysing similar examples in which the text portrays a sufferer wishing to die. He concludes that the Latin terminology and the specific expressions used make it impossible to determine whether these people actually considered (or were thought to consider) suicide.[52] As for the parents who testified about wishing for the death of their child, it is quite far-fetched to think that they would have actually considered killing their own children. Perhaps the question about the level of concreteness in these depositions is not even relevant. The primary purpose of the references to death wishes, whether the ill or disabled person was a child or an adult testifying about their own cure, was hagiographical: they were part of the narrative rhetoric, derived from difficult or unbearable real-life situations but primarily used to highlight the saint's power. This interlinking is even more pronounced in the cases in which the petition made to the saint included an explicit, occasionally even overt, death wish.

Praying for death

In the examples discussed above, the vows and implorings made to the saint are conventional and the wish that the infirm person would rather die than continue suffering was not directly referred to in the petition. At the same time, in most inquests reporting of the vows was quite standardised. It was crucial to investigate to whom the invocation was made; in other words, to find proof that it was precisely the saint under investigation who was the healer.[53] The Breton hearing of St Yves of Treġuier (Tréguier, 1331) is one of those in which the testimonies record the spoken words at the moment of the invocation. It is of course impossible to know if the reported words were exactly the same as had been said; they gave credibility to the account but also reflect the ideas of proper invocations and people's memories about them.[54]

Here again we have examples of parents wishing for their child's death rather than them staying disabled. A woman named Lavina had a two-and-half-year-old daughter who was blind. She testified that she took the girl to St Yves' shrine and prayed there that the saint would liberate her through death or would keep her alive but healed. She added that if he did this, she would bring him a denar every year ('dicto sancto Yvoni vovit, ipsum invocando per hunc modum: "O sancte Yvo, vobis voveo filiam meam, ut liberetis eam aut

52 A. Murray, *Suicide in the Middle Ages: The Violent against Themselves* (Oxford, 1998), pp. 319–20.

53 Krötzl, 'Prokuratoren, Notare und Dolmetscher', p. 128.

54 For the usage of direct quotations, see M. Goodich, 'The Use of Direct Quotation from Canonization Hearing to Hagiographical *Vita et Miracula*', in *Oral History of the Middle Ages. The Spoken Word in Context*, ed. G. Jaritz and M. Richter (Budapest, 2001), pp. 177–87. The other fourteenth-century Breton process, that of Charles of Blois, also often records direct quotations of the witnesses' prayers.

per mortem aut per vitam; et promitto vobis unum denarium reddere annuatim"'). After this, the girl received sight in one eye.[55] In another case, the starting point was similar to the end of Lavina's testimony. A woman named Mahauta testified about the cure of Margillia, the daughter of Petrus de Lamur, 'legum professor' (professor of law) and 'miles', whose nurse she had been. Margillia remained blind in one eye after an illness that the witnesses defined as 'vayrolhe'.[56] According to Mahauta, Margillia's mother had made a vow to St Yves, promising that she and Petrus would take an offering to his shrine.[57] According to Petrus de Lamur, the mother had said: 'We vow her to St Yves, because we much prefer her to be dead than to remain like this' and then promised a pilgrimage to Yves' shrine if her daughter was healed ('"Voveamus eam sancto Ivoni, quia magis vellem quod esset mortua quam quod ita remaneret." Et tunc voverunt eam dicentes: "Sancte Ivo, si detis sibi sanitatem, ibimus nudi pedibus ad sepulcrum vestrum"').[58] The commissioners asked Petrus for how long the girl had had the 'macula' ('spot' in her eye), to which he replied eight days. Margillia's miracle is the only one I have found in which any kind of death wish is recorded in the case of a seemingly mild, short-term impairment. The testimonies do not reveal why for these parents blindness in one eye was such a grave disability, while in Lavina's testimony a similar situation was interpreted as a miracle.[59]

Such a prayer could also be made by the parent of an adult child. Johannes Guilloti Textoris testified that he was severely paralysed by 'gutta' (likely gout) for two years. In his own prayer he asked Yves to heal him, but he also testified that his mother had prayed that the saint would restore her son to health or to death ('dicta mater testis loquentis ibidem existens subsequenter dixit: "Et ego rogo te, beate sancte Yvo, quod tu reddas michi filium meum ad sanitatem vel ad mortem"').[60] Another man from the same village explained how Johannes had been completely unable to walk or help himself and that his mother had to take care of all his needs. He did not mention the vow but presented the situation as very severe to both mother and son, despite Johannes' adulthood. Nobilia, Johannes' grandmother, by contrast, said that she and Johannes' mother had made the vow together; in her testimony the vow did not include any death wishes. Nobilia's deposition sheds light

55 'Processus de vita et miraculis Sancti Yvonis', in *Monuments originaux de l'histoire de Saint Yves*, ed. A. de La Borderie, J. Daniel, R. P. Perquis and D. Tempier (Saint-Brieuc, 1887), pp. 1–299 (p. 269).

56 This might be variola, but without further information it not possible to know.

57 'Processus de vita', ed. de La Borderie et al., p. 168.

58 Ibid., p. 210.

59 Miracles that were somehow 'partial', leaving the beneficiary with remnants of the symptoms of which they had been cured, were somewhat common. Sometimes the remaining marks of the healed infirmity could even be considered precisely as a sign of the divine grace received. See J. Kuuliala, 'Heavenly Healing or Failure of Faith? Partial Cures in Later Medieval Canonization Processes', in *Church and Belief in the Middle Ages: Popes, Saints, and Crusaders*, ed. S. Katajala-Peltomaa and K. Salonen (Amsterdam, 2016), pp. 171–99.

60 'Processus de vita', ed. de La Borderie et al., pp. 247–8.

on the family's situation, as she said that after the vow she went out to ask for alms.[61] It therefore seems that in this particular case the burden of taking care of an adult man fell on two elderly women; it is quite possible that with Johannes falling ill, they had also lost their financial support if he previously had earned enough as a weaver to help his family members. Still, the man's suffering was the primary way of constructing the severity of the case with long descriptions about his 'contracted' legs and disability.

In one case, the patient himself made the prayer. Fifteen-year-old Johannes Alani testified that a couple of years earlier a grave infirmity named 'guta' had struck him, causing major pain and preventing him from walking except curved, holding his hands on his thighs. It also prevented him from working or sitting. Eventually he was taken to St Yves' shrine, where he stayed for two days before being cured. His mother had made a 'votum' for him, but he also added that while he was at the shrine, he said frequently: 'Saint Yves, give me the grace of God, so that you liberate me from this infirmity to death or to being alive, as it pleases you' ('addidit se frequenter dixisse dum erat juxta ejus sepulcrum: "Sancte Yvo impetretis mihi graciam a Deo, ut me liberet de ista infirmitate per mortem vel per vitam, prout sibi placuerit"').[62] Two other people testified about the cure as well: a woman in whose house Johannes and his brother had stayed during their pilgrimage, as well as a man named Parvus Bonus. Parvus testified that he had seen Johannes at the church, 'praying that St Yves would give him health' ('rogantem sanctum Yvonem ut sibi sanitatem impetraret'). No exact words were recorded in his testimony, so it is left unclear whether his memory about the prayer was similar to that of Johannes.[63]

According to Parvus Bonus, there were more than one hundred people present at the church while Johannes was there, while Johannes himself said that there were many healthy and infirm people present. Popular pilgrimage destinations were busy, with a flow of devotees coming and going.[64] Making a pilgrimage was a public act, by which the pilgrim could perform his or her religiosity to other devotees and to the sacred.[65] Approaching the saint with humility and tears, emphasising one's suffering and the need for a grace,

61 Ibid., pp. 249–51.

62 Ibid., p. 152.

63 Ibid., p. 153.

64 The popularity of St Yves's cult, as was the case with other saints, was investigated in the canonisation inquest. The commissioners of Yves' process also recorded that they had seen approximately twenty-seven silver ships and more than ninety wax ships hanging above the shrine as well as numerous wax images of heads, eyes, arms, hands, legs and feet, napkins, waxen breasts, wooden crutches and other votive gifts. Ibid., pp. 5–6. For a life-cycle of a cult, see Finucane, *Miracles and Pilgrims*, pp. 181–8; Goodich, '*Mirabilis Deus in Sanctis Suis*', p. 142.

65 For the performative side of pilgrimage, see J. Dubisch, *In a Different Place. Pilgrimage, Gender and Politics at a Greek Island Shrine* (Princeton, 1995); R. Maniura, *Pilgrimage to the Images in the Fifteenth Century. The Origins of the Cult of Our Lady of Częstochowa* (Woodbridge, 2004), especially pp. 90–4; S. S. Morrison, *Women Pilgrims in Late Medieval England. Private Piety as Public Performance* (London, 2004 [2000]).

belonged to the ritual.[66] Damien Boquet and Piroska Nagy have written about the chain reaction of emotions: when one person expresses their emotion, others share it and pass it on. Furthermore, people within a social group interact in an intensive way when they experience emotions or emotional events together.[67] Pierre-Andrè Sigal, for his part, has called the atmosphere and interplay between clerics and pilgrims at a medieval shrine a 'dynamique miraculeuse' (miraculous dynamic).[68] Prayers like that of Johannes Alani are a fine example of that dynamic. Expressing an emotional plea that was both eager and powerful was not just a way to strongly highlight his personal need for a cure among the many petitioners, but also made his situation evident for the others lodging at the shrine. As the sacred was part of the dynamic at the shrine, perhaps these cases can also be read as bargaining with the saint. An old man with badly trembling hands wanted to go to St Louis IX of France's shrine in Saint Denis. A local woman told him that he was too old to be cured there, to which he replied that he would stay at the shrine for so long that he would either die or be cured.[69] The examples in which a saint is actually reported as having killed someone are sporadic punishment miracles.[70] Therefore, if such a prayer was successful, it could only result in a healing. At the same time, of course, personal devotion and firm hope that the saint could help was needed for a plea to succeed.[71]

It is an open question why the few examples we have of such prayers come from just one process – was it perhaps a notarial preference in that particular area or in St Yves of Tréguier's cult? At least we may see a cult as one type of emotional community; Barbara H. Rosenwein, for example, defines emotional community as a group of people who adhere to the same emotional experiences and values and who devalue the same emotions,[72] and this holds true of a cultic community as well. At the same time, when compared with the other miracles recorded in St Yves's process, it is impossible to detect any particular reasons why precisely in the cases discussed above the prayer included a death wish, while in many other cases that appear to be equally severe and full of grief and other sentiments such wishes were not recorded. As an example, several people testified about the cure of a man who had travelled to Tréguier from Guérande, hoping to be cured from a paralysis that completely prevented him from moving. The daughter of the house testified that the man,

66 Morrison, *Women Pilgrims*, pp. 137–8.

67 D. Boquet and P. Nagy, *Medieval Sensibilities. A History of Emotions in the Middle Ages*, trans. R. Shaw (Cambridge, 2018), p. 217.

68 P.-A. Sigal, *L'homme et le miracle dans la France médiévale (XIe–XIIe siècle)* (Paris, 1985), pp. 165–225. See also Finucane, *Miracles and Pilgrims*, pp. 90–1.

69 G. de Saint-Pathus, *Les Miracles*, pp. 30–1.

70 On punishment miracles, see Klaniczay, 'Miracoli di punizione e *maleficia*'.

71 R. Bartlett, *Why Can the Dead Do Such Great Things? Saints and Worshippers from the Martyrs to the Reformation* (Princeton, 2013), p. 364; M. Wittmer-Butsch and C. Rendtel, *Miracula: Wunderheilungen im Mittelalter. Eine historisch-psychologische Annäherung* (Cologne, 2003), pp. 182, 199.

72 Rosenwein, *Emotional Communities*, p. 2.

called Nicolaus, had frequently prayed for Yves 'full of feeling and devotedly' ('affectuose et devote'). After five weeks at the shrine in vain, he again returned to the house, 'sad, suffering and crying' ('tristis, dolens et lacrimans') because he did not regain his health. He also talked to the witness's parents, calculating the cost of his stay and saying that in the morning he would leave. The parents told him to stay, however, and at midnight he had a vision of St Yves and was finally healed.[73] Again, we see a situation in which the most difficult, even most desperate, moment precedes the miracle; here, the witness even gives up on the saint, but still it is not recorded whether he expressed any death wish. His distress, pain and need for a cure were reconstructed in another way.

Canonisation records are not statistically representative, and especially when studying people's sentiments and expressions it is dangerous to even attempt to estimate their prevalence across wider lived realities. The depositions also lack moral undertones, but it is likely that if praying for death or wishing that someone would die rather than suffer from a grave illness or disability had been considered highly questionable, the witnesses would have left it unmentioned. At the same time, one might also expect such prayers to have been more common, so effective are they in demonstrating the need for saintly help. It is, however, possible that including or omitting death wishes from the depositions simply reflected the preferences of those recording them – this would explain why they are somewhat frequent in John Buoni's inquest.

A rare possibility for examining different versions of the same story appears in the documents concerning St Louis of Toulouse. The edition of his process also contains a *Liber miraculorum*, a document penned by the custodian of Louis's shrine in Marseille. It includes a much larger selection of miracles than the canonisation document, although it also describes some of the same ones.[74]

One concerns the cure of Dulcesa, who became severely ill and disabled after a midwife removed a dead foetus from her womb. According to the *Liber miraculorum*, she decided that it would be better to die than live like that, which is why she asked a surgeon to come to operate on her – a situation completely opposite to that of the Italian boy Gulliermus discussed earlier. The risky operation was postponed because the surgeon refused to do it unless Dulcesa's husband, who was returning home the following day, or another family member was present. Fearing the operation, the following night Dulcesa made a vow to St Louis and was miraculously healed.[75] Although the depositions of Dulcesa and three other people in the canonisation records contain some of the same details, like her having to drag her bedclothes with her teeth, they do not refer to her thoughts about death or about calling for a surgeon.[76] Dulcesa made a pilgrimage to Louis's shrine as a sign of gratitude and told her story to the custodian there. She was a

73 'Processus de vita', ed. de La Borderie et al., pp. 253–4.

74 'Prolegomena', in *Analecta Franciscana*, ed. Collegio S. Bonaventura (Florence, 1951), pp. i–lxix (pp. xlviii–xlix).

75 'Liber miraculorum', in *Analecta Franciscana*, ed. Collegio S. Bonaventura, pp. 275–331 (p. 301).

76 'Processus canonizationis', ed. Collegio S. Bonaventura, pp. 165–9.

poor woman, so, unless the surgeon was willing to treat her as a charity case, her decision to call for him was drastic both economically and corporally. She had not yet given up completely on the idea that a medical professional could help her, but undoubtedly considered the operation extremely risky.

According to this version of the story, Dulcesa's decision caused the saint to heal her. Therefore, her willingness to undergo such a drastic operation proved the need for a miracle. Why her death wish and the surgeon are missing from the canonisation inquest testimonies is impossible to deduce, but perhaps here the surgeon did not have an important role for proving the case, as he had not yet operated nor concluded that Dulcesa's condition was incurable. As in all miracle cases here, she too had to make up her mind and decide what she could hope and expect and what could be the result of her suffering. Unlike in some other types of writings of the time, the 'miraculée's' pain was not valorised but described as something debilitating, leading to rather extreme sentiments and wishes.[77] Yet, when the suffering was erased due to God's grace, its significance changed and it became one of the many epitomes demonstrating the divine's presence on Earth.

Conclusion

The sentiments and death wishes surveyed here had a dual purpose in canonisation testimonies. Together with symptoms and diagnoses, they helped to prove the miraculous nature of the cure: they demonstrated the futile nature of mundane help and the medical, communal or familial consensus that nothing other than a miracle could heal the patient. They also helped to underline the severity of the patient's situation, which was needed for a miracle narrative to be credible.

At the same time, death wishes and the sentiments that prompted them were an important element of the invocation. When imploring a saint, the devotee had to make the need for their intervention explicit. Asking for a saint's assistance was a ritualistic act packed with emotions; the very same emotions could be what made the saint show his or her grace. Mentioning that the situation was so hopeless that the infirm person's death was desired more than their living with their infirmity was a powerful way of demonstrating the need for a saintly cure. When the same sentiment was expressed as a part of the invocation, it underlined the emotions – suffering, pain, grief – of the supplicant even more profoundly. At the same time, however, the death wishes contain a paradox, at least when reported after the fact. In order to receive a miracle, the petitioner had to have firm belief in the saint's ability to help; therefore the lack of hope was related to the possibility of mundane help. When a death wish was placed in its proper place in the narrative structure, right before the invocation, it strengthened the witness's deposition: adhering to the established narrative structure made the case more credible.[78]

77 E. Cohen, *The Modulated Scream: Pain in Late Medieval Culture* (Chicago, 2010), especially pp. 32, 139–41.

78 See Smoller, 'Defining the Boundaries'.

Disability did not need to be a tragedy in medieval society. The cases analysed are a selection of situations in which it did cause severe physical and social problems. Especially the testimonies in which death wishes are linked with shame demonstrate the issues caused by an inability to fulfil one's social role or the inability to raise children to fulfil theirs. Shame and honour were linked with public opinion about one's ability to live by norms and status.[79] The saints could thus heal not only a person's suffering but also the whole family's ability to fulfil their social expectations. Members of a cult, interpreted as an emotional community, could therefore express or even invoke certain emotions and sentiments to reach this goal. These sentiments and reactions were publicly accepted and valued, especially when they resulted in a miracle. In these narratives, the future has two forms: death and the miraculous. The petitioners were negotiating between the two, giving the ultimate power of decision to the sacred.

[79] See B. Hanawalt, *'Of Good and Ill Repute'. Gender and Social Control in Medieval England* (Oxford, 1998), pp. 1–3.

8

Bubo Men? Repurposing Medieval Anatomic Illustrations for Plague Therapy in the Fifteenth and Sixteenth Centuries

LORI JONES[1]

Medieval artistic images most commonly used today to depict the Black Death are not, in fact, illustrations of plague. Rather, they are contemporary images of other diseases or of biblical analogues.[2] This misidentification raises several questions, including why so few contemporary images exist with recognisable clinical symptoms of plague and when clinically relevant images first appeared. Initial answers to those questions – that artists focused more on the social chaos of disease than its symptoms and only in the later fifteenth century – now needs adjustment. We may have been looking in the wrong place for medical images of plague.

Medical and art historians are giving renewed attention to and asking new questions about the presence and function of diagrams in medieval and early modern medical manuscripts and printed books. In the 1960–70s, Loren C. MacKinney and Robert Herrlinger interpreted these diagrams as straightforward medical illustrations, but recent work has taken a more nuanced approach that considers them within a broader interdisciplinary context of the production and use of health and healing information.[3] Surviving sketches

1 I am grateful to Jack Hartnell, Sara Öberg Strådal, Teresa Tavormina and Nükhet Varlık for their insightful comments on early drafts of this chapter and to Monica H. Green for suggesting years ago that I write it. I also thank attendees at the International Congress on Medieval Studies and the New York University Medieval and Renaissance Center conference *The Worlds that Plague Made* for offering thought-provoking questions following my presentations on this topic.

2 On the misidentification of medieval plague images, see L. Jones and R. Nevell, 'Plagued by Doubt and Viral Misinformation: The Need for Evidence-Based Use of Historical Disease Images', *The Lancet Infectious Diseases* 16 (2016), e235–40; M. H. Green, K. Walker-Meikle and W. P. Müller, 'Diagnosis of a "Plague" Image: A Digital Cautionary Tale', *The Medieval Globe* 1 (2014), 309–26.

3 Among others, see P. M. Jones, *Medieval Medicine in Illuminated Manuscripts* (London, 1998); J. A. Givens, K. Reeds and A. Touwaide, ed., *Visualizing Medieval Medicine and Natural History, 1200–1550* (London, 2006); J. Hartnell, 'Medicine's Image', in *The Routledge Companion to Medieval Iconography*, ed. C. Hourihane (London, 2016), pp. 322–9; J. Hartnell, *Medieval Bodies: Life, Death and Art in the Middle Ages* (London, 2018); P. M. Jones, 'Visualization in Medicine between Script and Print, c. 1375–1550', in *The Visualization of Knowledge in Medieval and Early Modern Europe*, ed. M. Kupfer, A. S. Cohen and J. H. Chajes (Turnhout, 2020), pp. 341–60; S. M.

of surgical tools and procedures, urine wheels and flasks, Zodiac, Bloodletting and Wound Men, medicinal plants and therapies and medical practitioners at work are now being considered in a wider context that not only cuts across socio-economic, professional and intellectual strata, but also dismantles cultural, linguistic, geographical and medieval–early modern divides. This broader perspective lets diagrams 'speak' about the practical side of medicine.[4]

Some surviving medieval medical manuscript images also show people suffering from disease. A treatise in London, British Library (hereafter BL), Sloane MS 2276, for example, provides short textual descriptions of several disorders – including leprosy, gout, podagra and alopecia – accompanied by marginal sketches of people afflicted by these conditions. An even more fully illustrated example is an early fifteenth-century copy of John of Arderne's *De Arte Phisicali et de Cirurgia* preserved in Stockholm, National Library, X118; here one finds images of people afflicted with a wide range of illnesses, including leprosy, falling sickness, consumption and dysentery.[5]

Images of plague signs and symptoms, plague therapies and plague patients, by contrast, are notably absent from medical manuscripts before the fifteenth century and remain rare in both manuscript and print thereafter. The human toll of the Black Death (1346–53) was devastating, yet there is little contemporary pictorial evidence of it. Even the ubiquitous plague tract – a regimental/therapeutic genre of medical text that emerged during the Black Death to explain the disease and offer remedial and curative advice – is typically devoid of images or drawings, despite the fact that plague was diagnosed ultimately, at least in part, by visual notice of its most tell-tale sign, the bubo. This absence of plague-related images stands in stark contrast to a modern perspective that imagines disease visually, rather than just textually. Perhaps for the readers and users of plague tracts – physicians, surgeons, clerics and literate laypersons – textual descriptions sufficed, given their intimate familiarity with the disease. While the lack of plague imagery complicates modern attempts to visualise plague victims through the eyes of medieval and early modern witnesses, though, parsing the language that medical writers used tells us an increasingly graphic story.[6]

Öberg Strådal, 'Utility beyond Function: Practical and Social Uses of Diagrams in Late Medieval English Medical Manuscripts', in *The Diagram Paradigm*, ed. D. Roxburgh, J. Hamburger, L. Safran (Dumbarton Oaks, 2022). I thank Sara Öberg Strådal for allowing me to read her chapter before its publication. For earlier works, see L. C. MacKinney, *Medical Illustrations in Medieval Manuscripts* (London, 1965) and R. Herrlinger, *History of Medical Illustration from Antiquity to A.D. 1600*, trans. G. Fulton-Smith (London, 1970).

4 F. Wallis, 'What a Medieval Diagram Shows: A Case Study of *Computus*', *Studies in Iconography* 36 (2015), 1–40 (p. 33).

5 T. Svenberg and P. M. Jones, *De Arte Phisicali et de Cirurgia by John Arderne* (Stockholm, 2014). A digital facsimile is found at https://dl.wdl.org/11631/service/11631.pdf.

6 On the late emergence of artistic representations of plague's clinical signs and the evolution of textual descriptions that verged on the visual, see L. Jones, '"Apostumes, Carbuncles, and Botches": Visualizing the Plague in Late Medieval and Early Modern Medical Treatises', in *Asclepius, the Paintbrush, and the Pen: Representations of Disease in Medieval and Early Modern Art*

When we stop looking for images of plague symptoms and look instead for images of contemporary medical practice, something new appears: an adaptation of the iconic Phlebotomy/Bloodletting Man and Wound Man diagrams to this specific disease. We might plausibly call this the Bubo Man or the 'Pest-Aderlaßmann' (plague bloodletting man).[7] This chapter examines the emergence and function of these practical therapeutic illustrations in the early fifteenth century. Only ten such images have been identified thus far: they appear in five fifteenth-century manuscripts from southern Germany and England (München, Universitätsbibliothek (hereafter UB), 4° Cod. MS 885; München, Bayerische Staatsbibliothek Cgm 28; Stuttgart, Württembergische Landesbibliothek (hereafter WLB), MS HB XI 10; Vienna, Österreische Nationalbibliothek (hereafter ÖNB), MS 5184; and BL Egerton MS 1624), in printed plague tracts from Basel, Venice and Lyon in the sixteenth century and on a mid-sixteenth-century German broadsheet.[8] In exploring the interrelationship between the Bubo Man image and the accompanying texts, this chapter asks: How did illustrators intend to depict plague by repurposing existing didactic diagrams? What might these images indicate about late medieval efforts to understand and manage plague? And what does the imagery suggest about the process by which visual representation of plague found its way into plague treatises, a primarily textual tradition?

Medical responses to the Black Death: the textual tradition

Medical responses to plague circulated largely through the textual genre of plague tracts. These treatises – which combined the existing medical-textual genres of the 'regimina sanitatis' (health regimens) and 'consilia' (case studies on causes of and treatments for disease) – first appeared as university-trained physicians attempted to reckon with the Black Death, the preliminary wave of the multi-century Second Plague Pandemic. Whether they sought to explain the disease or simply to recommend suitable preventatives and therapies, physicians found little in the classical medical canon to prepare them for the visual and medical reality of plague. Traditional medical authorities had addressed painful

and Literature, ed. M. Ciavolella and R. F. Canalis (Turnhout, 2021), pp. 173–200. For a recent examination of plague art, see S. Barker, 'Painting the Plague, 1250–1630', in *Plague Image and Imagination from Medieval to Modern Times*, ed. C. Lynteris (Cham, 2021), pp. 37–67.

7 The German term comes from H. Bergmann and G. Keil, 'Das Münchner Pest-Laßmännchen. Standardisierungstendenzen in der spätmittelalterlichen deutschen Pesttherapie', in *Fachprosa-Studien: Beiträge zur mittelalterlichen Wissenschafts- und Geistesgeschichte*, ed. G. Keil (Berlin, 1982), pp. 318–30.

8 J. Vadianus, *Ein kurtz und trüwlich underricht wider die sorgklich kranckeyt der Pestilentz* (Basel, 1519); Anonymous, *Regime contro la pestilence per les medecins de Basle* (Venice, 1519); Anonymous, *Regime contre la pestil[enc]e ce faict et compose par messieurs les medecins de la cite de Basle en allemaigne* (Lyon, 1519); E. Ydeley, *Des secrets souverains et vrais remedes contre la peste* (Lyon, 1581). The woodcut by Michael Ostendorfer appears on a plague bloodletting broadsheet printed by Hans Kohl in Regensburg, c. 1555.

'apostemata' (abscesses or swellings), but not in the catastrophic form that physicians and other medical practitioners now witnessed.[9]

The tracts were largely formulaic, typically organised into three distinct sections. The first part elaborated on the causes and prognostic signs of plague and was typically grounded in traditional theoretical and/or astrological frameworks. The second part provided guidance for avoiding the disease, focused primarily on maintaining the six non-naturals (that is, the external factors that affected health: food and drink, sleep and wakefulness, exercise and rest, passions and emotions, air and excretion) and keeping a clean home environment. The third section offered a range of therapies, including herbals, cordials, plasters and phlebotomy. As devastating outbreaks recurred regularly over the following centuries, plague treatises circulated by the hundreds as original, copied, translated or adapted versions in manuscript and then in print. Some were short and devoted largely to offering straightforward prevention and treatment advice, while others considered the meaning, nature and cause of plague at length and in some detail.

Plague tracts contained few graphic descriptions of the disease's signs and symptoms before the sixteenth century, and even fewer diagrams. Regardless of any mention of signs, such as the presence of abscesses or buboes in the armpit, on the neck or in the groin, tract writers generally did not describe what they witnessed; few even initially presented the bubo as a unique and distinctive marker of plague.[10] There were some exceptions: the Perugino medical faculty lecturer Gentile da Foligno, for example, 'briefly referred to the back of the ears, the left armpit, and the right groin as the usual places where [undefined] "signs" (*signa*) of the disease [might] appear'.[11] Ibn Khātimah, a fourteenth-century Muslim author in Almería (Andalusia), wrote of glandular swellings, while Johannes Jacobi, chancellor at Montpellier's medical faculty, noted that a 'tumor magnus' (large tumour) developed on the emunctories. Several other writers in fourteenth- and early fifteenth-century Montpellier explained the location of buboes in terms of humoral pathology: an excess of humours in the brain generated a swelling behind the ear, they said, while a surplus in the liver caused one in the groin and superfluity in the heart gave rise to one in the armpit. Even so, these writers provided little description of plague signs, other than to vaguely list 'buboes, erysipelas, carbuncles, and other different kinds of abscesses'.[12]

9 For a comparative study of English and French tracts, see L. Jones, *Patterns of Plague: Changing Ideas about Plague in England and France, 1348–1750* (Montreal, 2022). Nahyan Fancy's chapter in this volume demonstrates, by contrast, that Arabic commentaries discussed plague in some detail between the ninth and mid-fourteenth centuries.

10 This changed dramatically in the later sixteenth and seventeenth centuries, when plague tract writing became more literary and graphic. Jones, '"Apostumes"'.

11 J. Arrizabalaga, 'Facing the Black Death: Perceptions and Reactions of University Medical Practitioners', in *Practical Medicine from Salerno to the Black Death*, ed. L. García-Ballester, R. French, J. Arrizabalaga and A. Cunningham (Cambridge, 1994), pp. 237–88 (p. 267).

12 'ex quibus humoribus sit dispositus causabuntur bubones, herisipili, carbunculi, et alia diversa genera apostematum'. Bernard Alberti, quoted in M. P. Chase, 'Fevers, Poisons, and Apostemes:

Even when they did not mention or describe the visual signs of plague, many tract writers included therapies or cures that addressed buboes in some way. Gentile da Foligno, for example, offered phlebotomy as a curative measure, arguing that bleeding provided 'an exit for the collected venomous matter' found in the 'apostemata' that would otherwise putrefy the organ in which it had accumulated and ultimately reach the heart, causing death.[13] Unlike most of his contemporaries, da Foligno also recommended scarifying, cauterising or cupping the apostemes directly to attract and to evacuate their poisonous matter and then covering wounds with plasters to dissolve the accumulated pus. In the 1360s, Guy de Chauliac offered similar advice, suggesting that he too had survived plague by opening the buboes and then cauterising them.[14]

Most plague treatises included phlebotomy instructions. Phlebotomy, or bloodletting, was the practice of opening a vein to draw blood in order to remove excessive or unhealthy humours. It had a long tradition in medicine, and the Ancient Greeks added a theoretical rationale to the practice, including the ideas that it was useful for both preventive and therapeutic purposes and that it should be conducted only under particular circumstances. Early medieval guides on the subject circulated widely, in Latin, Hebrew and Arabic versions, followed by vernacular editions in later centuries. As a preventive measure, phlebotomy ensured a healthy humoral balance that protected against disease; as a curative measure, it removed accumulated poison or corruption from the patient's body. It was in many ways a cure-all, as a fifteenth-century English almanac explains:

> Flebotomy clears the mind, strengthens the memory, cleanses the guts, dries up the brain, warms the marrow, sharpens the hearing, curbs tears, encourages discrimination, helps the stomach, develops the senses, promotes digestion, produces a musical voice, dispels sleepiness, drives away anxiety, feeds the blood, rids it of poisonous matter, and gives a long life. It eliminates rheumatic ailments whilst getting rid of pestilent diseases, it cures pains, fever and various sicknesses and makes urine clear and clean.[15]

Authority and Experience in Montpellier Plague Treatises', *Annals of the New York Academy of Sciences* 441 (1985), 153–70 (p. 165 n. 21).

13 Arrizabalaga, 'Facing the Black Death', p. 284.

14 G. de Chauliac, 'Bubonic Plague', in *A Source Book in Medieval Science*, ed. E. Grant (Cambridge MA, 1974), pp. 773–4.

15 C. H. Talbot, 'A Mediaeval Physician's Vade Mecum', *Journal of the History of Medicine and the Allied Sciences* 16 (1961), 213–33 (p. 231): 'Fleobotomia mentem sincerat, memoriam prebet, uesicam purgat, serebrum exsiccat, medullam calefacit, auditum aperit, lacrimas stringit, fastidium colit, stomacho proficit, sensum dirigit, digestionem inuitat, leniorem uocem producit, fugat sompnum, anxietate caret, proprium sangu inem nutrit, extraneum eicit, longiorem uitam ministrat. Incatesuras et collecciones et pestiferas [valetudines] et reumaticas passiones deponit dolores, febres et uarios morbos curat, caligines urinarum et turpitudinem tollit'. The translation from Latin is Talbot's. Teresa Tavormina kindly noted to me that the original text is found in the mid-twelfth-century *Flebotomia Archimathei*, itself compiled from even older sources. Personal correspondence, 19 July 2020. On this and a related text, see M. T. Tavormina, 'Supplementary Text II: *Liber fleobotomie*', in *Sex, Aging, and Death in a Medieval Medical Compendium. Trinity*

Determining which vein to open for bloodletting generally depended on the condition being treated or the site of the problem: the cephalic vein in the arm was typically opened for conditions above the neck, while the basilic (or hepatic) vein in the inner elbow was more suitable for conditions below the neck. The median (or cardiac) vein in the arm was also used frequently. In practice, each vein in the body was associated with specific illnesses and opened as appropriate: opening veins under the tongue relieved throat problems, saphenous veins on the ankles addressed problems in the genitals and the womb, veins in the head treated mental disorders and so on. Key to the proper practice of bloodletting were the twin concepts of derivation, or letting blood from a vein close to the affected body part, and revulsion, the letting of blood from the furthest possible vein. Which vein and which method were selected depended both on careful diagnostics – indications of particular illnesses or conditions and affected body parts, as well as the age and condition of the patient – and prudent consideration of the hour of the day, seasons, time of year and astrological factors.[16]

Some plague tract authors specifically noted the veins suitable for bleeding plague patients. In doing so, they adapted the long-standing method of managing and controlling humoral imbalances by setting aside phlebotomy's traditional head-to-toe anatomical sequence and focusing instead just on the sites (and thus organs) affected by plague buboes. The purpose of bloodletting in cases of plague was to evacuate accumulated poison (corruption) from the affected site. Da Foligno listed six suitable veins, according to the location of the 'apostemata'. The most dangerous locations for an 'apostema' to appear were under the left armpit, behind the ears or in the right groin, since these positions corresponded to the evacuation points of the three principal members of the body: the heart, brain and liver.[17] A fifteenth-century English translation of a tract written by the Liègois physician John of Burgundy around 1365 likewise noted that the pestilential sores associated with plague erupted in the emunctories or purging spots of the body's three main organs: in the 'armeholes' (armpits) for the 'hert' (heart), in the 'gryndes' (groin) for the 'lyvre' (liver) or 'undir the ij eyrs & undre the tunge' (under the two ears and under the tongue) for the 'brayn' (brain).[18] More so than some of his contemporaries, John's treatise contained a rather long section on phlebotomy in which he discussed the specific veins from which to let blood: the 'cardiaca or cordiall' vein was suitable for a bubo in the armpit, while the cephalic vein ('that is the hede veyne') was for a bubo in the neck. Either

College Cambridge MS R.14.52, Its Texts, Language, and Scribe, 2 vols., ed. M. T. Tavormina (Tempe, 2006), II, 277–86.

16 On medieval phlebotomy, see L. E. Voigts and M. R. McVaugh, 'A Latin Technical Phlebotomy and Its Middle English Translation', *Transactions of the American Philosophical Society* 74 (1984), 1–69, and P. Gil-Sotres, 'Derivation and Revulsion: The Theory and Practice of Medieval Phlebotomy', in *Practical Medicine*, ed. García-Ballester et al., pp. 110–55.

17 Arrizabalaga, 'Facing the Black Death', p. 284.

18 BL Sloane MS 3449, fol. 8v.

the 'basilica veyne … undir the veyne cardiaca' or the vein in the foot between the big and second toes were bled for a bubo in the groin.[19]

These three purging spots (also called cleansing places by some tract writers) correlate with the location of the three lymph nodes – cervical, axillary and inguinal – that characteristically become swollen following infection by the *Yersinia pestis* bacterium and the development of the bubonic form of plague. Like his contemporaries, John noted that special care should be taken to let blood only on the same side of the body as the bubo itself:

> or ellis ther is two harmes: oon, if thow bleede on that other side, the goode bloode and cleene in thi side nat corrupt nat venymed shal be drawen out of, and the evil bloode shal dwel stil ther. And than the body is fiebler for defaute of goode bloode … and the harme is more, for than the bloode that is venymed shal passe overthwert the herte and venymeth it and hastith a man to his endyng.[20]

It was important to know not just the proper vein from which to bleed a plague victim, but also the time frame within which to do so. Bleeding needed to be started as soon as the patient felt the 'prickyng of bloode or flakeryng' that indicated infection and, especially, within the first one to six hours, since (as a later version of John's tract stated) 'lettinge blood in tyme is a specyall meanes of cure'.[21] Waiting too long, by contrast, would cause mortal danger: if 'ther passe xxiiij houres the matier than is gadred and harded and wil nat passe out of the veyne [even] if it be striken'.

Similar advice appeared in plague tracts over the centuries, in some accounts only briefly and in others with extensive detail. Some treatises advised regular, preventative bleeding, while others counted more on phlebotomy's curative potential. A few tract authors, however, definitively rejected the suitability of phlebotomy for plague treatment. In 1521, the Munich city physician Alexander Seitz argued that blind recourse to therapeutic bloodletting as a plague treatment was dangerous, having been improperly understood from ancient practice and poorly taught.[22] The mid-seventeenth-century English physician George Thomson likewise attacked Galenist reliance on humoral medicine and all therapies that accompanied it, ultimately engaging in a pamphlet war about the value of medical bloodletting.[23] For the most part, however, the same basic therapeutic recommen-

19 Ibid., fol. 9v.

20 Cambridge, Trinity College, MS R.14.52, fols. 157r–v. Lister Matheson provides an edition of this copy of the treatise in 'John of Burgundy: Treatises on Plague', in *Sex, Aging, and Death*, ed. Tavormina, II, 569–606. Matheson also discusses an adapted version of the treatise that contains a different discussion of the virtues and dangers of bloodletting on pp. 574–5.

21 London, Wellcome Collection (hereafter Wellcome Collection) MS 674, p. 32 (the first half of this manuscript is paginated). See L. Jones, 'Unrecorded Versions of John of Burgundy's Plague Tract and Identifying "Lost" Copies of the Same', *Notes & Queries* 65 (2018), 14–17.

22 E. A. Heinrichs, *Plague, Print, and the Reformation: The German Reform of Healing* (London, 2018), p. 85.

23 Acceptance of the therapeutic value of phlebotomy waxed and waned during the early modern era. In 1720, Monsieur D. M. Pons, a physician in Montpellier's Faculty of Medicine, admitted

dations remained in place between the mid-fourteenth and the mid-eighteenth centuries: manage the six non-naturals, use plasters, cold electuaries, cordials and herbs mixed with wine and rely on phlebotomy.

This emphasis on phlebotomy, among other plague prophylaxes and therapies, is relevant not just because of its long-standing purpose to manage and control humoral balances, but also because its appropriate practice required some knowledge of human vein anatomy. Pertinent as well is the fact that while physicians (university trained or not) wrote the majority of plague tracts, the practice of bloodletting was more commonly (but not exclusively) the purview of surgeons and barber-surgeons, who engaged with the more manual aspects of medical practice. Canonical surgical texts like the thirtieth volume of Abū al-Qāsim Al-Zahrāwī's (Albucasis) eleventh-century *Kitāb al-Taṣrīf* and Ibn Sīnā's (Avicenna) eleventh-century *Al-Qānūn fī al-Ṭibb* – translated into Latin from their original Arabic as *Chirurgia* and *Canon medicinae*, respectively, and taught in European medical faculties – further entrenched phlebotomy into learned medical practice. Al-Zahrawi's work presented the most comprehensive theoretical discussions of venesection, noting thirty different veins suitable for bloodletting and the many techniques for opening them; it was a critical source for university-trained practitioners engaged in the diagnostic, prognostic and therapeutic aspects of phlebotomy. The fourteenth-century emergence of diagrams of what today are called Phlebotomy/Bloodletting Man, alongside shorter practical treatises sometimes found in verse, point to the vernacularisation of the practice of bloodletting beyond the academically trained.[24] The significance of this development and its adaptation to plague tracts is treated later, but first it is helpful to explore the development of these diagrams, as well as the associated imagery of the Zodiac Man and Wound Man and their association with plague.

Phlebotomy Man, Zodiac Man and Wound Man imagery

Recent work on the multifaceted meanings and purposes of Phlebotomy Man, Zodiac Man and Wound Man diagrams emphasises the intertwining of humans, the natural world and the cosmos that underscored medieval medical thought.[25] Humoral theory did

he had believed previously that buboes and other plague-related swellings were nothing more than the result of medical prejudice against using phlebotomy and purging to release the body's accumulated impurities ('n'étoit qu'une suite de leurs prejugés à ne point saigner ni purger … [dont] il arrivoit des Parotides, des Bubons, des Charbons, des Éxanthémes, & toutes les autres efflorescences qu'on observe dans la Peste'). D. M. Pons, in J. Boecler, *Recueil des observations qui ont étées faites sur la maladie de Marseille* (Strasbourg, 1721), 14.

24 Voigts and McVaugh, 'Latin Technical Phlebotomy', pp. 4–6. On English versified phlebotomy texts, see T. Hunt, 'The Poetic Vein Phlebotomy in Middle English and Anglo-Norman Verse', *English Studies* 77 (1996), 311–22.

25 S. M. Öberg Strådal, 'Depictions of Physical Order: Diagrams in Late Medieval English Medical Manuscripts' (unpublished Ph.D. dissertation, University of Glasgow, 2015), p. 124. Other medieval anatomical diagrams, such as those comprising a series that sketched out the internal

not exist in isolation, but was integrally linked with nature, astrology and cosmographic influences; in this light, the diagrams acted as a framework or map on which theoretical 'iatromathematical ideas' could be more simply presented to medical practitioners who operated, perhaps, outside learned university circles. Furthermore, '[a]natomical imagery mingled with consistently replicated physiological texts that elucidated their forms and comparative workings; zodiacal and bloodletting schemes [for example] relied on adjacent tables of text and numbers that aided in the calendrical calculation of lunar and solar cycles'.[26] In other words, the images both emerged from a textual tradition and generated new texts of their own. Image and text worked in tandem to explicate a theoretical understanding of man's place in the universe.

Also known as the Man of Signs ('homo signorum'), the Zodiac Man has a long history, as a surviving astrological table of signs and body parts in cuneiform suggests.[27] More commonly attested in Western Europe after the thirteenth century for medical purposes, copies and diverse versions of the image appeared in a wide range of medieval religious, astrological, medical and philosophical texts, offering a visual representation of the relationship between astrological signs – the cosmos – and the parts of the human body. In short, it visualised in a relatively straightforward and didactic way the belief that, as they moved across the universe, the stars, moon and planets directly affected the workings of the human body. The names and/or pictures of the star signs overlaid or appeared beside the parts of the (usually) male body they were believed to influence. The Aries ram, for example, ruled the head, while the Capricorn goat dominated the knees and the Pisces fish affected the feet. For medieval medical practitioners, these connections influenced both the nature and timing of recommended therapies, including phlebotomy.[28]

First attested in the fourteenth century, the Phlebotomy/Bloodletting Man diagram is linked both intellectually and iconographically to the Zodiac Man image.[29] The two appear together in numerous medieval manuscripts and are, at times, even combined into a single image. This was possible because their 'structure and appearance … are often very similar and they are expressions of the same medical practice'.[30] They could also be linked through their 'appearance, placement on the page and the content of the text surrounding'

organs and network systems (skeletal, arterial/venous, nervous, muscular, etc.) or that visualised the gestation of foetuses played a similar role.

26 J. Hartnell, 'Wording the Wound Man', *British Art Studies* 6 (2017), http://dx.doi.org/10.17658/issn.2058–5462/issue-06/jhartnell.

27 J. Z. Wee, 'Discovery of the Zodiac Man in Cuneiform', *Journal of Cuneiform Studies* 67 (2015), 217–33. On the image's multiple purposes, see C. W. Clark, 'The Zodiac Man in Medieval Astrology', *Journal of Rocky Mountain Association* 3 (1982), 18–38.

28 For examples, see Wee, 'Discovery' pp. 217–18 n. 1. See also see R. French, 'Astrology in Medical Practice', in *Practical Medicine*, ed. García-Ballester et al., pp. 30–59.

29 Images showing cautery points are older, such as the early-twelfth-century images in BL Sloane MS 2839.

30 Öberg Strådal, 'Depictions of Physical Order', p. 126. For a cross-cultural comparison of such images, see J. Hartnell, 'Bloodlines: Medicine and Cosmology in France, China, and Mexico',

them. In some ways, the two images acted as counterweights: the Zodiac Man represented outside or celestial influences on the body, while the Phlebotomy Man indicated which veins should be opened to effectively manage one's internal humoral balance and/or to treat specific ailments or conditions. The two diagrams also acted together in another sense: the Zodiac Man had a largely prognostic–therapeutic function – telling the physician or surgeon when (or not) to treat a given limb or organ – while the Phlebotomy Man offered an explanatory support.

Some sketches are devoid of text or simply name the veins without offering additional information. In many cases, though, text and image worked in tandem through the Phlebotomy Man: lines and word bubbles linked the bloodletting site on the image to marginal text that discussed the condition for which each vein was indicated, as seen in figure 8.1 On a Phlebotomy Man diagram contained in the later fourteenth-century manuscript belonging to astrologer John Somer (figure 8.1), for example, the text circle at the top left explains that 'The cardiac vein, i.e. of the heart or the "coralis" [vein], is cut for diseases of the spiritual members' ('vena cardiaca i[d est] cordis uel corrallis incidit[ur] pro passionib[us] sp[irit]uali[b]u[s]) membro[rum]'.[31] The fourth from the top on the right reads 'We cut two veins on the neck for headache and rheumy eyes' ('In collo duas venas incidim[us] p[ro]p[ter] dolore[m] capiti[s] & oculos reumatizantes'). Several of the bloodletting points on this diagram would have been especially familiar to medical practitioners dealing with plague patients, since they address the same veins mentioned in plague tracts: 'The cephalic vein, i.e. of the head, which is cut for diseases of the head and brain' ('Vena cephalica i[d est] capitis que p[ro] passionibus capitis inciditur et cerebri) and 'The basilic vein, i.e. from the liver, is usually opened for diseases of the liver and spleen' ('Vena basilica i[d est] epatica solet aperiri pro passionib[us] epatis et splenis'). Plague tract authors repeated similar phrases, demonstrating how traditional venesection advice was easily incorporated into therapy for this 'new' disease.

A small number of Phlebotomy Man diagrams, including an elaborate one in the fifteenth-century BL Harley MS 3719, contain sketches of bloodletting tools, such as the bowl used to collect the drawn blood. Numerous manuscripts contain images of both the Zodiac Man and the Phlebotomy Man; some – like BL Harley MS 3719, Cambridge, Trinity College MS 943, München, Staatsbibliothek Cod. Lat. 4394 and Paris, Bibliothèque nationale de France (hereafter BnF), Hebreu MS 1181 – are notable in that they combine the Phlebotomy Man and the Zodiac Man into a single image: here the vein identification and descriptions are augmented with zodiac labels written or drawn on the figure's body to remind the viewer which sign ruled what body part.[32] While the

---

in *Illuminating the Middle Ages: Tributes to Prof. John Lowden from his Students, Friends and Colleagues*, ed. L. Cleaver, A. Bovey and L. Donkin (Leiden, 2020), pp. 446–68.

31 Oxford, Bodleian Library MS Savile 39, fol. 10r.

32 BnF Hebreu MS 1181 contains the only known duo Zodiac Man/Phlebotomy Man image on which all the bloodletting locations are labelled in Hebrew. Interestingly, the 'absence of any specifically Jewish features in the iconography of the signs of the zodiac indicates that this

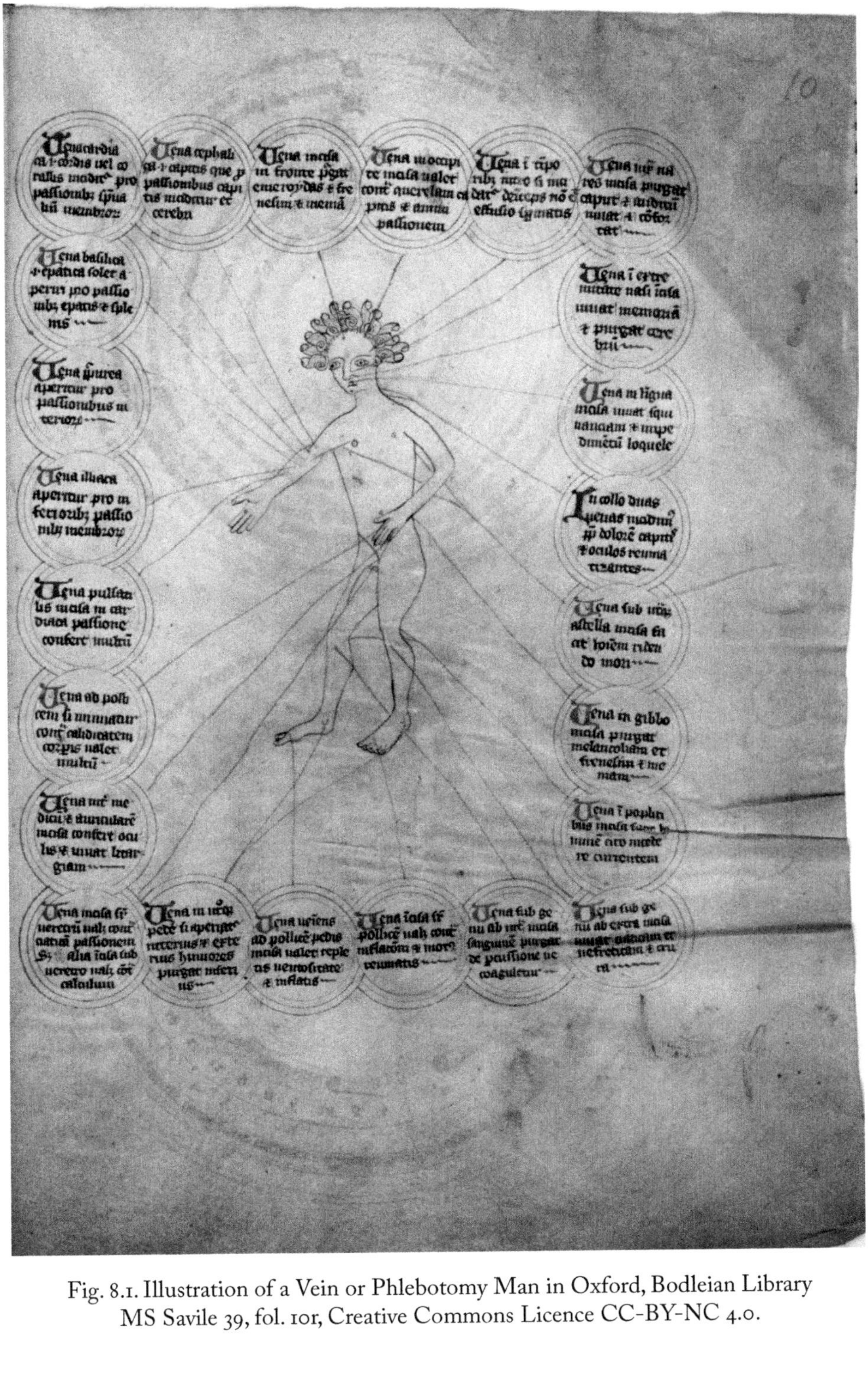

Fig. 8.1. Illustration of a Vein or Phlebotomy Man in Oxford, Bodleian Library MS Savile 39, fol. 10r, Creative Commons Licence CC-BY-NC 4.0.

diagrammatic descriptions and tools were adapted for plague therapy, however, they and the humoral logic on which they were based applied equally well to a much wider range of ailments. The standard Phlebotomy Man, then, aided and informed plague medicine, but it was neither created nor intended solely for addressing plague.

Recent work on the origins and afterlives of the later fourteenth-/early fifteenth-century Wound Man ('Wundenmann') diagrams suggests that this image could have been more closely linked to plague than either the Zodiac Man or the Phlebotomy Man, at least in their original conceptions.[33] Like its counterparts, though, the Wound Man diagram served a didactic function, in this case to advise surgeons of treatments and cures for each of the illustrated wounds. In its earliest form, in the fourteenth-century Lobkowicz Library and Archives, Nelahozeves Castle, MS Cod. VI Fc. 29, the locations of diseases and injuries were simply noted on the Wound Man diagram, linked by a line or arrow to text indicating their curability or incurability. Plague does not appear explicitly on these 'proto-Wound Men', but then neither does any diagnostic label. Sites located on the image close to the neck/behind the ears, armpit and groin concern fistulae and cancers. While they could denote plague, they appear to be labelled incurable, rendering the association plausible but not definitive.

Later fifteenth-century iterations of the diagram were far more expansive, both visually and textually. Alongside the 'multitude of graphic wounds' indicated on the man's body – often colourised and including cuts and lesions inflicted by a number of still-present weapons, animals and insects – many extant copies such as is found in Wellcome Collection MS 49 clearly show numerous rounded blue-green swellings in the armpit, neck and groin, suggesting that in addition to his injuries the man has contracted plague (see figure 4.4). Although they are never labelled specifically as plague buboes, the precise location of these swellings in the same cleansing or purging spots that attracted the attention of plague tract writers cannot be coincidental. Short textual phrases and paragraph numbers

---

well-executed figure was copied from a non-Jewish model'. G. Bos, C. Burnett and T. Langermann, 'Hebrew Medical Astrology: David Ben Yom Tov, Kelal Qaṭan: Original Hebrew Text, Medieval Latin Translation, Modern English Translation', *Transactions of the American Philosophical Society*, n. s. 95 (2005), i, iii, v–vii, ix, 1–61 and 63–121 (p. vii). I thank Gerrit Bos for this notice. Jack Hartnell points out, however, that the figure is circumcised, a sign of his Jewishness. Personal correspondence, 8 July 2020. I also thank Mary Yearl for alerting me to J. Isserles, 'Bloodletting and Medical Astrology in Hebrew Manuscripts from Medieval Western Europe', *Sudhoffs Archiv* 101 (2017), 2–41. Although a broad set of anatomical diagrams does appear in the Islamicate tradition, the Phlebotomy and Wound Men do not. On Islamic anatomical diagrams, see E. Savage-Smith, 'Anatomical Illustration in Arabic Manuscripts', in *Arab Painting: Text and Image in Illustrated Arabic Manuscripts*, ed. A. Contadini (Leiden, 2007), pp. 147–60. On earlier Sino-Tibetan cautery images that appear to have served much the same purpose, see V. Lo and R. Yoeli-Tlalim, 'Travelling Light: Sino-Tibetan Moxa-Cautery from Dunhuang', in *Imagining Chinese Medicine*, ed. V. Lo and P. Barrett (Leiden, 2018), pp. 271–90. I thank W. A. McGrath for this notice.

33 Hartnell, 'Wording the Wound Man'.

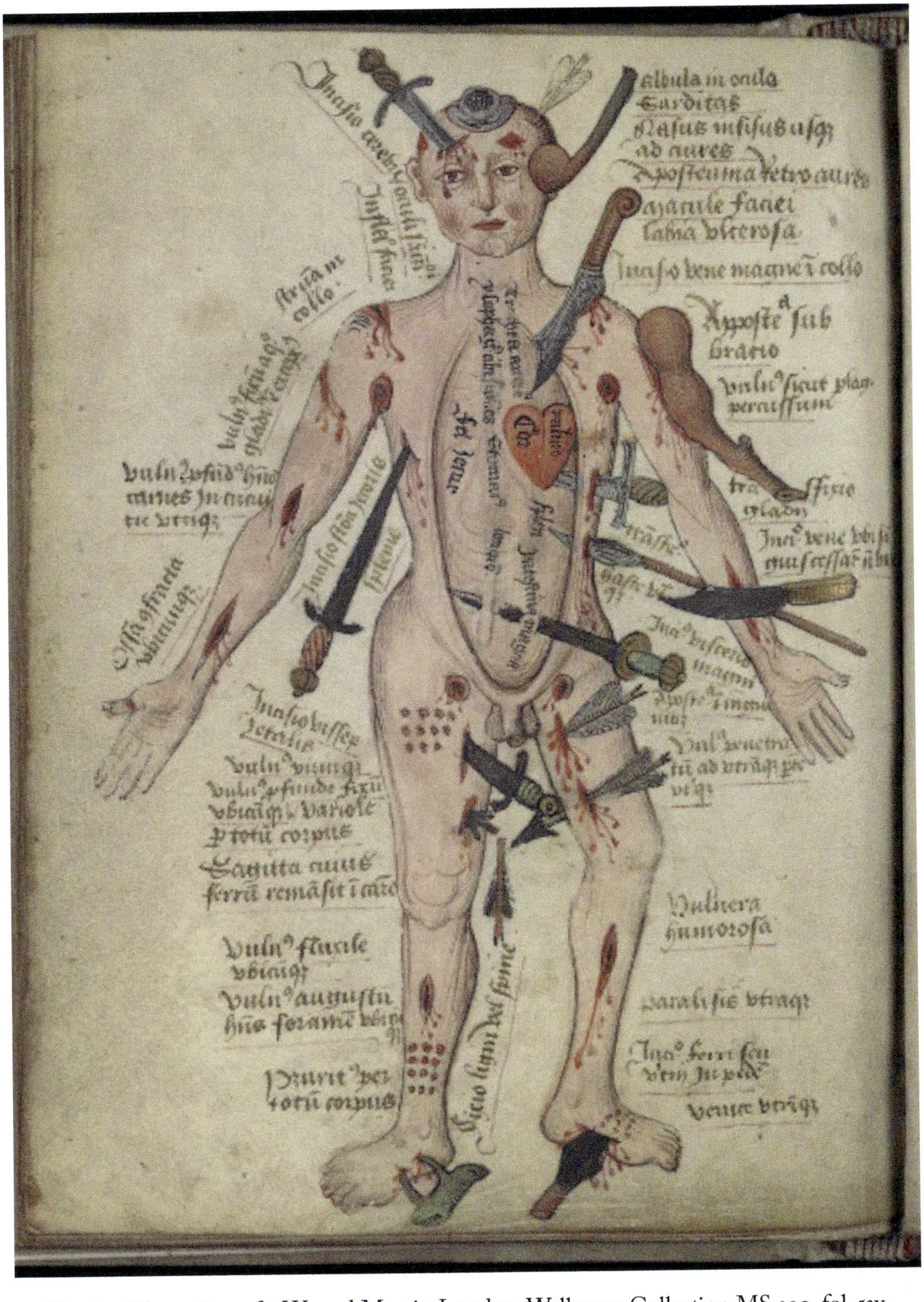

Fig. 8.2. Illustration of a Wound Man in London, Wellcome Collection MS 290, fol. 53v, available under a Public Domain Mark.

direct the viewer/reader to the appropriate place in the associated surgical treatise for more information.

In addition to directions on how to remove embedded arrow heads or to remove spider venom, Wellcome Collection MS 49's Wound Man includes numbered labels 8, 9, 30 and 36 that point to 'Bresten an den halse vor den kropf' (botches on the neck), 'Bresten hynder den Oren' (botches behind the ears), 'Bresten undir den armen' (botches under the arms) and 'Bresten by der scham' (botches near the groin – literally, private parts).[34] Shifting one's eye to the instructive text on the preceding pages reveals the associated instructions: for botches under the arm, bleed the median or lung vein or one on the finger on the opposite side; for botches in the groin, bleed the vein that runs between the thigh and the foot that is called the menstrual vein of women ('der frawe[n] me[n]strual[i]s adir'); for botches behind the ears or on the neck, bleed the cephalic vein on both arms. Accompanying these instructions is a familiar phrase found in regimens of health: 'Et sunt pensanda inedito [sic] curare volenti / Ars etas virtus regio complexio fforma (Nec) non simpthona [sic] commixtio temporum et aerum' ('These are the things which must be considered by a doctor wishing to cure: Occupation, age, strength, habitat, complexion, physique, as well as the symptoms and the balance of seasons and airs').[35]

What appear to be plague buboes, whether brightly coloured or in a less startling flesh tone – as they are in München, Bayerische Staatsbibliothek Cgm 597 – do not appear on all manuscript copies of the Wound Man. The diagram in a later seventeenth-century manuscript compiled for a southern German Franciscan house, for example, shows no such swellings.[36] They do appear on the only known English Wound Man image, found in the fifteenth-century Wellcome Collection MS 290 (figure 8.2). Here, the buboes – labelled 'apostema behind the ears' ('aposteuma retro aures'), 'apostema under the arm' ('apposte[m]a sub bracio') and 'apostema at the groin' ('aposte[m]a ingui[nalis]'), respectively – are deep red and vividly weeping, reminiscent of the plague bubo that appears on St Roch's inner thigh, rather than green-blue and fully engorged as they appear in other instances.[37] Unlike its German counterparts, however, this English Wound Man appears without the accompanying surgical text or more detailed therapeutic instructions.[38]

Wound Man diagrams survive in a smaller number of manuscripts than the Zodiac or Phlebotomy Man: twelve late medieval manuscripts and some twenty copies of early

[34] Wellcome Collection MS 49, fol. 35r. I have translated the German word 'bresten' here as botch; it can likewise mean 'relic', a term used by some plague tract writers to denote the bubo.

[35] Wellcome Collection MS 49, fols. 34r–v. I thank Lucy Barnhouse for her help with transcription and Winston Black for his with the Latin translation.

[36] Wellcome Collection MS 990, fol. 572.

[37] For a discussion of colour and plague buboes, see Jones, '"Apostumes"' and Nükhet Varlık's chapter 4 in this volume.

[38] Hartnell, 'Wording the Wound Man'. Hartnell convincingly suggests that this manuscript image was adapted, with some confusion and mistaken assumptions, from the printed version in the *Fasciculus medicinae.*

modern printed books contain the image – the latter being famous surgical compilations such as Giovanni and Gregorio De Gregori's multi-edition *Fasciculus medicinae* (which had circulated in manuscript for nearly a century before appearing in print in multiple languages) and popular surgery books written by well-known medical writers of the late fifteenth through later seventeenth centuries, including Hieronymus Brunschwig, Hans von Gersdorff, Thomas Gale, William Clowes, Ambroise Paré and John Browne. These early modern printed woodcut versions of the Wound Man updated the injurious weapons and refashioned the very presentation of the maimed man to meet modern tastes. Yet, aside from the late fifteenth-century printed edition of the *Fasciculus medicinae* – which dutifully noted in the Italian version 'apostema behind the ear' ('Aposte[m]a drieto all'orechia'), 'apostema under the arm' ('Apostema sotti el braccio') and 'apostema near the groin' ('Apostema nelle anguinagle'), along with a more detailed discussion of the corresponding bloodletting veins and a plague treatise by Pietro da Tossignano – plague buboes largely disappeared from the Wound Man by the sixteenth century.[39] The explanatory text surrounding the Wound Man also disappeared from printed versions of the diagram inserted into surgery books; here, the diagram became less about identifying potential wounds and injuries than 'stand[ing] as an embodiment of the very craft of surgery, proudly displaying the grievous injuries that the owner of such a surgical book was qualified to treat'.[40] Perhaps by this point, familiarity with plague made oozing buboes a less interesting reflection of the early modern surgeon's handiwork than limbs destroyed by cannon balls, rapiers and battle-axes.

As interesting as the medieval Wound Man's apparent link to plague – a link that is absent or barely acknowledged in the paired Disease Man and Disease Woman images that join the Wound Man in the fourteenth- and fifteenth-century surgical *Dreibilderserie* (three picture series) group – is its place of origin in southern Germany.[41] This is where the

39 *Fasciculo de Medicina* (Venice, 1495), p. 24. One of the veins indicated for buboes in the groin is the 'virginal vein', also called the 'menstruous vein of women' ('Ma se sara la apostema nelle anguinagle allora minuiscasi el sangue dala vena virginale la quale e soto el calcagno et chiamasi vena menstruosa delle donne o vero vena virginale'). I thank Ann Carmichael for verifying my transcription of the Italian text. Aside from the vague notation that bleeding certain arm or foot veins is suitable 'against old pustules' ('contra pustulas antiquas'), the Phlebotomy Man diagram in the *Fasciculus medicinae* makes no connection to plague.

40 J. Hartnell, 'The Many Lives of the Medieval Wound Man', *The Public Domain Review* (7 December 2016), https://publicdomainreview.org/essay/the-many-lives-of-the-medieval-wound-man. On the separation of medical images from their text, see P. M. Jones, 'Image, Word, and Medicine in the Middle Ages', in *Visualizing Medieval Medicine*, ed. Givens, Reeds and Touwaide, pp. 23–46. For the ways in which text–image relationships reveal images' practical function, textual origin and social utilitarian purpose, see Öberg Strådal, 'Utility'.

41 Aside from the earlier 'proto' images and the English copy, all other medieval copies of the Wound Man diagram accompany the surgical text *Wundartznei* that was adapted from the thirteenth-century *Artzneibuch* by the Würzburg surgeon Ortolf von Baierland. Hartnell, 'Wording the Wound Man'.

unique Bubo Man image also first emerged in the early fifteenth century, not to accompany a surgical text but, rather, to guide the therapeutic aid of plague victims.

Bubo Man images

Despite their common appearance in texts about phlebotomy or surgery and the sometimes long discussion about bloodletting and the surgical management of buboes in plague treatises, no Phlebotomy Man or Wound Man appears in the tracts. Instead, writers relied on their readers' familiarity with the proffered instructions, perhaps assuming that the primary audience for their work was other medical practitioners and a lay clientele that included wealthy patrons and literate readers who could be counted on to turn to the medical profession for treatment.[42]

The few exceptions to this rule, however, are intriguing. Alongside a copy of the Chronicle of Scheyern, the early fifteenth-century UB 4° Cod. MS 885 contains numerous texts about plague, including a plague tract, a preventative plague regimen, a list of medicines and foods suitable in times of plague and detailed bloodletting instructions for plague victims.[43] The seven-chapter plague tract has been traced to Jakob Engelins von Ulm, a physician or surgeon who possibly wrote it at the Viennese Habsburg court of Duke Albrecht IV of Austria at the turn of the fifteenth century.[44] Accompanying the plague texts is a unique diagram that looks like typical Phlebotomy Man drawings found in German manuscripts, except that multiple plague buboes are distinctly shown on the neck, armpits and groin (figure 8.3).[45]

The curly-haired man in the diagram faces forward, eyes averted to his left as if the large buboes on his neck make him uncomfortable. His arms are held away from his body, impeded by the large red abscesses under his arms. The backs of his hands and the tops of his feet are marked with venesection points. More importantly, the text that surrounds the image does not offer the usual wide-ranging bloodletting instructions. Instead, it provides direction for bloodletting specifically associated with the location of the clearly marked buboes, drawing from the more expansive instructions found in the manuscript's phlebotomy text that is appended to the plague tract.

German scholars have examined the bloodletting text and its accompanying diagram, but to date both largely have been ignored in English scholarship. The text itself can be dated to around 1400 and attributed to an Upper German ('oberdeutschen') – that is

42 Numerous tract writers nevertheless claimed to have written their work for the benefit of the poor who could not afford a physician's help and/or those who could use the advice directly.

43 The chronicle was likely the early thirteenth-century *Chronicon Shirense* written by Abbot Conrad von Scheyern, head of a Benedictine abbey in the southern German diocese of Freising.

44 H. Bergmann, 'Neufunde zum Pesttraktat Jakob Engelins von Ulm', *Sudhoffs Archiv* 62 (1978), 282–93 (p. 283). Bergmann has identified at least twenty-eight extant copies of Engelin's tract.

45 I thank Rodo Pfister and Thomas Gloning for their assistance in tracking down the German manuscript images and the sources in the following footnotes.

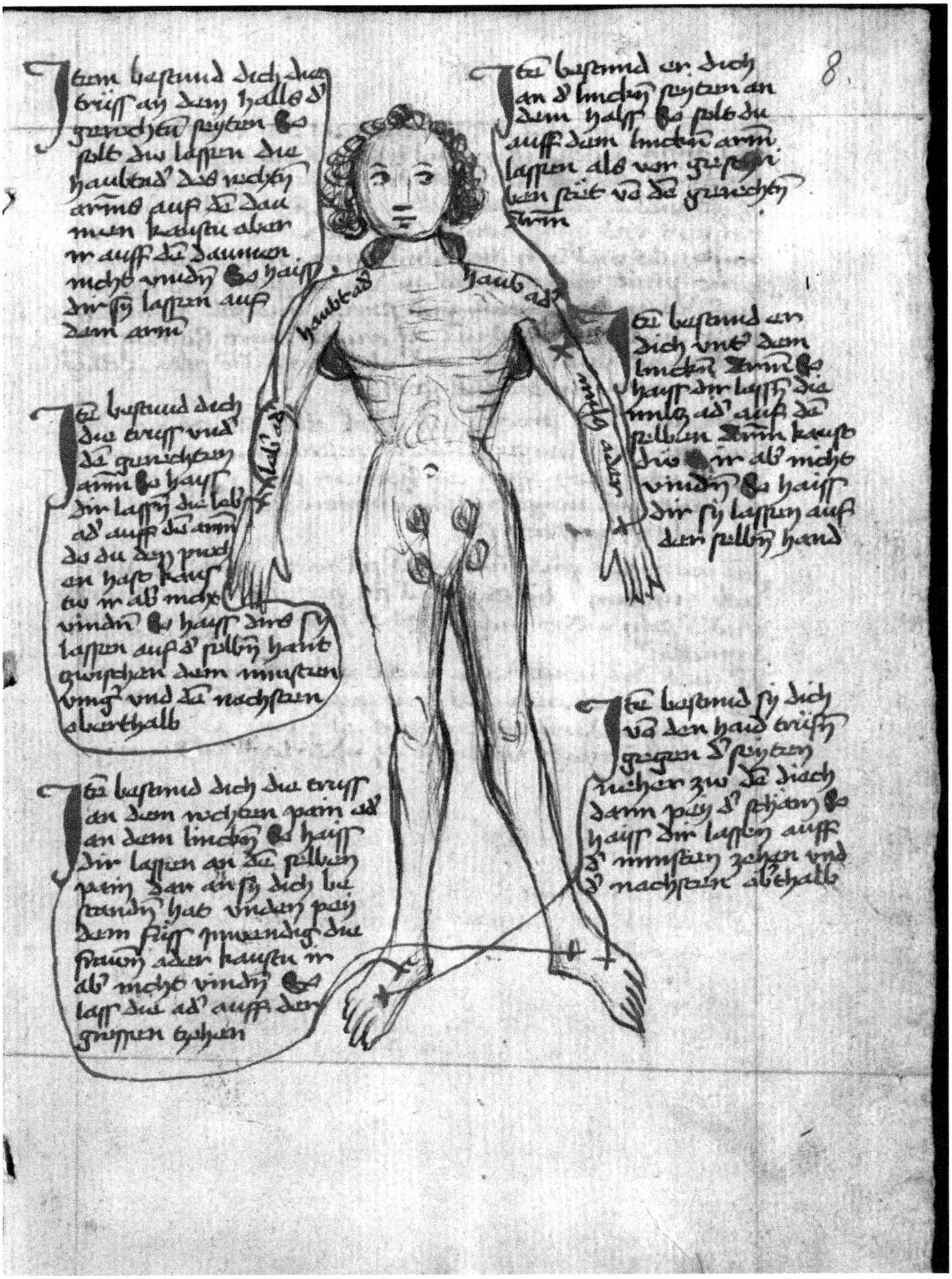

Fig. 8.3. Illustration of a Phlebotomy Man with buboes in Ludwig-Maximilians-Universität München, 40 Cod. MS 885, fol. 8r, available under a Public Domain Mark.

southern, High German-speaking – writer. It was likely derived from the popular *Pest-'Brief an die Frau von Plauen'* (plague letter from Mrs von Plauen) that included bloodletting instructions for plague victims meant for a lay audience.[46] The text on the diagram appears in six groups, representing the three main bleeding sites on each side of the body that correspond to the three main bubo locations. These six sites are the same as those typically discussed in plague tracts, including in Engelins' treatise that appears in UB 4° Cod. MS 885. The diagram's captions come from the phlebotomy text itself, though, which appears as a stand-alone, collected with but not part of the plague tract.

The phlebotomy text is systematic and orderly, discussing bloodletting separately from cupping, noting astrological influences and calendric prohibitions and equally balancing discussion of the two sides of the body. While largely didactic, the text also acts as a kind of dialogue, wherein both the physician's and plague patient's voices are present.[47] This formula is then carried over into the diagram, with the phlebotomy instructions starting at the head and working their way down.[48] If the gland at the right ear is affected, the main vein on the right arm should be bled at the thumb; if this is not done, poison will remain in the arm. If the gland under the right arm is affected, then the liver (i.e., hepatic) vein on the right arm should be opened; if this is not possible, bleed the vein between the small finger and the one next to it. Whether the affected gland is in the right or left groin or thigh, it is crucial to let blood on the same side, either on the foot – from the woman's vein ('inwendig die frauen ader') – or from the vein on the big toe. Similar instructions follow for the left side of the body 'as written for the right' ('als vor geschriben stet von dem gerechten'). In addition to the bleeding points, the locations of the veins are also marked with text on the man's body: cephalic vein ('haubt ader') on the shoulders, basilic or hepatic vein ('leber ader') on the right forearm and median or cardiac vein ('milcz ader') on the left forearm. The feet veins are left unlabelled.

It is not clear whether Jakob Engelins is linked to the other plague texts in UB 4° Cod. MS 885, or even to the bloodletting instructions and diagram. Seven copies of the bloodletting text survive, all in German, but aside from UB 4° Cod. MS 885 only two manuscripts contain the diagram (WLB Hs. HB XI 10 and ÖNB Cpv. 5184); of these two, only the Stuttgart manuscript also contains Engelins' plague tract.[49]

46 Bergmann and Keil, 'Das Münchner Pest-Laßmännchen', pp. 325, 329.

47 Ibid., p. 329.

48 UB 4° Cod. MS 885, fol. 8r. A transcription is found in H. U. Schmid, 'Austernrotz und Opodeldok: Medizinische Sprache im Mittelalter', in *Sprache und Medizin: Interdisziplinäre Beiträge zur medizinischen Sprache und Kommunikation*, ed. S. Bechmann (Berlin, 2017), pp. 157–80 (pp. 169–70).

49 Bergmann and Keil, 'Das Münchner Pest-Laßmännchen', p. 330 for surviving copies of the bloodletting text and diagram and Bergmann, 'Neufunde zum Pesttraktat', pp. 228–9 for the corresponding copies of Engelins' plague tract. WLB Hs. HB XI 10 unfortunately has not been digitised and I was unable to consult it as, indeed, Bergmann and Keil were unable to do. They note that a fourth manuscript, München, Bayerische Staatsbibliothek Cgm 28, contains a possibly 'contaminated' version of the diagram ('Zuordnung noch ungewiß; überliefert Laßmännchen

The 'Pest-Aderlaßmann' found in ÖNB Cpv. 5184 is dated to the early 1480s. This man is longer haired, wild ('verwildertem') and certainly more awkwardly drawn than the earlier version found in UB 4° Cod. MS 885.[50] Red lines lead from each bleeding point on the right arm to its respective text, overwritten with the name of the vein; the veins are also named on the left arm and hand. Some of the man's buboes are in the correct places, but other red spots appear to have been randomly placed on his forehead, breast and shoulders and under his chin. The artist may have been drawing additional bloodletting points. Two folios later (fol. 71r) is another more detailed (and also long-haired) Phlebotomy Man diagram; here, the same round red circles denote bleeding spots and the circles on the forehead, chin and ribcage are given explanatory and descriptive labels.[51] The text on the Bubo Man has also been modified from its earlier version and is not symmetrically arranged, although the intent and contents are largely similar.

What appears to be a further manuscript adaptation of the Bubo Man diagram accompanies a mid-fifteenth century English verse version of the plague tract attributed to John of Burgundy, found in BL Egerton MS 1624 (figure 8.4). More than 130 copies survive of that plague tract, but this is the only one that contains a therapeutic diagram.[52] It is also the only verse adaptation of the text. The manuscript itself has received attention recently for its inclusion of Henry Daniel's *Liber Uricrisiarum*.[53] It includes four anatomical diagrams: a Latin parchment booklet contains a planetary man (showing planetary influences on body parts), a Zodiac Man accompanying a series of astrological and liturgical texts and tables and a Phlebotomy Man; the Middle English paper section contains the Bubo Man, who sits embedded within the plague tract. There is little in the manuscript that suggests a connection to southern Germany and word forms in the plague text using 'qw' and 'lk' (e.g., 'qwylk' for 'which') clearly suggest that the text was copied in a northern location in England. Until more is known about its provenance and the people involved in

---

mit kontaminierten Beischriften') along with a Zodiac Man, while a fifth, ÖNB Cpv. 2967, contains the bloodletting text and part of Engelins' plague treatise, but not the diagram.

50 Bergmann and Keil, 'Das Münchner Pest-Laßmännchen', p. 330; ÖNB Cpv. 5184, fol. 69v.

51 Between the two diagrams in the manuscript, on fol. 70r, there is also an unusually drawn Zodiac Man, who likewise has red circles drawn on his body to link the zodiac signs to their respective body parts.

52 The earliest known copy of John of Burgundy's treatise (BnF NAF MS 4516), commissioned for France's King Charles V in 1371, contains a miniature of a robed physician sitting at a lectern consulting a large manuscript, possibly the treatise itself. Several professionally made deluxe copies of the same tract produced in England are lavishly decorated and a copy made for Lady Margaret Beaufort includes elements of Margaret's arms and badge together with the red dragon and silver greyhound found on King Henry VII's arms (Cambridge, Fitzwilliam Museum, MS 261). For more on John of Burgundy's tract, see L. Jones, 'Itineraries and Transformations: John of Burgundy's Plague Treatise', *Bulletin of the History of Medicine* 95 (2021), 277–314.

53 M. T. Tavormina, 'The Heirs of Henry Daniel: The Fifteenth- and Sixteenth-Century Legacy of the *Liber Uricrisiarum*', in *Henry Daniel and the Rise of Middle English Medical Writing*, ed. S. Star (Toronto, 2022). I thank Professor Tavormina for sharing her research on the Egerton manuscript.

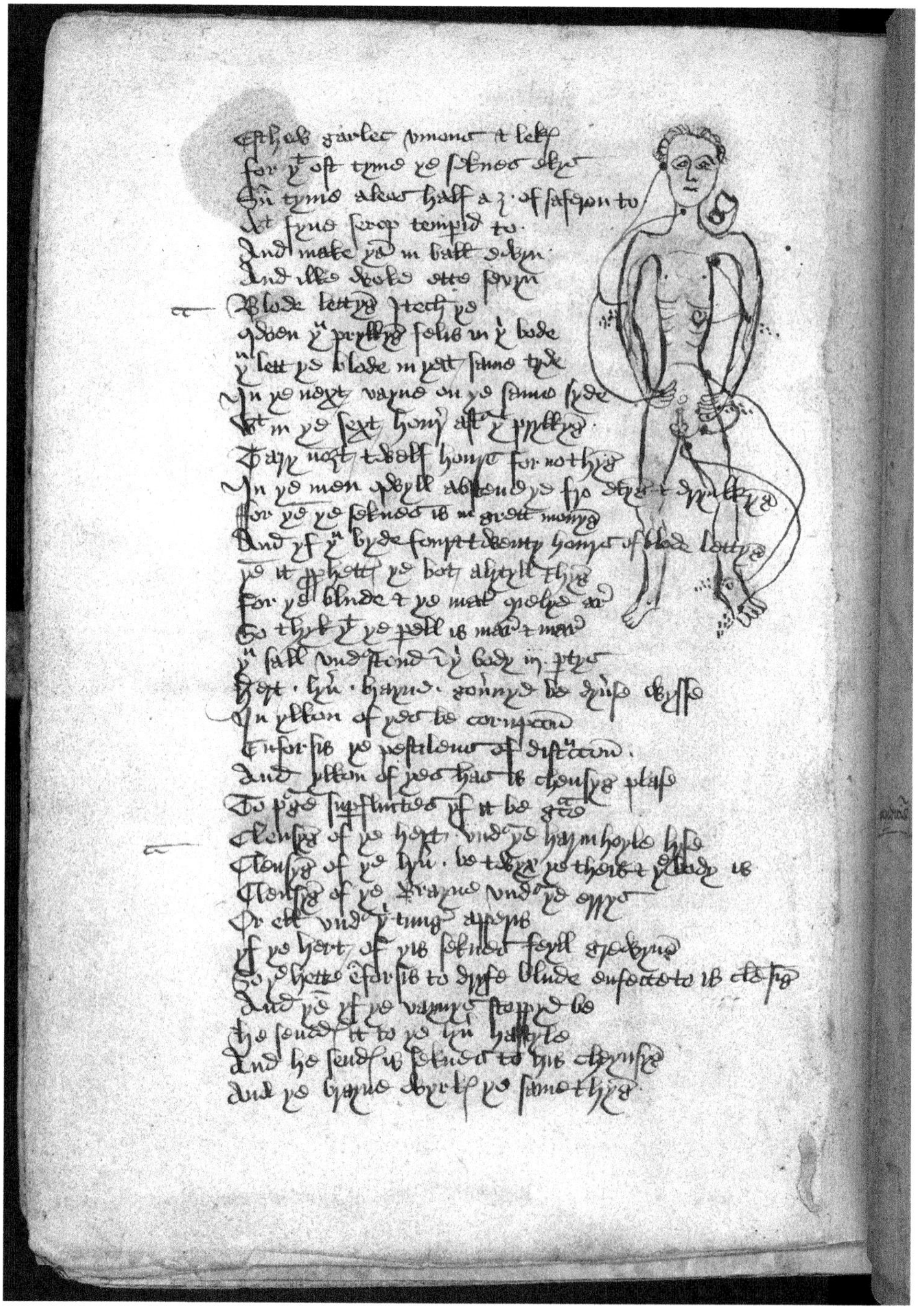

Fig. 8.4. Illustration of Phlebotomy Man with buboes in a versified version of John of Burgundy's plague tract, in London, British Library, Egerton MS 1624, fol. 216v. The British Library Board.

its production, it remains an open question whether the scribe received inspiration from a sketch that he saw elsewhere or this diagram is another one-off original.

The treatise itself, called *De Pestilencia* in this version, takes the four-chapter version of John of Burgundy's popular tract and turns it into a mnemonic didactic poem. Although the scribe claims to have 'Made [it] in Y[n]glis owt of Latyne', John's tract had already been circulating in Middle English since the late fourteenth century.[54] The verse more or less follows the content of its source, which focuses on the preventive and therapeutic measures necessary to avoid and treat plague. These include eating and drinking in moderation, avoiding bathing, sweating and sex and being bled for both prophylactic and curative reasons. The phlebotomy advice is of most relevance here, for it is in this section that the verses' didactic purpose is clearest:

> Blode letty[n]g I tech þe / Wen þ[o]u prykky[n]g felis in þi bode / þ[o]u lett þe blode in þat same syde / in þe next vayne on þe same syde / W[i]t[h] in þe sext hours aft[er] þ[a]t prykky[n]g / Tary noȝt twelf hours for nothy[n]g / … For þe þe [sic] seknes is in grett mouy[n]g / and yf þ[o]u byde four & twenty hours of blode lettyng / þe[n] it p[ro] phettes þe bot a lytyll thy[n]g / for þe blude & þe mat[er] [con]ielyd ar[e] / so thyk þ[a]t þe p[er]ell is mar[e] & mar[e].[55]

These words envelop the diagram on the left and across the bottom, a few lines even running across the man's legs. The subsequent text discusses the three main parts of the body – the heart, the liver and the brain – and their respective 'clensing plase(s)', followed by the appropriate vein to bleed depending on the bubo's location. Departing from the wordier prose version on which it is based, the instructions are straightforward: 'And yf þe boch appeyre und[er] the harme hoyle / On þe hart vayne of þe harme þ[o]u blode thoyle'.[56] Likewise, a bubo in the outer groin ('Betwyx þe the & þe body') calls for bleeding the vein between the little finger and the one beside it, while the vein between the big toe and the next one is better suited for a bubo in the inner groin ('Ynwarde nere toward þe p[ri]vete'). The vein between the ankle and the heel targeted a bubo higher on the body, on the side or the back, as did cupping between the shoulders. Cupping was likewise suitable for buboes under the ears or on the throat, although so too was bleeding 'the heyd vayne of þe harme'. After bloodletting, the heart should be comforted with cold electuaries.

54 In addition to Jones, 'Itineraries and Transformations' and Jones, *Patterns of Plague*, see A. Honkapohja and L. Jones, 'From *Practica Phisicalia* to *Mandeville's Travels*: Untangling the Misattributed Identities and Writings of John of Burgundy', *Notes & Queries* 67 (2020), 18–27; L. M. Matheson, 'Médecin sans frontières? The European Dissemination of John of Burgundy's Plague Treatise', *ANQ: A Quarterly Journal of Short Articles, Notes and Reviews* 18 (2005), 19–31.

55 BL Egerton MS 1624, fol. 216v. A transcribed but somewhat faulty copy of the verse appears in R. H. Bowers, 'A Middle English Mnemonic Plague Tract', *Southern Folklore Quarterly* 20 (1956), 118–23. I have re-transcribed the manuscript rather than use Bowers's work.

56 BL Egerton MS 1624, fol. 217r.

The short-haired Bubo Man in BL Egerton MS 1624 stands at the top of the verso folio in the inner margin, enabling the reader to consult the diagram while reading the phlebotomy instructions. He stares directly at the reader, his hands on his hips. Small round circles indicate the numerous bubo sites mentioned in the text, joined by lines to their respective bleeding spots. The venesection points on the arms, hands, feet and toes are themselves further indicated by numerous spots drawn outside the lines of the body, likely representing draining blood. A cup sits just above and behind his shoulder. The man's heart is drawn on his chest, behind his ribs, linked by a line to the bubo in his armpit and to his inner elbow – supplementing the text by demonstrating that buboes in the armpit are associated with the heart and can be mitigated by letting blood from the basilic vein in the arm. Similar lines link other buboes to their associated organ and appropriate bloodletting vein.

Versions of the Bubo Man illustration subsequently appeared in at least four printed plague tracts, one each from Basel and Venice and two from Lyon. The earliest ones from Basel, Venice and Lyon all appeared around 1519 and are found in vernacular translations of the same plague tract. The Swiss author, humanist, Protestant reformer and self-proclaimed 'doctor of medicine and the seven liberal arts' ('der syben fryen künsten und Ertzny Doctor') Joachim von Watt claimed, in the Basel edition, to have translated the tract from Latin ('Züsamen bracht als dem Latin durch den hoch gelerten') into German.[57] The French and Italian versions are attributed to unnamed physicians from Basel.[58] A recent study on German plague tracts situates the appearance of the printed Bubo Man squarely in the Reformation, casting it as both a novel and subtle shift away from images of saints and a reimagining of the image of St Sebastian.[59] It is far more probable, however, that this printed work from Basel and its image were simply adapted from a copy of the southern German manuscript tract and image from the previous century. In other words, by the time it appeared in print, this Bubo Man image was neither new nor was it meant to have any religious connotations at all. Its adaption into print was not out of the ordinary, as the manuscript-to-print transition of the illustrated *Fasciculus medicinae* also attests.

In the printed Basel tract, the Bubo Man appears alone on the final page, along with the phrase 'you will find the passages about how, when, where and to whom this [the bloodletting] should be done in the sixth chapter' ('von den lässen wie / wen / wo / und an wem die geschehen söllent / findest du gnügsam am sechsten Capitel').[60] There is no text on the diagram itself, just multiple bubo sites (including on the front of the knees and

[57] J. Vadianus, *Ein kurtz und trüwlich underricht*, title page.

[58] Anonymous, *Regime contro la pestilence*; Anonymous, *Regime contre la pestil[enc]e*. The French tract was reprinted numerous times: five editions in Lyon (1519–30) and at least once in Toulouse (1532) on its own and then again in Paris (possibly c.1530 and c.1570), Lyon (1575) and Rouen (1578), the latter editions attached to a treatise on the properties and virtues of water. The diagram was omitted in the later copies, in some cases replaced with other images.

[59] Heinrichs, *Plague, Print, and the Reformation*, p. 78.

[60] Vadianus, *Ein kurtz und trüwlich underricht*, D3v.

back of the shoulders – sites not usually associated with buboes) joined by lines to their respective bleeding sites on the arms, hands and feet. The curly-haired man stands on a rocky landscape, his arms held away from his body and his head tilted as if to ease pain caused by a bubo on the neck. His genital area is covered by what in today's world looks like a small bathing suit or underwear, similar to what one commonly finds in both Wound Man and Phlebotomy Man diagrams of the same era. In the Lyon tract, the same image appears on the title page with no textual instructions, although the tract itself (like the Swiss one) offers bloodletting directions depending on the buboes' location. Later editions of the same French tract omit the image all together. In the Venetian version, the Bubo Man's placement likewise does not appear to be directly associated to the text that speaks to bloodletting and buboes. Here, uniquely, the Bubo Man is seated, his arms held up at an awkward distance from his body and his head again tilted to one side.

The fourth printed Bubo Man image associated with a plague tract appeared in 1581. Like its earlier Lyonnais counterpart, this image appears on the plague tract's title page, rather than alongside the relevant text. In this case, though, the author of the text was a cleric, not a physician. Although Estienne Ydeley discusses the importance of letting blood from the appropriate veins, depending on where the bubo ('bosse') is located, his text focuses much more on spiritual than on physical therapies for plague. Indeed, his image reflects a decidedly religious perspective because it includes a seemingly angry god above the man who is surrounded by the words 'The plague is not an illness but a rod of God' ('La peste n'est pas une maladie, mais une verge de Dieu') – meaning a punishment or chastisement for people's sins.[61] In this context, bloodletting might help to cure the body, but it does not in any way cleanse man's soul of plague. This reading is further attested by the fact that the tract's printer, Jean Stratius, focused on producing Catholic religious works.

Finally, a fully bearded Bubo Man appears on a mid-sixteenth-century German broadside dedicated to the art of bloodletting for plague victims. Printed in Regensburg, this image has much in common with the earlier German manuscript diagrams in that it includes bloodletting instructions that surround the image. Here, the lines on the body used to link the buboes to their appropriate bloodletting veins are lettered A to G, matched to the same letters in the instructions. Given the level of detail in the instructions, such broadsheets had a clear didactic function in the early modern world.

Conclusion

In 1482, the Nuremburg barber-surgeon, printer and playwright Hans Folz used a woodblock image of a surgeon lancing an axillary plague bubo in the *Pestregimen in Versen*, which he wrote and printed himself (figure 8.5). Folz intended the bubo-lancing image to serve as a technical instruction both for his fellow (but, he said, inexperienced) practitioners and for the unlearned layperson, based on his own experience providing treatment

[61] Ydeley, *Des secrets souverains*, title page.

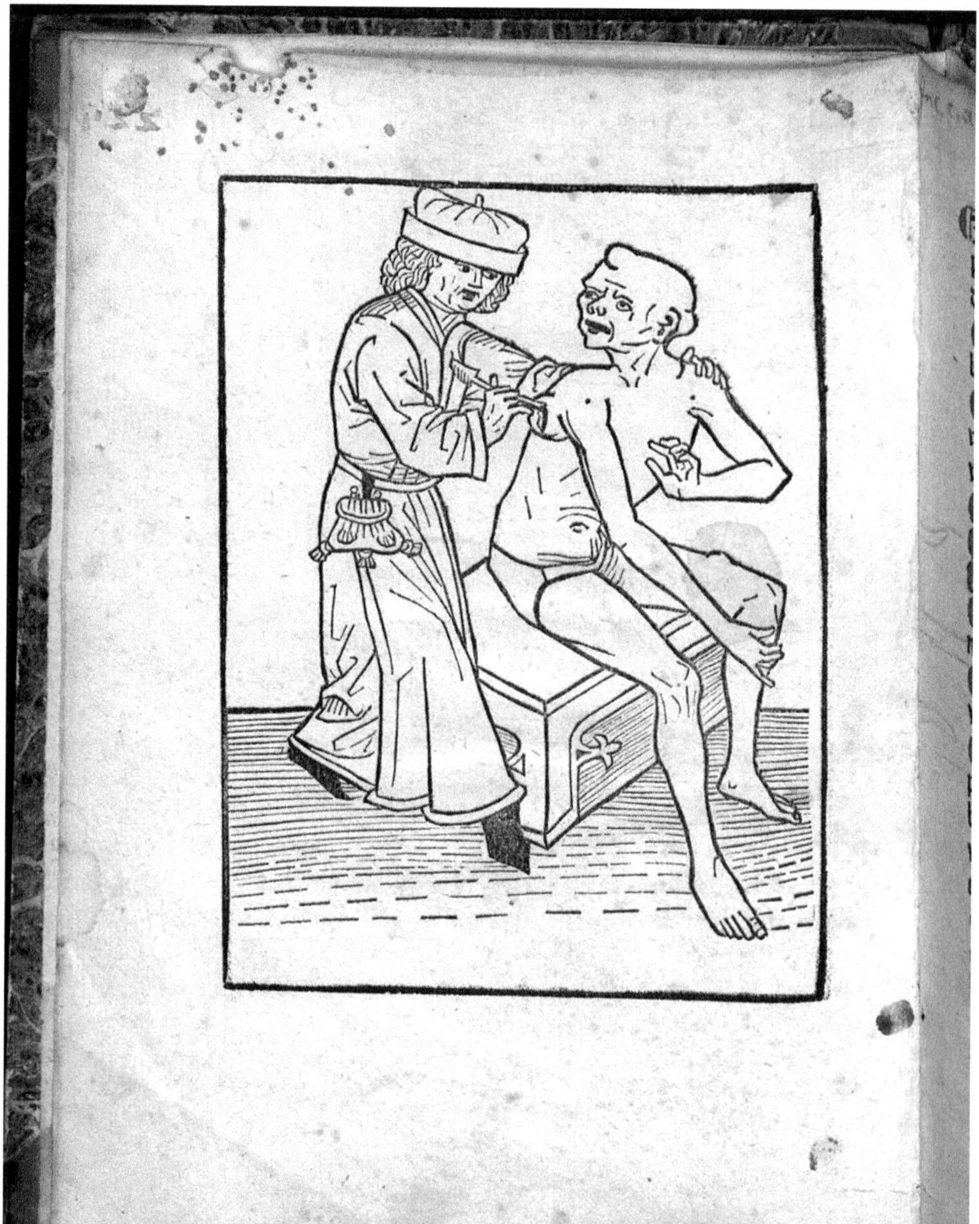

Fig. 8.5. Doctor lancing a plague bubo, frontispiece in Hans Folz, *Item ein fast köstlicher spruch von der pestilencz un[d] anfenglich von den zeiche[n] die ein künfftige pestilencz beteuten* (Nuremburg: Hans Folz, 1482). Bayerische Staatsbibliothek, Attribution–NonCommercial–ShareAlike 4.0 International (CC BY-NC 4.0).

to plague victims.[62] Barber-surgeons were far more likely than physicians to treat plague patients and it was critical that they be aware of the disease's recognisable signs and how to deal with them. Folz's image of the bubo is little more than a line drawing, but it gives the impression of a large, cavernous abscess. Despite the fact that illustrated anatomy treatises appeared before the mid-sixteenth century, though, medical and surgical treatises included almost no other illustrations of plague patients or their physical signs of disease before Thomas Bateman's illustrated *Delineations of Cutaneous Disease* in 1817.[63] In this context, the Bubo Man, while certainly not widespread, filled a niche in plague treatment. More copies of the diagram may have once existed than have survived, its didactic value lying in its rather novel representation of plague not for diagnostic or descriptive purposes but for treatment.

Even though bloodletting remained one of plague's primary therapies for centuries, plague treatises remained largely unillustrated. They were, first and foremost, textual instructions for understanding and managing the disease. Largely formulaic in their structure and layout, they offered the same basic medical explanations and advice across the centuries. Nevertheless, the emergence of the vernacular Bubo Man in the early fifteenth century demonstrates that novelty and innovation was possible and that the tract's didactic purpose could be taken a step further. The image might have been drawn for the benefit of one person – the southern German writer of a text specifically dedicated to bloodletting for plague victims – but its value extended further when it was copied into other German manuscripts and then adapted into a German printed plague tract. The national and international networks of early modern print then led to its appearance in Italy and France. The appearance of a remarkably similar diagram in a mid-fifteenth-century English manuscript, however, is more difficult to reconcile without knowing who created BL Egerton MS 1624 and on what source manuscript it relied.

The paucity of medical diagrams of plague before the nineteenth century complicates our attempts to conceptualise what late medieval and early modern medical practitioners saw when they looked at and attempted to treat their stricken patients. Plague – the disease caused by *Yersinia pestis* – may not have appeared significantly different to those who witnessed it in the fourteenth century than it did to those who saw it centuries later. Its most telling signs remained relatively constant across time. For a relatively short period, however, between the early fifteenth and later sixteenth centuries, we do get a glimpse of how physicians and surgeons envisioned treating it.

62 C. Huey, *Hans Folz and Print Culture in Late Medieval Germany: The Creation of Popular Discourse* (Farnham, 2012), p. 86.

63 D. Bertoloni Meli, *Visualizing Disease: The Art and History of Pathological Illustrations* (Chicago, 2018), p. 135. George Thomson's mid-seventeenth century plague tract describes his dissection of a plague victim and contains an image demonstrating this dissection in progress. G. Thomson, *Loimotomia, or the Pest Anatomized* (London, 1666).

9

Psalm 38 as Plague Diagnostic and Prophylactic in Abraham Yagel's *Moshi'ah Ḥosim* (1587)

ANDREW BERNS[1]

Introduction

Twentieth-century scholarship on premodern writing often distinguished 'medical' from 'spiritual' approaches to healing. When a premodern physician emphasised the spiritual state of a patient, explored connections between sin and disease or suggested prayer and penitential acts as treatment for illness, many scholars relegated such writings to the ignominious realm of 'pseudo-science'.[2] Even today, the study of medicine is often associated with material interventions, chiefly dietary recommendations and prescriptive therapeutics. Abraham Yagel's *Moshi'ah Ḥosim* (henceforth MH), a Hebrew plague treatise published in Venice in 1587, challenges this misleading binary. Yagel, a Jewish banker and medical doctor, wrote this work in the wake of sixteenth-century Italy's most devastating plague outbreak as confidence in the medical establishment ebbed markedly.[3] In MH, traditional advice common in Galenic medicine sits comfortably aside a detailed description of how to use biblical incense to treat plague. Naturalistic explanations and religious practices are so closely related in Yagel's text – and in his cosmology – as to be nearly

1 Warm thanks to Lori Jones and Nükhet Varlık for the invitation to contribute to their volume and for their help in improving this piece. Susan Einbinder also provided welcome feedback and comments. Thanks are also due to David Ruderman, Matthew Melvin-Koushki and Yaacob Dweck.

2 P. Preto, *Peste e società a Venezia nel 1576* (Vicenza, 1978) distinguishes between 'dispute scientifiche' (pp. 47–57) and 'pseudo-medicina' (pp. 90–7). This distinction was enshrined in classic works such as L. Thorndike's *History of Magic and Experimental Science*, 8 vols. (New York, 1923–58). With regard to premodern medicine, such Enlightenment binaries were celebrated by eighteenth-century physicians and are sometimes unwittingly adopted by their modern students, as in G. B. Risse, 'Medicine in the Age of Enlightenment', in *History of Medicine in Society: Historical Essays*, ed. A. Wear (Cambridge, 1992), pp. 149–95 (p. 154). This concept has a distinguished pedigree in Jewish Studies as well. See, for example, H. S. Lewis, 'Maimonides on Superstition', *Jewish Quarterly Review*, o. s., 17 (1905), 474–88 and J. Trachtenberg, *Jewish Magic and Superstition* (New York, 1979).

3 Preto, *Peste e società*, 91.

symbiotic. This chapter joins a new wave of scholarship that seeks to revise and recast narratives stressing the 'pseudo-scientific' properties of premodern healing.[4]

Sixteenth-century medical science from the world of northern Italian universities – itself predicated on a blend of long-standing medieval practice and a humanist emphasis on empiricism – was one feature of this Jewish physician's healing practice.[5] Another was a rich blend of kabbalistic doctrines, appeals to non-physical worlds and psalm recitations. One function of Yagel's MH, as we shall see, is to medicalise a spiritual text and treat liturgy as prophylaxis against the plague. Although Yagel and his works are known to historians of premodern Jewry, he and his plague treatise are virtually unknown to scholars of the Second Pandemic. This chapter endeavours to bring Yagel's work into dialogue with current scholarship on plague. In so doing, it builds on work that strives to recast the enduring and misleading scholarly dichotomy between premodern science and religion.

Background to Yagel's treatise

Abraham ben Hananiah Yagel was born in 1553 in Monselice, part of the Venetian *terra-ferma*. His life did not follow the sort of trajectory common to other medical doctors of his time and place, however: he was itinerant; left no record of matriculating at, or graduating from, a university medical faculty; and none of his major works was published during his lifetime.[6] From his own writings one gets the sense that he devoted as much time and energy to banking and other business enterprises as he did to the practice of medicine. Yet Yagel saw himself mostly as a physician.

Despite his lack of university education and, likely, a formal medical licence like those acquired by his Christian counterparts, a document in a Roman archive testifies that on 9 February 1593 Yagel was granted permission to care for Christian patients, in the absence of qualified Christian physicians, in the *terra rubiera* (between Reggio and Modena).[7]

4 For a recent example, see N. Cohen-Hanegbi, *Caring for the Living Soul: Emotions, Medicine and Penance in the Late Medieval Mediterranean* (Leiden, 2017). An earlier instance of this more reasonable approach to premodern categories may be found in M. McVaugh, 'Treatment of Hernia in the Later Middle Ages: Surgical Correction and Social Construction', in *Medicine from the Black Death to the French Disease*, ed. R. French, J. Arrizabalaga, A. Cunningham and L. Garcia-Ballester (Aldershot, 1998), pp. 131–55.

5 On the shift to empiricism in early modern medicine and medical teaching, see L. Jones, 'Experience over Education or Education over Experience? Pre-Modern Medical Writing on the Plague' and M. Stolberg, 'Training Future Practitioners: Medical Education in Sixteenth- and Early-Seventeenth-Century Padua and Montpellier from the Students' Perspective', both in *Transforming Medical Education: Historical Case Studies of Teaching, Learning, and Belonging in Medicine in Honour of Jacalyn Duffin*, ed. S. Lamb and D. Gavrus (Montreal, 2022), pp. 86–111, 112–35.

6 D. B. Ruderman, *Kabbalah, Magic, and Science: The Cultural Universe of a Sixteenth-century Jewish Physician* (Cambridge MA, 1988), pp. 8–26.

7 Rome, Archivio di stato, Fondo camerali I: Diversorum del camerlengo, filza 407, fol. 158b, as cited by Ruderman, *Kabbalah*, p. 179 n.8.

Such permission was explicitly granted because he had earned the title of *artium et medicinae doctor*. He is best known today for an autobiography entitled *Ge Ḥizzayon* (Valley of Vision), which describes a heavenly journey, as well as two sizable encyclopaedias: *Bet Ya'ar Ha-Levanon* (House of the Forest of Lebanon) and *Be'er Sheva*.[8] The encyclopaedic works display the eclecticism of Yagel's interests and feature much engagement with medicine and natural philosophy.

In 1575, some years before he published his plague treatise MH, Yagel penned a brief description of the plague outbreak in Luzzara, near Mantua. Venetian Jews had been temporarily expelled from Venice in 1571–72 and Yagel, along with others, took refuge in the Mantovano.[9] Yagel's description is minimal, focused more on the economic and social impact of the outbreak than on the public health threat that it posed. He lamented 'a person will do anything to rescue himself' from plague and that as a consequence 'all the matters of the bank came to a standstill'.[10] Despite his medical practice, banking, it seems, was still among his first priorities.

But this brief description of plague was a mere prelude to his enduring composition on this theme: *Moshi'ah Ḥosim* (Figure 9.1). That work, of which two manuscripts survive, was dedicated to a banker: Or Shraga Sanguini of Venice.[11] This dedication may reflect Yagel's ongoing business concerns, although the work itself never mentions finance or trade of any kind. It is likely that Yagel wrote his treatise in the wake of the devastating plague epidemic that struck Italy in 1575–77.[12] By one account, more than 50,000 Venetians died in that outbreak – nearly one-third of the city's population.[13] Among the by-products of this deadly epidemic was a sense of life's inherent precarity,[14] as well as a wellspring of literary energy. As Samuel K. Cohn has argued, this large-scale epidemic 'hardly killed off creativity. Instead, it unleashed a wave of plague writing'.[15] While most plague tracts were written in the vernacular by this point in time, including another known Italian-Jewish response to this particular epidemic, Yagel chose Hebrew, a lingua franca among literate

8 On all three texts see Ruderman, *Kabbalah*, especially pp. 25–42.

9 D. B. Ruderman, ed. and trans., *A Valley of Vision: The Heavenly Journey of Abraham ben Hananiah Yagel* (Philadelphia, 1990), p. 6.

10 Ruderman, *Valley of Vision*, p. 131.

11 Washington, Library of Congress, Hebr. MS 115; Oxford, Bodleian Library, MS Mich. 179.

12 Preto, *Peste e società*, p. 48 for the identification of this contagion as bubonic plague.

13 R. J. Palmer, 'Girolamo Mercuriale and the Plague of Venice', in *Girolamo Mercuriale: medicina e cultura nell'europa del cinquecento*, ed. A. Arcangeli and V. Nutton (Florence, 2008), pp. 51–65 (p. 51).

14 Preto, *Peste e società*, p. 102, drawing on the work of A. Tenenti, '"Ars moriendi": quelques notes sur la problème de la mort à la fin du XVe siècle', *Annales E. S. C.* 6 (1951), 433–46.

15 S. K. Cohn, *Cultures of Plague: Medical Thinking at the End of the Renaissance* (Oxford, 2010), p. 294.

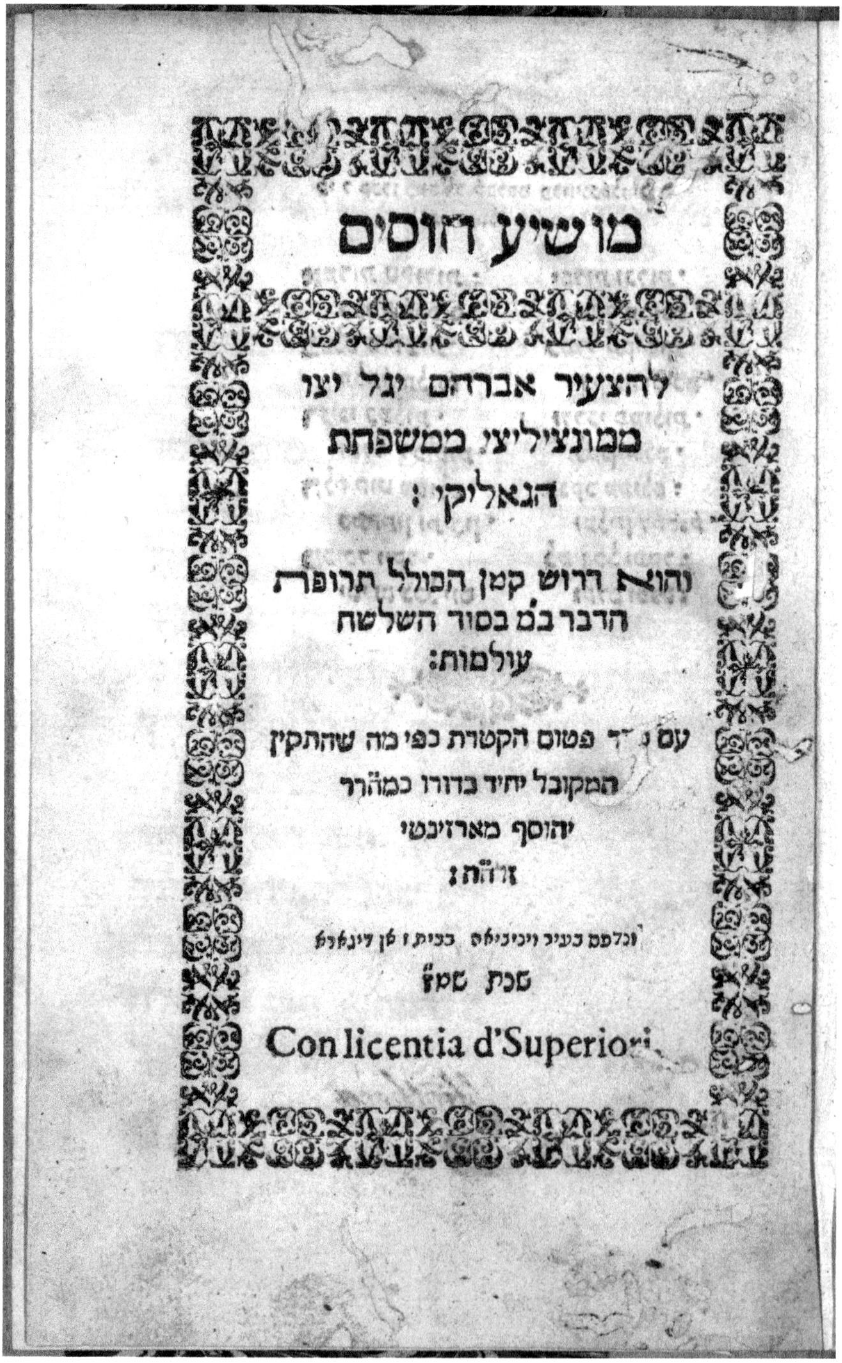
מושיע חוסים

להצעיר אברהם יגל יצו
ממונציליצי ממשפחת
הגאליקי:

והוא דרוש קטן הכולל תרופת
הדבר בֿמ בסוד השלשה
עולמות:

עם סדר פטום הקטרת כפי מה שהתקין
המקובל יחיד בדורו כמהר״ר
יהוסף מארזיניטי
זצ״ל:

ונדפס בעיר ויניציאה בבית זואן די גארה
שנת שמ״ז

Con licentia d'Superiori.

Fig. 9.1. Cover page of Abraham Yagel's plague treatise *Moshi'ah Hosim* (Venice, 1587). Allard Pierson, University of Amsterdam, PH3213 A.

Jews, as his language of expression.[16] The book's title, 'savior of those who take refuge', is a quotation from Psalm 17. 7; Yagel chose it because, as he put it, 'anyone who takes refuge in God will be saved by means of the matters stated here. For through them God performs his message and he will surely be healed [Ex. 21. 19], since he gave permission to the physician to heal.'[17] For Yagel, medicine was a spiritual practice.

Scientific and cosmological premises

This nexus of the physical and metaphysical expresses itself throughout MH. The treatise is predicated on and displays Yagel's belief in a triadic universe consisting of natural, astral and divine realms.[18] While many Christian plague tracts distinguished between two realms – the upper and lower – Yagel states that 'The root of everything [rests] on the manner and rotation of the three worlds we have mentioned.'[19] The structure of MH reflects this preoccupation. The book is divided into nine chapters, at the end of which is a *pittum haQetoret* addendum: a prescribed recitation of the list of ingredients in biblical incense.[20] Recitation of those passages was thought to have salubrious effects.[21] The nine chapters, appropriately, demonstrate Yagel's triadic scheme. The first three chapters address

16 D. de Pomis, *Brevi discorsi et efficacissimi ricordi per liberare ogni città oppressa dal mal contagioso* (Venice, 1577) included originally dated letters presented to the health board of Venice – they are the earliest precisely dated reactions to the outbreak in Venice, 1575–77. Cohn, *Cultures of Plague*, pp. 172–3.

17 A. Yagel, *Moshi'ah Ḥosim* (Venice, 1587), p. 4v.

18 Ruderman, *Kabbalah, Magic, Science*, p. 32 n. 35. For more detail see pp. 110–11 and M. Idel, 'The Magical and Neoplatonic Interpretations of Kabbalah in the Renaissance', in *Jewish Thought in the Sixteenth Century*, ed. D. B. Cooperman (Cambridge MA, 1983), pp. 186–242 (pp. 224–6) for an explicit comparison of Yagel and Agrippa. See also Idel, 'Differing Conceptions of the Kabbalah in the Early Seventeenth Century', in *Jewish Thought in the Seventeenth Century*, ed. I. Twersky and B. Septimus (Cambridge MA, 1987), pp. 137–200 (p. 169 n. 154), where Idel notes a medieval source for Agrippa.

19 Ruderman, *Kabbalah, Magic, Science*, p. 32. The fourteenth-century Liège physician John of Burgundy, for example, had noted in his plague tract that 'Everything below the moon, the elements and the things compounded by the elements, is ruled by the things above, and the highest bodies are believed to give being, nature, substance, growth and death to everything below their spheres'. Cited in R. Horrox, *The Black Death* (Manchester, 1994), pp. 184–5. Medieval Christian plague tract writers had little to say about divine influences; although religiosity played a greater role in their sixteenth- and seventeenth-century treatises, none divided the universe into a triadic nature as Yagel has done. For this discussion as it pertains to English and French treatises, see L. Jones, *Patterns of Plague: Changing Ideas about Plague in England and France, 1348–1750* (Montreal, 2022), chapter 1.

20 See Exodus 30. 34–8.

21 A. D. Berns, *The Bible and Natural Philosophy in Renaissance Italy* (Cambridge, 2015), p. 12. See also the recent contribution of E. Reichman, 'Incensed by Coronavirus: Prayer and Ketoret in Times of Epidemic', *Lehrhaus*, Tuesday, 8 June 2021, at https://www.thelehrhaus.com/timely-thoughts/incensed-by-coronavirus-prayer-and-ketoret-in-times-of-epidemic/. See also

the causes of plague in the natural, astral and divine realms. The fourth, fifth and sixth chapters concern the signs by which plague is known – and can be prevented – in the astral world. The final three chapters propose cures and secrets for mitigating the plague's severity in the upper, divine realm.

Underlying this hierarchical presentation is a cosmology according to which all three worlds are interconnected. Actions in the lower, 'natural' realm affect the celestial and divine realms. The reverse is also true. In his Introduction, immediately following his presentation of the triadic system, Yagel notes that 'every lower thing' – meaning tangible, earthly substances – 'receives and admits the force and influence of the higher realm'. As support he quotes a well-known passage from midrashic literature: 'as our sages of blessed memory hinted in Bereshit Rabbah, there exists no blade of grass from below without a constellation in the sky that beats it and tells it to grow'.[22] Crucial to this conception is the notion that actions on earth influence celestial and divine behaviour: 'according to the awakening of the lower realm, so does the upper realm provide abundantly'.[23] Yagel reminds his readers that 'ancient philosophers', an expression denoting non-Jewish authorities, knew how to use natural means to connect heaven and earth. Incense is his principal example of this expertise, but herbs and stones that are burnt may accomplish it as well.[24]

Many of Yagel's ideas concerning the origin of plagues, as well as their signs and potential treatments, are found in other plague tracts written by Christians and Muslims of his period. Beautification of the home is important: people should live in nice, spacious dwellings. Yagel tells his readers not to eat or sleep too much, not to dress in a way that makes them overheated and to avoid pulse crops and, in general, nutriment that produces excessive heat. One should anoint oneself with oil and eat sour things.[25] There is even basic advice about daily routine: stretching first thing in the morning is advised, as is

S. Einbinder, *Writing Plague: Jewish Writing, Memory, and the Great Italian Plague (1630–31)* (Philadelphia, 2022).

22 MH, p. 3r. Quoted in Ruderman, *Kabbalah, Magic, Science*, p. 32. See *Bereshit Rabbah* 20. 7.

23 MH, p. 3r. This is also an axiom of Lurianic Kabbalah. See J. Garb, *Manifestations of Power in Jewish Mysticism* [in Hebrew] (Jerusalem, 2005), pp. 185–7; A. Bar-Levav, 'Ritualization of Jewish Life and Death in the Early Modern Period', *The Leo Baeck Institute Yearbook* 47 (2002), 69–82; U. Safrai, '"Worship of the Heart" in the Kabbalah of the Sixteenth Century' [in Hebrew] (unpublished Ph.D. dissertation, Ben Gurion University, 2016). My thanks to Dr Safrai for sharing his dissertation with me.

24 MH, 3v, where Yagel also cites Ibn Ezra, *Sefer ha-Atzamim*, which claims that incense ascends from earth to the heavens, like a ladder set up on the earth (cf. Gen. 28. 12).

25 MH, p. 14r–v. For similar recommendations in English and French plague tracts, see Jones, *Patterns of Plague*, chapter 1. On oil, see the remarks of the Sephardi convert to Islam İlyas bin İbrahim, who recommended the use of almond and violet oil to preserve health in times of plague, as well as chamomile and rose oil in preparing ointments to treat plague buboes. See also N. Varlık, *Plague and Empire in the Early Modern Mediterranean World: The Ottoman Experience* (New York, 2015), p. 36.

combing one's hair and cleaning one's teeth.[26] Clearly, some of Yagel's advice for how to avoid or mitigate the effects of plague comes from a common stock of knowledge and medical recommendation.[27]

One difference is that Yagel approaches his subject from the perspective of Hebrew literature. This not only opens the riches of rabbinic and kabbalistic texts but also provides Yagel with an opportunity to assess the language of plague in his chosen medium of literary expression. For example, he expatiates upon three of Hebrew's main terms for plague. They are, he writes, '*magefah*, *mashḥit*, and *dever*'. *Magefah*, Yagel reminds his readers, is a general term for any sudden death brought about by transgressions. As an example, he quotes three biblical verses in which the root *n-g-f*, from which *magefah* is derived, appears: 'And the Lord smote [*va-yigof*] the people', [Ex. 32. 35] because they had constructed the Golden Calf; 'and those that died by the plague [*magefah*]' were twenty-four thousand' [Num. 25. 9]; and 'the plague [*ha-negef*] was begun among the people' [Num. 17. 12]. The common denominator in these episodes is that Israelites were punished for their sins and struck down immediately, without warning. *Mashḥit*, by contrast, can be either spiritual or physical. It can affect animals as well as plants.[28] *Dever*, in turn, 'comes from the mist of the earth' and does not derive from the four elements. Rather, it comes from a hidden quality whose nature is to invert things, according to the changing of seasons. In terms of human suffering, blood is first infected, then other parts of the body.[29]

Yagel's discussion of Hebrew's terms for plague illustrates the holistic way in which he approached medicine, as did many other writers in an age in which strictly medical ideas and understanding of plague circulated alongside and in combination with non-medical ideas. His analysis of *dever* as free from the four elements is predicated on solid Galenic learning, while his notion of *mashḥit* as either corporeal or psychological testifies to a more capacious understanding of affliction. All of this is based both on Yagel's biblical erudition and on his medical training. Above all, the semantic range of Hebrew's three main words for plague demonstrates one of Yagel's cosmological axioms: that the physical and spiritual interpenetrate to the point of indistinguishability.

The centrality of spiritual practice in any medical treatment was commonplace to Jews, Christians and Muslims in the sixteenth century. Yagel's Christian neighbours in northern Italy frequently invoked spiritual life in their medical writings and plague tracts. A popular plague treatise by the Bolognese physician Leonardo Fioravanti advised people to above all entrust their souls to God.[30] During the plague outbreak of 1575–77, no less a figure than the archbishop of Milan, Carlo Borromeo, advocated piety, penance and prayer for those

26 MH, p. 15v.

27 On similar recommendations elsewhere, see Cohn, *Cultures of Plague*; Jones, *Patterns of Plague*; and S. Cavallo and T. Storey, *Healthy Living in Late Renaissance Italy* (Oxford, 2013).

28 MH, p. 5r.

29 Ibid., p. 5v.

30 Fioravanti, *Il reggimento della peste*, p.p. 135–7 in the 1626 edition [1571], cited in Preto, *Peste e società*, p. 71.

Christians afflicted by plague. Such a pious stance was on display in Venice, too: there was much prayer for the cessation of the plague. In 1576, the state itself recommended and sponsored fasts and prayers, such as the one on 3 August.[31]

Similar tendencies were at work in the Islamicate world. For example, a mid sixteenth-century Ottoman plague treatise written by Taşköprüzāde Aḥmed entitled *Treatise on Healing Epidemic Diseases* blends medical and occult science. It is 'the most comprehensive of all known and extant early modern Islamicate' plague treatises and it too places much emphasis on prayer, including a substantial 'Prayer for the Removal of Plague'.[32] In the early modern Islamicate world, prayer, communal or otherwise, was recommended by the righteous forebears (*salaf*) to free oneself from pain or punishment, especially when combined with herbs and stones. Such practices are predicated on occult scientific insistence that prayer, incense and mineralogy can both prevent and treat disease. As they had done in other traditions, however, scholars until recently have typically dismissed such practices as superstitious and of little scientific worth.[33]

Unfortunately, even the best-informed scholars on this subject have denigrated these religious practices as superstitions, claiming that they flourish only in times of grave psychological trauma. To understand how people in the sixteenth century (Jewish, Muslim or Christian) understood and experienced plague epidemics, we must examine these notions as they were understood and lived by our historical actors, 'for whom occult science was often simply good natural and mathematical science, predicated on and conducive of both physical and spiritual health'.[34]

Psalm 38: Torah as medicine

An effective way to underscore Yagel's synthesis of the spiritual and the scientific is to focus on a specific passage in MH. One under-appreciated aspect of this plague tract is its contribution to a genre well known to sixteenth-century Italian Jews: biblical commentary. Some Italian Jews of this period engaged in biblical exegesis in relatively conventional formats: some offered glosses on specific verses and terms within verses, as can be seen in the work of Ovadiah Sforno, while others took a more topical view, as in the sermons

[31] Preto, *Peste e società*, p. 76–7, 81.

[32] M. Melvin-Koushki, 'Taşköprüzāde on the (Occult) Science of Plague Prevention and Cure', *Nazariyat* 6 (2020), 133–68 (p. 139).

[33] Ibid., p. 135.

[34] Ibid.

of Judah Moscato.[35] Still others pursued their biblical analysis in genres less familiar to modern scholars: antiquarian treatises, dictionaries, encyclopaedias and medical writings.[36]

Yagel's approach to the Bible belongs to this later group. Although he never penned a commentary on scripture, he did engage in a form of biblical exposition, especially in his encyclopaedic work.[37] In MH, immediately prior to the better-known *pittum haQetoret* texts, Yagel engages in a line-by-line explication of Psalm 38.[38] While the *pittum haQetoret* readings had a long association with repelling epidemics, they gained new meaning by the early seventeenth century through their association with the fumigation practices recommended in plague regimens. Even with new research on the enduring use of ancient incense practices, the recitation of the sacred texts antecedent to the *pittum haQetoret* reading has received less attention in the context of Jewish responses to the Second Pandemic.[39] The same could be said of the prophylactic properties of psalm recitation. According to Yagel, the recitation of Psalm 38 functioned as a deterrent to plague, by strengthening one's immunity to infection. Most interestingly, MH features a medical interpretation of this single psalm that effectively medicalises a spiritual text and treats liturgy as prophylaxis.

In the wake of the Black Death, Jews and Christians alike made ample use of the psalms for intertwined medical and spiritual purposes.[40] Jewish writers between 1348 and

35 On Sforno see E. Finkel, *R. Obadja Sforno als Exeget* (Wrocław [Breslau], 1896). See also the editors' introduction to *Kitvei Rabbi 'Ovadyah Sforno*, 2 vols. (Jerusalem, 1983); R. Bonfil, 'Il Rinascimento: la produzione esegetica di 'O. Servadio Sforno', in *La lettura ebraica delle Scritture*, ed. S. S. Sierra (Bologna, 1995), pp. 261–77; S. Campanini, 'Un intellettuale ebreo del Rinascimento: 'Ovadyah Sforno a Bologna e i suoi rapporti con i cristiani', in *Verso l'epilogo di una convivenza: gli ebrei a Bologna nel XVI secolo*, ed. M. G. Muzzarelli (Florence, 1996), pp. 99–128. On Moscato, see G. Veltri and G. Miletto, ed., *Rabbi Judah Moscato and the Jewish Intellectual World of Mantua in the 16th–17th Century* (Leiden, 2012) and Veltri and Miletto, ed., *Judah Moscato: Sermons*, 4 vols. (Leiden, 2011–15).

36 Berns, *Bible and Natural Philosophy*.

37 See especially *Bet Ya'ar ha-levanon* and Ruderman's discussion in *Kabbalah, Magic, and Science*, passim.

38 MH, pp. 30r–1v.

39 S. Einbinder, personal correspondence. I thank Professor Einbinder for discussing this point and sharing her forthcoming work with me.

40 In general, on Jewish responses to the Black Death, see S. Einbinder, *After the Black Death: Plague and Commemoration among Iberian Jews* (Philadelphia, 2018); G. Bos and G. Mensching, 'The Black Death in Hebrew Literature: Abraham Ben Solomon Ḥen's *Tractatulus de pestilentia*. Edition of the Hebrew Text with Introduction, English translation and Supplement of the Romance Terminology', *Jewish Studies Quarterly* 18 (2011), 32–63; T. Barzilay, 'The Black Death in Aragon: A Look at a Jewish Chronicle', *Hayo Haya: A Young Forum for History* 8 (2011), 53–71; S. Einbinder, 'Physicians and Their Daughters: Memory and Medicine during the Plague Years', chapter 5 of *No Place of Rest: Jewish Literature, Expulsion, and the Memory of Medieval France* (Philadelphia, 2008), pp. 112–36; L. Raspe, 'The Black Death in Jewish Sources: A Second Look at "Mayse Nissim"', *The Jewish Quarterly Review*, n.s. 94 (2004), 471–89. For Jewish plague treatises, see G. Bos, 'The Black Death in Hebrew Literature: Ha-Ma'amar be-qaddahat ha-dever (Treatise on Pestilential Fever)', *European Journal of Jewish Studies* 5 (2011), 1–52.

1500 deployed two main sources: biblical methods of controlling plague and the Book of Psalms.[41] Reciting psalms to guard against the plague was, after all, a form of magic. The most important book of Jewish magic was the *Sefer Shimush Tehillim*, also popular in Latin as *de usu psalmorum*.[42] Closer to Yagel's own time and setting, a cleric at Forlì (where there happens to be no evidence of plague in the 1570s) published a digest of ordinances promulgated by Antonio Gionnotto, the city's bishop. To celebrate the Jubilee, Gionnotto organised processions of religious companies and 'many barefooted men and women' singing litanies and psalms.[43] The physician Castore Durante, in his *Tesoro della sanità*, notes that exercising the mind by singing psalms and listening to theological stories would delight and invigorate the soul and spirits, which in turn would help the body to better resist infirmity.[44]

Yagel's position was stronger: he believed in the Torah itself as medicine. At the beginning of the ninth chapter of MH, which concludes with the *pittum haQetoret* ritual and also includes the author's psalm commentary, there is a clear argument that the Torah 'is given as a keepsake for every matter'.[45] In other words, plague prophylaxis is one of the Torah's many possible applications. Furthermore, Yagel stresses that 'it is appropriate that you continue to read it [Scripture], and meditate on it day and night,[46] and surely no plague will approach your tents'.[47] Yagel's support for this concept, that the recitation of scripture has salubrious effects, is drawn in part from the Zohar: 'Our sages of blessed memory said in the *midrash* of Rabbi Shimon bar Yohai to the pericope *va-Yaqel* that man is saved from three death sentences: judgment in this world, the judgment of the angel of death, and the judgment of gehenom, etc.'.[48] The angel of death was, not surprisingly, associated with plague. Among the key biblical passages mentioned in the Zohar is one detailing the incense mixture: performative ritual concerning 'the elements in it [the *pittum haQetoret*] and the verses contained in [this passage] ward off and defend against' plague.

41 Barkai quotes an anonymous adjuration 'To Remove the Plague', written in the second half of the fourteenth century. Barkai, 'The Black Death,' p. 17.

42 A fifteenth-century Spanish-Jewish version specifically invoked Psalm 96 against plague. Barkai, 'The Black Death', p. 18.

43 Cohn, *Cultures of Plague*, p. 232. For more on plague processions see J. Henderson, *Florence under Siege: Surviving Plague in an Early Modern City* (New Haven, 2019).

44 Durante, *Il Tesoro della sanità* (Venice, 1586), pp. 45–6, cited in Cavallo and Storey, *Healthy Living*, p. 195. For more on Psalms and Christian practice at this time see R. Chiu, 'Singing on the Street and in the Home in Times of Pestilence: Lessons from the 1576–78 Plague of Milan', in *Domestic Devotions in Early Modern Italy*, ed. M. Corry, M. Faini and A. Meneghin (Leiden, 2018), pp. 27–44.

45 MH, p. 29v. My translation of *mesugelet* as 'given as a keepsake' follows M. Jastrow, *A Dictionary of the Targumim, the Talmud Babli and Yerushalmi, and the Midrashic Literature* (Leipzig, 1903), p. 955.

46 Joshua 1. 8.

47 Psalms 91. 10. Yagel adds the word 'surely', which is not part of this verse, as a point of emphasis.

48 MH, p. 29v.

They constitute 'a shield against divine punishment'.[49] If medicine's chief function is to preserve health, the best medicine of all is contained in the Torah, activated by intentional reading and focused recitation.

Psalm 38 was not among the biblical passages traditionally invoked as protection against contagion. Yagel chose it because 'in the recitation of this Psalm all afflictions of the plague and contagion and poisonous fever are mentioned'.[50] Listing these maladies was the first step towards gaining protection from them: perhaps King David, Yagel mused, intended to 'make known all types of plagues that come from God'.[51] Above all, he thought it crucial to know the 'primary reasons on account of which the plague arrives: these are [crimes deserving of] the death-penalty [enjoined in the Torah], and [transgressions of the laws concerning] the produce of the Sabbatical year, as is mentioned in the third chapter'.[52] These causes went beyond the canonical reasons listed in the Mishnah and include aggadic tales from later rabbinic literature. Yagel mentions Nahum Ish Gamzu, whose story is related in the tractate *Ta'anit*. This eccentric personality asked for his whole body to 'be covered with boils'[53] in recompense for his sinful actions. Although the author of the thirty-eighth psalm specifically implores God not to rebuke him in His anger, Yagel's commentary presupposes that plagues – and sickness more generally – are indeed punishments for transgression.

Beyond this theological framing, Yagel is committed to a medical explanation of a sacred text. The psalm's third verse exclaims 'for Thine arrows are gone deep into me' and the commentator takes this as an opportunity to specify what the Psalmist meant by the term 'arrows': these are 'poisonous fevers', which constitute 'God's arrows and God's flaming fire'.[54] The arrow as metaphor for illness appears frequently in both Christian and Muslim theological discussions of plague. And in Yagel's immediate surroundings, Christian iconography of the early modern period that featured St Sebastian – a third-century martyr later recognised as a plague saint – often depicts him being pierced by arrows.[55] The first association Yagel has with arrows is fever, but his exegesis becomes even more specific: these 'arrows' can 'manifest in the body as stains, as when one sees them as pale

49 Ibid. Yagel draws from Zohar 2. 218b–19. For a fifteenth-century example, see also Moshe Idel, 'Investigations into the Methodology of the Author of Sefer haMeshiv' [in Hebrew], *Sefunot* 17 (1983), 185–286.

50 MH, p. 30r.

51 Ibid.

52 Ibid., pp. 10r–12v. See specifically p. 11r and Mishnah *'Avot* 5. 8. On the produce of the Sabbatical year being prohibited, see Leviticus 25. 1–7.

53 Babylonian Talmud, *Ta'anit* 21r.

54 MH, p. 30r.

55 C. M. Boeckl, *Images of Plague and Pestilence: Iconography and Iconology* (Kirksville, 2000). On Saint Sebastian more generally see H. C. González, 'San Sebastián, mártir y protector contra la peste', *Revista digital de iconografía medieval* 7 (2015), 55–65.

green or red, as if arrows pierced there, and this is the illness called *petechiae*'.[56] This mention of *petechiae*, a skin rash, is perhaps the clearest evidence that Yagel had maladies of his own time in mind as he read and explicated this psalm.

Another point in Yagel's exegesis of Psalm 38 that may reflect the specific symptoms of the plague outbreak of 1575–77 appears in his explanation of the term loins. 'Loins', Yagel writes, refer to 'that which is under the pubic bone[57] above the base of the upper thighs, and they fill with abscess and pus,[58] and the rest of the body is not spared, for [the body] does not expel[59] [the illness], as there is no soundness in it'.[60] This passage may draw on Yagel's exposure, as a medical professional, to the plague buboes that often appeared in the groin area of those suffering from bubonic plague. And we should not lose sight of the massive toll this outbreak took on Venice's population: suffering would have surrounded Yagel, as it would have any other physician – Jewish or Christian. Between 1575 and 1576, at least fifty-six doctors died from plague in Venice.[61] When Yagel remarked that the psalmist's utterance 'I groan'[62] indicates 'I shout with my own voice because of the moaning of my heart'[63] and notes that this is brought on by the 'agony of my sickness', or when he commented that the phrase 'my heart fluttered'[64] means that the sufferer was 'surrounded by grief' and 'overcome with weakness', this may reveal a practising physician's own experience in northern Italy during the mid-1570s. While some of these comments could describe common symptoms for a variety of afflictions not necessarily particular to plague, Yagel's motivation to gloss this psalm in the first place – as a defence against plague itself – indicates otherwise.

The explanation of this psalm from a medical perspective reflects and accomplishes several goals. One is to underscore that the biblical text contains within itself full knowledge of plague afflictions: this is likely what Yagel meant when he noted that the Torah was 'given as a keepsake for every matter'. This perspective shares an intellectual genealogy with Judah Messer Leon's *Sefer Nofet Zufim* (Book of the Honeycomb's Flow), in which a fifteenth-century Italian Jewish writer set out to prove that the laws of classical rhetoric elaborated most famously by Cicero and Quintillian could be identified in the Bible,

56 See also Leon Modena's mention of this malady, which afflicted his wife in the spring of 1594, as discussed in M. R. Cohen, ed. and trans., *The Autobiography of a Seventeenth-Century Venetian Rabbi: Leon Modena's Life of Judah* (Princeton, 1988), p. 96. For the definition of *petechiae* as 'a skin rash, which can be a sign of various diseases' see p. 204 n. i.

57 Kimhi on Psalm 38: 8.

58 Literally 'mouldering' or 'decay'.

59 Cf BT *Hulin* 108v.

60 Isaiah 1. 6.

61 As Preto notes, this is probably a low estimate. *Peste e società*, p. 69.

62 Ps. 38. 9.

63 Ibid.

64 Ps. 38. 11.

centuries before those Roman writers lived.[65] Emphasising medical knowledge in a psalm was a way for Yagel and his audience to relate more intimately to a scriptural tradition purported to contain all knowledge: it was another way to invest a sacred text with contemporary meaning. Furthermore, the conceptual expansion of individual verses so that they detail medical symptoms accentuates and strengthens the prophylactic efficacy of scriptural recitation. Armed with a fuller knowledge of what King David meant, the reciter finds himself in a stronger position to summon the sacred force of scripture and harness it for his own ends, chiefly the recuperation or preservation of health. Ultimately, Yagel deepens the Bible's descriptive language in order to enhance its power of medical diagnosis and therapeutics.

Yagel's commentary on Psalm 38 is, for the most part, original. The most obvious source base for him – medieval Hebrew commentaries – would not have been of much help as he embarked on his medicalised interpretation of Psalm 38. Three Hebrew commentaries would have been readily available to him as he wrote: Rashi, David Kimhi and Abraham Ibn Ezra. All three were easily found in the Rabbinic Bible of 1517, and Rashi and Ibn Ezra were reprinted in the 1525 edition of that work. All three of these commentaries were relatively terse compared to Yagel's more luxurious writing style, however. Rashi has very little to say of any medical nature: he does give Old French definitions for a variety of terms, but with little to no elaboration.[66] Abraham Ibn Ezra occasionally amplifies the medical content of this psalm. On verse 4, where the psalmist writes, 'there is no soundness in my flesh', Ibn Ezra adds, 'regarding health'. On verse 7, where the psalmist laments, 'I am bent', Ibn Ezra notes, 'I have no strength to stand with straight, upright stature'. These brief glosses may have piqued Yagel's curiosity regarding the medical nature of this psalm, but Rashi and Ibn Ezra provided minimal detail. Yagel does seem to have borrowed freely from David Kimhi's comment on verse 8, in which he specifies that the term 'loins' refers to the region 'underneath the pubic bone',[67] but otherwise does not draw on the work of the medieval French glossator. In general, Yagel's commentary includes much more detail and medical specificity than those of his medieval predecessors.[68]

65 I. Rabinowitz, ed. and trans., *The Book of the Honeycomb's Flow* (Ithaca, 1983). On Messer Leon, see R. Bonfil, 'The Book of the Honeycomb's Flow by Judah Messer Leon: The Rhetorical Dimension of Jewish Humanism in Fifteenth-Century Italy', *Jewish History* 6 (1992), 21–33.

66 See, for example, Rashi to Ps. 38. 4 and 7. On Rashi's use of Old French, see D. Blondheim, *Les parlers judéo-romans et la vetus latina: étude sur les rapports entre les traductions bibliques en langue romane des juifs au moyen âge et les anciennes versions* (Paris, 1925) and *Les gloses françaises dans les commentaires talmudiques de Raschi* (Baltimore, 1937).

67 MH, p. 31r.

68 This is not the proper occasion for a full exploration of Christian psalm commentaries to which Yagel had access. I have not found any Latin or vernacular commentaries on this psalm that approach the degree of medical specificity in Yagel's work. The well-known Latin commentary of Agostinus Steuchus, for example, to which Yagel almost certainly had access, while detailed and philologically precise, does not mention plague. See *Augustini Steuchi Eugubini Episcopi Kisami, sedis apostolicae bibliothecarii, enarrationem in psalmos pars prima* (Lugduni, 1548), pp. 339–50.

Conclusion

Yagel's MH is worthy of study not only in terms of the historical and intellectual experience of the Jews in premodern Europe, but also for the sake of its contribution to the voluminous plague literature of the Second Pandemic – especially the crippling epidemic of 1575–77. Its unique triadic scheme demonstrates how mind and body, spirituality and health were inextricably linked in Yagel's cosmology and, presumably, in that of his readers. Although the final act of his opus has received some attention, with its startlingly detailed presentation of the *pittum haQetoret* ritual, the propaedeutic to that passage is equally informative and important. Biblical commentary, in all of its genres and expressions, played many roles on the stage of sixteenth-century intellectual life. In the case of MH, Yagel's commentary on Psalm 38 was no mere scholarly exercise; it was spiritual warm-up not only to intensified devotion but also to protection from the major public health scourge of Yagel's day. Rituals such as recognising – and even recreating[69] – the ancient incense mixture were paired with and enhanced by focused scriptural recitation. That recitation served two complementary functions: to impress upon the reader how truly all-encompassing biblical knowledge could be, if read from the proper scientific and theological perspective; and, just as importantly, meditation on this aspect of scripture could heal bodies as it could heal souls. For Yagel and others of his time, there was little difference between the two.

Appendix: Abraham Yagel on Psalm 38

fol. 30r

How good and how pleasant[70] is the institution that our ancient sages established when they preceded [the *pittum haQetoret* ritual] with [the recitation of] psalms: the song of plagues,[71] which protects against all afflictions;[72] and the psalm that begins 'the Lord answer thee in the day of trouble',[73] which we pray to God 'who will answer us on the day we call upon him',[74] and the Psalm that begins 'O Lord, rebuke me not in thine anger,'[75]

The 'arrows' in v. 2, which Yagel saw as ciphers for fever, Steuchus understands as symbols of spiritual pain (pp. 340–1). With regard to the 'loins', in v. 7, a frequent site of plague buboes, Steuchus explains this locution as yet 'another [instance of] hyperbole' (p. 342). On Steuchus, see R. K. Delph, 'Italian Humanism in the Early Reformation: Agostino Steuco (1497–1548)' (unpublished Ph.D. dissertation, University of Michigan, 1987) and C. B. Schmitt, 'Perennial Philosophy: From Agostino Steuco to Leibniz', *Journal of the History of Ideas* 27 (1966), 505–32.

69 See Abraham Portlaeone's work on biblical incense in his *Shilte Ha-Gibborim*, as discussed in Berns, *The Bible*, pp. 194–229.

70 Ps. 131. 1.

71 Ps. 91. 1–9.

72 This word (*nega'im*) can refer to plagues, evil spirits or affliction.

73 Ps. 20. 1.

74 Ps. 20. 10.

75 Ps. 38. 2.

which [King] David, peace be upon him, arranged to be recited by every person oppressed by illness. And if you open your eyes[76] you will see that in the recitation of this Psalm all afflictions of the plague and pestilence[77] and poisonous fever are mentioned. The psalmist acknowledges to God that they come as a result of his sins and transgressions and for these he begs pardon and forgiveness. Incline thine ear[78] and hear a psalm of David, *lehazkir*. Perhaps he said ['*lehazkir*'] to mention and make known all types of plagues that come from God. And if so, it is proper to chant all of them, as the sages of blessed memory said in *Perek HaRoeh*:[79] one must bless the evil as one blesses the good.[80] The commentators say of '*lehazkir*' that one should recite this according to its musical inflection.[81] And now he [King David] begins to pray to God, that God not rebuke him out of His anger due to his sins, nor chasten him in his rage.[82] The verse is doubled,[83] and perhaps it comes to hint regarding the primary reasons on account of which the plague arrives: these are capital crimes [enjoined in the Torah], and [transgressions of the laws concerning] the produce of the Sabbatical year, as is mentioned in the third chapter.[84] And when he says 'thine arrows are gone deep into me',[85] he begins to explicate the types of afflictions and disease. 'Your arrows' these are pestilential fevers, which are God's arrows and God's flaming fire. And also

fol. 30r–v

spots are visible on the body, and yellowish or reddish splotches, as if arrows pierced there, and this is the illness called *petechiae*.[86] 'Thine hand is come down upon me':[87] from your blow does this descend upon me. 'There is no soundness in my flesh': now he mentions a symptom that is precious to those suffering from pestilential fevers and which precedes affliction and great pain. He says 'all of this indicates that it came to me because of [your]

76 Prov. 20. 13.

77 On this distinction between *dever* and *mashḥit* see MH Chapter 1, 5r–v.

78 Prov. 22. 17.

79 The ninth chapter of BT *Berakhot*, 54r–64r. On music and chanting the psalms, see K. Golden, 'An Italian Tune in the Synagogue: An Unexplored Contrafaction by Leon Modena', *Revue des Études Juives* 177 (2018), 391–420; C. Roth, 'L'accedemia musicale del Ghetto Veneziano', *Rassegna mensile di Israel* 3 (1928), 152–62.

80 Mishnah *Berakhot* 9. 5.

81 See D. Kimhi on Ps. 38. 1.

82 Ps. 38. 2.

83 In other words, there is an apparent redundancy.

84 Of MH. See 11r. See also *'Avot* 5. 8. On the produce of the Sabbatical year being prohibited see Leviticus 25. 1–7.

85 Ps. 38. 3.

86 See also Leon Modena's mention of this malady that afflicted his wife in spring 1594, in *Life of Judah*, 96. Editors define this as 'a skin rash, which can be a sign of various diseases' (p. 204 n. i).

87 Ps. 38. 3.

indignation'[88] from the primary cause among the transgressions – namely the law of the four forms of capital punishment,[89] specifically regarding the matter of incest, which is related to what Rabbi Oshiah said in the chapter 'With what may one light?'[90] 'He who devotes himself to sin, wounds and bruises break out over him, as it is said, "stripes and wounds are for him that devoteth himself to evil".'[91] [Concerning the verse] 'neither is there any health in my bones because of my sin',[92] this refers to the second transgression: the [transgression of the laws regarding] produce of the sabbatical year. We have already mentioned how [this sin] opposes[93] and prevents one from performing [acts of] righteousness and mercy.[94] You shall surely remember[95] that it was on account of a similar [transgression] that Nahum Ish Gamzu wished to be punished, as our sages said in *Pirka dehaside*,[96] his mind was not at rest until he said, 'may my whole body be covered with boils',[97] and there was no health in his bones,[98] for he knew that the punishment for this sin was such, and he wished to bear his sin in this world so that there would be future hope for him in the world to come, as he said to Rabbi Akiva who saw him in such a state, 'if you did not see me in such a state my righteousness would not be upheld'.[99] And when he finished mentioning each category, he began to confess that his wickedness engulfed him, and he said 'for mine iniquities are gone over my head', etc.[100] Following this he proceeds to explain one kind of affliction, and he says 'my wounds stink, they fester'.[101] These are the discolorations[102] that precede the onset of a fever, or afterwards, as we mentioned in Chapter 7.[103] Due to their great pain [they say] 'I am bent and bowed down.'[104] The body is bent and afflicted, and the face darkens and

88 Ps. 38. 4.
89 BT *Sotah* 8v.
90 BT *Shabbat*, chapter 2.
91 BT *Shabbat*, 33r. See Prov. 20. 30. Soncino translation.
92 Ps. 38. 4.
93 I translate *temurah* following J. Klatzkin, *Thesaurus Philosophicus Linguae hebraicae*: 'entgegengesetzt; oppositum'.
94 Prov. 21. 21.
95 Lam. 3. 20.
96 BT *Ta'anit*, chapter 3.
97 *Ta'anit* 21r.
98 Ps. 38. 4.
99 This passage may be found in *Ta'anit* 21a, but Rabbi Akiva is not mentioned there.
100 Ps. 38. 5.
101 Ps. 38. 6.
102 The word *ḥaburah* can mean both wound and discolouration.
103 See MH, 26r.
104 Ps. 38. 7.

fol. 31r

ceases to shine.[105] All day he is stooped, he walks with discomfort, and finds no rest. He continues to explain, saying 'for my loins are filled with burning'.[106] 'Loins' refers to that which is under the pubic bone[107] above the base of the pelvis, and they fill with abscess and pus,[108] and the rest of the body is not spared, for [the body] does not expel[109] [the illness], as 'there is no soundness in it'.[110] He says that on account of these illnesses 'I am benumbed and sore crushed',[111] meaning, I am extremely weakened. 'I groan'[112] [indicates that] I shout with my own voice, 'because of the moaning of my heart'[113] that moans at him due to the agony of the sickness: 'Lord, all my desire is before Thee.'[114] After he remarks that his heart and his bowels confound him[115] he asks for refuge and revival from the healer of all flesh,[116] and says that before Him he places his heart's desire,[117] his hope, and faith, not in any Other[118] for He knows the secrets of the heart[119] and its murmurings: [they] are not hidden from Him. After this he proceeds to explain another type of affliction and says 'my heart fluttered'.[120] This means [that he is] surrounded by grief[121] due to the poison that approaches the heart, and he is overcome with fainting, so that his strength and the 'light of his eyes'[122] leave him, and no longer reside in him. And he said that no one arises to strengthen and gladden him and restore his spirit with apples and with cakes made from scented wine, for all his friends and companions[123] stand aside out of fear lest the evil [plague] infect them: his writhings and throes of agony, which are his enemies,

[105] Joel 4. 15.
[106] Ps. 38. 8.
[107] Kimhi on Psalm 38: 8.
[108] Literally 'mouldering' or 'decay'.
[109] Cf. BT *Hulin* 108v.
[110] Isaiah 1. 6.
[111] Ps. 38. 9.
[112] Ibid.
[113] Ibid.
[114] Ps. 38. 10.
[115] Cf. Song of Songs 5. 4.
[116] BT *Berakhot* 60v.
[117] Ps. 10. 3.
[118] Cf. Ps. 146. 5.
[119] Ps. 44. 22.
[120] Ps. 38. 11.
[121] See Rashi to Ps. 38. 11.
[122] Cf. Ps. 38. 11.
[123] Ps. 38. 12.

place a snare before his life[124] to sweep it away:[125] his hand is powerless. Due to all this pain he becomes like a man who cannot hear, and who has no pleas[126] to make regarding what might aid him and restore his soul from the agony he has mentioned. And he says 'for in Thee, O Lord, is all my hope',[127] and in your mercy you shall answer. For I said to you, God, 'you shall answer',[128] for the hour is urgent, and 'there is but a step between me and death',[129] lest my enemies rejoice at my expense[130] when I stumble[131] at my death. For my sickness gathers strength over nature, and I am ready and prepared[132] for this, as my sickness is continually before me,[133] and 'would not allow me to take my breath'.[134]

fol. 31v

My strength continually weakens, and the enemies who are battling against my nature are 'strong in health'.[135] 'Those that repay evil for good'[136] – these are the wicked thoughts that oppress him, and [encourage him] to turn away from God [due to] his constrained circumstances, and on account of this [he says] 'abandon me not'[137] into their hands lest I stumble in work and thought: make haste to help me, God,[138] for I know that you are close to all who call upon you.[139]

124 Prov. 18. 7.
125 Ps. 40. 15.
126 Ps. 38. 15.
127 Ps. 38. 16.
128 Ps. 17. 6.
129 I Samuel 20. 3.
130 Cf. Ps. 35. 19.
131 Ps. 38. 17.
132 See Rashi to Deut. 32. 35.
133 Ps. 38. 18.
134 Job 9. 18.
135 Ps. 38. 20.
136 Ps. 38. 21.
137 Ps. 38. 22.
138 Ps. 38. 23.
139 Cf. Ps. 86. 5.

10

The Protection of Innocents: Red Coral as a Lapidary Cure for the 'Children's Disease' and Conditions Related to Childbirth in Medieval and Early Modern England

NICHOLA E. HARRIS[1]

In *Discoverie of Witchcraft*, first published in 1584, English Member of Parliament Reginald Scot offered the following observation about the popularity of paediatric coral amulets in contemporary English society:

> Coral ... preserveth such that beare it from fascination or bewitching, and in this respect they are hanged about children's necks. But from whence that superstition is derived, and who invented the lie, I know not: but see how readie the people are to give credit thereunto by the multitude of corrals that way employed.[2]

Scot's early modern denunciation of amulets might not be entirely unexpected in a Calvinist excoriation of superstition, witches and the devil. Yet his scepticism of this custom appears within a chapter that actually *affirms* the practical and medicinal virtues of stones. 'The excellent vertues and qualities in Stones, found, conceived and tryed by this Art, is wonderful,' he wrote, thereafter providing a list of lapidary materials and their corresponding therapeutic applications.[3] In this chapter, I explore how the object of Scot's scorn – the

1 This chapter is dedicated to the life and memory of Rudolph Bell, the best possible academic advisor, whose work on medieval women and children influenced a generation of medievalists. I wish to thank the editors of this volume, Lori Jones and Nükhet Varlık, for their vision and diligence in bringing this project to fruition. I am particularly indebted to Lori for her help in locating and obtaining archival sources as well as for her advice, guidance and support, which greatly helped to clarify my arguments and resulted in innumerable improvements to the final version of the chapter. I am grateful to Winston Black and Beth Petitjean for their valuable insights and suggestions. I also wish to thank Marla Gruner and Tess Hartman-Cullen, librarians at Macdonald Dewitt Library, for their considerable efforts in obtaining sources for me during a global pandemic.

2 R. Scot, *Discoverie of Witchcraft* (London, 1584), p. 293.

3 Scot lists Ludovicus Coelius Renodaeus, Bartholomaeus Anglicus and Albertus Magnus as his sources. Also noted within this chapter are selected excerpts (lines 1–14, 14–21) from Marbode of Rennes's Latin hexameter poem entitled *De lapidibus*, attributed to 'one, who professed

use of red coral for children's amulets – was not, in fact, simply the popular superstition that he labelled it. Instead, it was a physical manifestation of paediatric and obstetric medical theories that had endured and evolved in Western pharmacology for nearly two millennia to ultimately find wide acceptance among early modern English medical consumers, much to Scot's consternation. My examination traces the development of coral-based treatments for children and their labouring mothers and draws upon a variety of written and iconographic sources, from mineralogical and medical treatises to early modern popular advice manuals, apothecary inventories and works of art.

From the ancient world to early modern Europe, coral was prized not only for its beauty as a precious ornament, but also as a valuable therapeutic for addressing numerous medical conditions. Premodern remedies sought to utilise the healing virtues of coral through external applications, such as branches fashioned into amulets, ligatures or suspensions (i.e., bound to a body part or hung around the neck), or by means of internal cures received in the form of lozenges, troches, tonics, syrups, tinctures, oils, salts or quintessences. Twentieth-century scholarship on medicinal jewellery and mineral pharmacology often sought to separate the methodology of these approaches into apotropaic (having the power to avert harm or sickness) versus medicinal classifications. However, little distinction was made in most historical lapidaries, pharmacopoeias or popular advice manuals between a topical application (whether in a plaster or as an amulet) and ingestion in terms of a natural object of healing's purpose or function. Indeed, authoritative medical writers across the centuries such as Dioscorides, Hildegard of Bingen, Albertus Magnus and Nicholas Culpeper regarded methods such as compresses or ligatures as simply alternative ways to transfer or wield the natural healing powers of stones. The *Pharmacopeia Londinensis*, a catalogue that governed the production and sale of pharmaceutical products sold in England for more than two centuries, likewise prescribed numerous suspensions or ligatures, listing them alongside and amongst other recommendations for applying animal, vegetable or mineral pharmaceuticals. Following my sources, I do not consider amuletic and pharmaceutical uses of coral separately, but, rather, explore them as equivalent therapies that existed across the broad spectrum of premodern medical possibilities.

In this chapter, I focus on the use of coral to treat illnesses and ailments related to birth, infancy and early childhood. From the fifth century BCE, following the works attributed to Hippocrates, Western medical practitioners wrote about several common paediatric medical concerns: stomach pains, diarrhoea and other bowel issues, eye disorders, earaches, skin complaints, fevers and convulsions.[4] This last, the occurrence of seizures

---

himself a very skilful and well experimental lapidary', and a corresponding English translation by 'Abraham Fleming'. Marbode's lapidary did not appear in English print in its entirety before the mid-nineteenth century. See C. W. King, *Antique Gems* (London, 1860).

4 The terms 'epilepsy' and 'epileptic' are Greek in origin, derived from the verb 'epilambanein', meaning 'to seize', 'to take hold of' or 'to attack'. Premodern medical texts used the word when referring to symptoms (particularly seizures or convulsions) that could stem from several different diseases and conditions. While the Latin term 'epilepsia' was used to refer to symptoms

or convulsions in children, was often linked to the trauma of childbirth, teething or the presence of fever; it was long understood as a condition that had its specific origins in infancy and early childhood.[5] Indeed, the frequency with which infants and young children experienced convulsions led to the condition being called the 'Children's Disease' within the Hippocratic–Galenic medical tradition and later, during the medieval and early modern periods, by the term 'the Falling Sickness' ('morbus caducus').[6] A thirteenth-century Latin translation of work by Islamicate philosopher-physician al-Rāzī, entitled *Liber continens*, considers the presence of chronic and intermittent fevers resulting in paediatric convulsions as a 'disease' affecting children ('morbus infantilis').[7] Fourteenth-century Montpelliérain physician Bernard de Gordon further stressed that many of the childhood medical conditions noted in the Hippocratic corpus accompanied the cutting of first teeth, an observation that was frequently repeated by subsequent medieval and early modern medical authors.[8] This critical period in life was, for example, recognised by Michele Savonarola, a fifteenth-century professor of medicine at the University of Padua, who suggested that the age of two represented a milestone in children's mortality risk.

Among other remedies, Savonarola endorsed the effectiveness of wearing coral around the neck to cure paediatric convulsions.[9] Certainly by this point in time, coral – and red varieties in particular – had become a widely accepted cure not only for the 'Children's Disease' but also for other related health concerns in children. My discussion begins with the general theory behind the medicinal use of coral and the specific properties traditionally ascribed to it by ancient, medieval and early modern authors. Thereafter, I examine how ideas based in classical mineralogy and Galenic pharmacology developed into Salernitan paediatric and obstetric medicine. These ideas were then disseminated through the circulation of mendicant encyclopaedias and humanist lapidaries, eventually finding widespread

associated with various illnesses, its use in the paediatric sense was largely understood to mean convulsions. O. Temkin, *The Falling Sickness: A History of Epilepsy from the Greeks to the Beginnings of Modern Neurology* (Baltimore, 1971) pp. 21, 28–9, 225.

5 Ibid., p. 193.

6 Ibid., pp. 29, 86, 115–16, 225.

7 Al-Rāzī (known in the West by the Latinised versions of his name, Rhazes or Rasis) is credited with the composition of the first treatise on paediatric medicine, known in its Latin translation as *De curis puerorum*. His translated works circulated widely beginning in the late thirteenth century and his influence extended into the fifteenth and sixteenth centuries. See S. Zarrina, A. Shannaee and S. Aslanabadi, 'Rhazes (AD 865–925) and His Early Contributions to the Field of Paediatrics', *Child's Nervous System* 34 (2018), 1435–8 and L. Demaitre, 'The Idea of Childhood and Childcare in the Medical Writings of the Middle Ages', *The Journal of Psychohistory* 4 (1977), 461–90 (p. 464). A critical edition of his text on children's medicine can be found in Al-Rāzī, *On the Treatment of Small Children* (*De curis puerorum*), ed. and trans. G. Bos and M. McVaugh (Leiden, 2014).

8 Demaitre, 'Idea of Childhood', p. 466.

9 Ibid., pp. 465–6. Savonarola's suggestion can be found in note 101.

acceptance as both an orthodox and popular – the latter underlying Scot's scorn – medical practice in seventeenth-century England.

The theory and practice of lapidary medicine in Western pharmacology

Within the Western medical and textual tradition, all natural pharmaceutical objects were grouped into three broad classifications based on their origin: plants, animals and stones. Lapidary medicine is a system of healing based on the therapeutic properties or virtues of stones.[10] Ancient, medieval and early modern treatises on the topic, known as lapidaries, typically included the physical descriptions and healing virtues of some forty to ninety substances, including minerals, metals, metalloids and fossilised substances, as well as some animal and plant-based products.

Ideas about the origins and specific physical and medicinal properties of a wide variety of stones appeared regularly in lapidaries, yet premodern authors were often at a loss to explain the exact natural origin of coral. Pliny the Elder, for example, includes coral in Book XXXII of his *Naturalis Historia* – within the topic of marine animals – yet describes it as having the form of a shrub or bush ('frutex') that hardens into stone once touched by human hands or removed from the sea.[11] In his work *Mineralia*, Albertus Magnus states that coral is produced from wood or plants.[12] Like those of many other natural pharmaceutical substances, the curative properties historically associated with coral often rested on a perceived sympathetic relationship between their physical appearance and their medicinal applications.[13] According to the natural philosophy of the ancient world, all products of nature possessed specific virtues ('virtutes') that, if known and understood, could be employed for the benefit of humankind. These theories included a doctrine of

[10] My definition of the term 'stone' consists of those substances that were traditionally included within this category in mineralogical treatises, natural encyclopedias, medical texts and popular advice manuals produced in medieval and early modern Europe. A more extensive description of lapidary medicine can be found in N. E. Harris, 'The Idea of Lapidary Medicine: Its Circulation and Practical Applications in Medieval and Early Modern England: 1000–1750' (unpublished Ph.D. dissertation, Rutgers University, 2009).

[11] Pliny, *Natural History*, xxxii.11; ed. H. S. Rackham and W. H. S. Jones, 10 vols. (Cambridge MA, 1938–83), VIII, 476–9.

[12] Albertus Magnus, *Book of Minerals*, trans. D. Wyckoff (Oxford, 1967), p. 28.

[13] Modern historians sometimes refer to this relationship as 'sympathetic magic'. In the nineteenth and twentieth centuries, historians of science and medicine often labelled antiquated medical practices, particularly those that were wholly or partially reliant on religious belief or pharmaceuticals drawn from animal or mineral products, as 'magical'. I reject such terminology when associated with lapidary medicine or the use of natural pharmaceuticals. Most ancient, medieval or early modern authors of lapidary sources clearly characterised the use of stones as medicinal, not magical. Rather than measuring premodern practices by modern standards, I employ the terminology used by contemporary authors in their texts. For an account of the doctrine of signatures and notions of sympathy, see K. Thomas, *Religion and the Decline of Magic: Studies in Popular Beliefs in Sixteenth and Seventeenth Century England* (New York, 1971), p. 190.

signatures in which Nature was thought to mark objects of the physical world with visual signs to indicate their use. The potential healing virtues of pharmaceutical substances were thus communicated through their physical appearance, which in turn supplied clues for their appropriate usage. For lapidary materials exhibiting a reddish hue, such as red coral, this meant assignment to complaints that involved blood.

The healing virtues of most lapidary products were deemed to be manifest ('manifestus'), meaning visibly clear and evident in their form. Natural objects could, however, also have virtues that were occult ('occultus'), meaning hidden, secret or not readily apparent to human perception.[14] Pharmaceutical substances could possess both manifest and occult virtues. In certain circumstances, occult virtues were valued over manifest ones, such as for illnesses or afflictions believed to be caused by poison, since occult qualities were thought to be most efficacious in countering toxins.[15] These ideas about the manifest and occult properties of healing objects persisted well into the seventeenth century, when scientific theories on the nature of matter led to their demise.[16]

Dioscorides' *De materia medica* and, later, the works of Galen, held that natural healing objects (simples) were instilled with specific virtues, determined by the qualities associated with their elemental complexion.[17] Ancient practitioners selected simples whose elemental composition would counteract a sick patient's humoral imbalance and thereby restore their balance and health.[18] Lapidary objects could be ingested or physically applied in direct contact with the skin; in the latter form, they could be used as hot or cold compresses or

14 Albertus Magnus provides an overview of this idea in regard to stones in his work *Mineralium Libri V* in his *Opera Omnia*, ed. A. Borgnet, 38 vols. (Paris, 1890–99), V, 1–116; see I.i.1 and III.i.8; *Book of Minerals*, pp. 10, 206. The Latin adjective 'occultus', meaning 'concealed from the eye', and its English equivalent 'occult', were used in medieval and early modern lapidaries to convey the notion that their practical applications could not be discerned from sight and were thus 'unseen' or 'hidden' from the senses. Lodestones, or natural magnets, are often cited as an example of a natural substance with occult virtues since the physical properties of the stone that worked to attract iron could not be detected through a visual observation of their material form. As these theories about nature were discredited through the scientific revolution, the meaning of the term 'occult' shifted to 'supernatural' and even became associated with demonic practices; see Thomas, *Religion*, p. 68. This topic is discussed further in G. Kornbluth, 'Early Medieval Crystal Amulets: Secular Instruments of Protection and Healing', in *The Sacred and the Secular in Medieval Healing: Sites, Objects, and Texts*, ed. B. S. Bowers and L. M. Keyser (New York, 2016), pp. 151–88.

15 Temkin, *Falling Sickness*, p. 103.

16 See J. Henry, 'Occult Qualities and the Experimental Philosophy: Active Principles in Pre-Newtonian Matter Theory', *History of Science* 24 (1986), 335–81 and K. Hutchison, 'What Happened to Occult Qualities in the Scientific Revolution?' *Isis* 73 (1982), 233–53 (p. 234).

17 865 For recent work on Galenism and its reception, see P. Bouras-Vallianatos and B. Zipser, ed., *Brill's Companion to the Reception of Galen* (Leiden, 2019).

18 P. S. De Vos, *Compound Remedies: Galenic Pharmacy from the Ancient Mediterranean to New Spain* (Pittsburgh, 2021), pp. 8, 20–5.

be incorporated into open-backed rings or amulets that would allow their healing virtues to pass into the wearer.

Byzantine physicians codified ancient works of pharmacology, while Islamicate authors added further simples to the established Galenic materia medica (medical material/substance) and formulated new compound remedies that mixed the qualities of simples to achieve the desired humoral balance for health.[19] As it does with most lapidary substances, a study of the pharmaceutical history of coral evidences the continuity of an idea over millennia while also demonstrating how medical ideas changed and evolved as intellectual traditions merged and interacted.

Coral pharmacology, immoderate fluxes and obstetric innovations

Classical mineralogical studies and Galenic pharmacology established the medicinal applications of coral within Western materia medica, introducing coral's usefulness as a paediatric talisman against a wide range of dangers. These included bleeding, issues of the bowels, spleen and bladder, ulcers, sores and scars, eye complaints and fear and nightmares. It also served as protection against demons, lightning, storms and hail.[20] In later centuries, Byzantine, Islamicate and Salernitan physicians formulated additional ideas about the pharmaceutical effectiveness of coral against menstrual fluxes, haemorrhages (particularly those related to pregnancy and childbirth), palpitations of the heart, stomach pains, conditions of the gums and teeth, fevers and convulsions. Starting in the late sixteenth century, the new theories and techniques of chemiatry, or chemical medicine, advocated by Paracelsus and his followers further expanded the paediatric applications of coral to include melancholy and diseases such as plague, measles and smallpox.[21]

While many ancient lapidary sources are lost to us, the earliest known Western work to expressly mention the properties of red coral and to classify it as a lapidary object is the Greek treatise entitled *Peri lithōn* ('On Stones'), written by Theophrastus circa 315 BCE.[22] Three centuries later, the work of Roman naturalist Pliny the Elder provided significant authority for the medicinal virtues of coral and, especially, its use as a paediatric amulet. In Book XXXII of his encyclopaedic *Naturalis Historia*, Pliny offers forty-three remedies and

19 De Vos, *Compound Remedies*, p. 9.

20 Works of natural philosophy, medicine and pharmacology connected the healing virtues of pharmaceuticals to the physical symptoms exhibited by a patient or to a specific part of the human anatomy, rather than to an underlying illness or disease, that was the cause of poor health.

21 While there was nothing new in the sixteenth- and seventeenth-century making of pharmaceuticals using lapidary substances, a different philosophical framework now guided those efforts. The term chemiatry is used to define the practice of preparing pharmaceuticals with alchemical methods within a Paracelsian framework and should not be confused with iatrochemistry, which refers to the school of medical thought founded by Franciscus (de la Boe) Sylvius. B. T. Moran, 'A Survey of Chemical Medicine in the 17th Century: Spanning Court, Classroom and Cultures', *Pharmacy in History* 38 (1996), 121–33 (p. 121).

22 Theophrastus, *De lapidibus*, trans. D. E. Eichholz (Oxford, 1965), p. 38.

observations about the origin, physical appearance and pharmaceutical applications of red coral ('curalium'), including:

> Branches of coral, worn as an amulet by babies, are believed to be protective, and reduced to powder by fire and taken with water are helpful in gripings,[23] bladder trouble and stone; similarly, taken in wine, or, if fever is present, in water, coral is soporific. Coral resists fire for a long time, but they say also that taken in drink repeatedly as medicine, it consumes the spleen. The ash of coral branches is good treatment for bringing up or spitting of blood. It is a component of eye salves, for it is astringent and cooling, fills up the hollows of ulcers, and smooths out scars.[24]

Pliny thus established coral as an effective cure for pain or spasms of the bowels, to stem blood, to counter issues in the spleen, to reduce fevers, to address eye complaints and to heal sores and ulcers. It also could act as a sleep aid. Pliny's suggestion that coral should first be calcined by fire to render it useful as an internal medicament later became a popular method of preparing coral in early modern remedies. Perhaps most significantly, his idea in *Naturalis Historia* that branches of coral offered amuletic protection for infants served to establish the legitimacy of the practice with future medical authors and audiences.

Pliny's contemporary, Greek physician Dioscorides, also detailed the properties of red coral in his compendium of Greco-Roman pharmaceutical knowledge, *De materia medica*.[25] In Book V, which includes wines, ores, earths, minerals, corals and salts, Dioscorides describes coral ('korallion') as therapeutic for the bowels, abnormal growths, painful urination, clearing scars on the eyes, filling hollow sores and cracks, treating the spitting up of

23 In English, this term signifies intense spasmodic pain in the bowels, or 'gripes'. See J. Norri, *Dictionary of Medical Vocabulary in English, 1375–1550: Body Parts, Sicknesses, Instruments, and Medicinal Preparations* (London, 2016), p. 478.

24 'Surculi infantiae adalligati tutelam habere creduntur, contraque torminum ac vesicae et calculorum mala in pulverem igni redacti potique cum aqua auxiliantur, simili modo ex vino poti aut, si febris sit, ex aqua somnum adferunt– ignibus diu repugnat – sed eodem medicamine saepius poto tradunt lienem quoque absumi. Sanguinem reicientibus excreantibusve medetur cinis eorum; miscetur oculorum medicamentis, spissat enim ac refrigerat, ulcerum cava explet, cicatrices extenuat'; Pliny, *Natural History*, xxxii.11; ed. Rackham and Jones, VIII, 478–9. Pliny states that the notion that red coral could be useful for warding off dangers stems from Indian tradition. Rome's outposts and history of trade with the western coast of India would certainly have allowed for the exchange of cultural practices and medical ideas as well as the trading of goods. In Book XXXVII of *Naturalis Historia* on precious stones, Pliny cites thirty-eight ancient authoritative sources on gemstones and minerals, any one of which might have provided additional insights into the origins and reasoning behind this idea; yet the only surviving source that he lists, Theophrastus, is silent on this topic.

25 *De material medica* was revered as a textual authority on the topic of pharmacology well into the seventeenth century. Its fifth book provides a description of the physical appearance, properties and medical usages of ninety-nine lapidary substances, including coral. D. Fausti, *Pedanius Dioscorides of Anazarbus: De materia medica*, trans. L. Beck (Hildesheim, 2005).

blood and (when taken as a drink with water) reducing the spleen.[26] *De virtutibus lapidum*, an early medieval verse lapidary attributed to Damigeron, recommends coral ('corallius') for its effectiveness against poison, fear, dreams ('somniorum ludibria' and 'vanis somniis'), demons ('umbris dæmoniorum'), lightning ('fulminum ictibus'), hail ('grando'), winds, storms and whirlwinds ('ventis et tempestatibus et turbinibus') and, particularly, for its ability to act as a safeguard by day and night for those who wear it.[27] While Damigeron's evaluation seemingly focuses on spiritual and environmental threats, several of the dangers that he lists (poison, fear, demons, lightning, hail and storms) were believed to be among the root causes of the 'Children's Disease' within the Hippocratic and Galenic traditions.

Classical authorities considered stones to be marvellous products of Nature that could be usefully employed for a variety of spiritual, physical and practical objectives. Medieval monastic writers then integrated this approach into a Christian cosmology that perceived all natural objects as gifts from God purposely created for the benefit of humankind. Ideas about the pharmaceutical applications of coral found in Pliny, Dioscorides and Damigeron were thus interpreted through this new paradigm as they were preserved, copied and expanded by Salernitan philosopher-physicians and integrated with the ideas found in Byzantine and Arabic texts.

Constantinus Africanus, an eleventh-century North African physician who contributed to the Salernitan medical school from the Benedictine monastery at Monte Cassino, brought ideas about the paediatric and obstetric applications of coral to the West through both his Latin versions of Arabic medical texts and his own works.[28] In the first book of his *Liber de gradibus*, Constantine recommended several compound Galenical remedies containing coral, citing Rufus of Ephesus and Galen among his sources. For example, he prescribed coral as a useful therapeutic for heart palpitations ('de tremore cordis'), stomach complaints linked with two types of fluxes – diarrhoea ('de lyenteria') and dysentery ('de dysenteria') – and fluxes of blood related to menstruation ('de fluxu sanguinis cum

26 Dioscorides, *De materia medica*, v.161.

27 The Latin text of *De virtutibus lapidum* begins 'Evax, King of Arabia' ('Evax rex Arabum'), which caused Damigeron to be cited as 'Evax' in later lapidaries. Damigeron, *De virtutibus lapidum: The Virtues of Stones*, ed. J. Radcliffe, trans. P. P. Tahil (Seattle, 1989), pp. 54–6. The origins of the text are obscure, although it appears to be based on the ancient Greek work *Lithica*, ascribed to a writer named Orpheus. Damigeron's version appears to be a fifth- or sixth-century Latin translation of a fourth-century copy of *Lithica*; see the introduction to Damigeron, *De virtutibus lapidum*, vi, and L. Thorndike, *A History of Magic and Experimental Science*, 8 vols. (New York, 1923–58), I, 293.

28 L. Ferre, 'The Multi-Cultural Origins of the Salernitan Medical School: A Historiographical Debate', *Journal of Mediterranean Studies* 27 (2018), 1–18. See also F. Newton, 'Constantine the African and Monte Cassino: New Elements and the Text of the Isagoge', in *Constantine the African and 'Ali ibn al-'Abbas al-Magusi: The 'Pantegni' and Related Texts*, ed. C. Burnett and D. Jacquart (Leiden, 1994), pp. 16–47 (pp. 20–3) and M. H. Green, 'The *De genecia* Attributed to Constantine the African', *Speculum* 62 (1987), 299–323.

menstruis' and 'de multitudine menstruorum').[29] Among the coral-based medicaments listed as effective against diarrhoea and dysentery, Constantine provided instructions for making troches or lozenges of coral calcined by fire ('coralli assati'), boluses or pills of coral and a coral electuary to bind the blood. He also noted that many of these remedies were similarly useful against the bloody flux ('fluxus sanguinis') of the upper chest and lungs as well as menstrual fluxes. Coral calcined by fire is also included in a compound Galenical that Constantine credited as efficacious for bloody flux of the liver ('de fluxu sanguinis ab epate'), an affliction that he discussed in relation to both convulsions and fever.[30]

These ideas conform to the Hippocratic and Galenic corpus, which taught that diarrhoea and flux of the blood were often the products of the same physical conditions that brought about convulsions.[31] They also represent a connection to the work of Alexander of Tralles, a sixth-century Byzantine physician who suggested that coral, peony and the root of strychnos gathered at the time of the waning moon and hung around the neck in a piece of linen could cure convulsions.[32] In the second book of *Liber de gradibus*, Constantine provide a further entry on the medicinal virtues of coral, suggesting its usefulness for eye salves, whitening teeth, healing gums ('gingiuas putridas sanat') and, when burnt, mixed with gum and ingested with water, its ability to comfort the stomach and restrain 'fluxus sanguinis'.[33] Additionally, he cites Galen for the suggestion that coral suspended around the neck is effective for healing pain in the stomach.[34]

29 *Constantini Africani … Opera*, 2 vols. (Basel, 1536–9) I, 77–82, 127, 129, 177–8, 183, 200–4. Winston Black provides an excellent historiographical overview of Constantine's *Liber de gradibus* in his article on Henry of Huntingdon's lapidary. See W. Black, 'Henry of Huntingdon's Lapidary Rediscovered and his *Anglicanus Ortus* Reassembled', *Medieval Studies* 68 (2006), 43–87. Black further notes (p. 66) that Henry of Huntingdon's use of Constantine demonstrates the far reach of this work and the implications for 'pan-European intellectual trends'. Rufus of Ephesus was a late first-century Greek physician often cited by Islamicate authors, such as al-Rāzī. Rufus is credited with multiple treatises on the treatment of women and children now lost to us but referenced in the works of medieval Islamicate medical writers. See M. Bujalkova, 'Rufus of Ephesus and his Contribution to the Development of Anatomical Nomenclature', *Acta Medico-Historica Adriatica* 9 (2011), 89–100.

30 *Constantini Africani … Opera*, I, 98–9.

31 *Constantini Africani … Opera*, I, 98.

32 Alexander credits this use of coral to the obscure Greek author Osthanes, writing in the first century BCE, but Galen discusses his own experiences and belief that the root of peony worked as an effective cure for convulsions. Temkin, *Falling Sickness*, pp. 13, 25. Constantine frequently mentions peony as a cure for convulsions, but not combined with coral or strychnos.

33 *Constantini Africani … Opera*, II, 354.

34 Ibid. 'Galenus dixit se probasse corallum suspensum in collo habentis dolorem in ore stomachi …'. This citation cannot be located within the extant works of Galen and may have been contained in one of his lost works. Other medieval authors, such as Albertus Magnus, also cite Galen as the source of this idea. John Riddle notes twelfth- and fourteenth-century Latin manuscript copies of ninth- and tenth-century writing by Qusṭā ibn Lūqā [Costa Ben Luca] that also credit Galen with this statement, but he too had no success locating it within Galen's known works. See

The virtues that Constantine ascribed to coral were widely adopted by later authors, and his ideas, remedies and authority served to expand the therapeutic applications of coral to include obstetric conditions and childbirth. However, Constantine's use of the term 'fluxus sanguinis' when referring to both dysentery and the flux of blood in women also introduced a level of confusion regarding the medicinal attributes of coral found in later lapidaries. Some authors interpreted the term to mean dysentery or bowel issues, while others understood it as bleeding in women, particularly with regard to menses and childbirth. Many subsequent authors drawing upon Constantine simply listed 'fluxus sanguinis' as a use for coral without any clarification or further explanation, while others stated that it might be used for any type of bleeding.

The *Trotula*, a later Salernitan text that stands as the most significant and influential treatise on women's medicine to circulate in medieval Europe from the late twelfth through the fifteenth centuries, includes the following obstetric use for coral: 'Likewise, it should be noted that there are certain physical remedies whose power is obscure to us, which are helpful when done by midwives. Therefore, let the patient hold a magnet in her right hand and it helps … Coral suspended from the neck is good.'[35] In 1300, English physician John of Gaddesden echoed this recommendation in *Rosa medicinae* (also known as the *Rosa anglica*), in which he discusses the suspension of coral paired with the use of a lodestone to aid childbirth.[36] At least one version of the popular fourteenth-century treatise *Regimen Sanitatis* – the regimen of health that emerged from dietetic doctrines translated from Arabic into Latin – also suggested that a piece of coral should be suspended over a woman's right hip during labour.[37]

J. M. Riddle, ed., *Marbode of Rennes' (1035–1123)* De lapidibus*: Considered as a Medical Treatise with Text, Commentary, and C. W. King's Translation, Together with Text and Translation of Marbode's Minor Works on Stones* (Wiesbaden, 1977), p. 110.

35 'Item notandum est quod sunt quedam phisicalia remedia quorum uirtus est nobis obscura, que ab obstetricibus facta prosuerunt. Teneat ergo patiens magnetem in manu dextra et confert … Corallus in collo suspensus prodest.' M. H. Green, ed. and trans., *The Trotula: An English Translation of the Medieval Compendium of Women's Medicine* (Philadelphia, 2002), p. 82 and M. H. Green, ed. and trans., *The Trotula: A Medieval Compendium of Women's Medicine* (Philadelphia, 2001), p. 106. Monica H. Green surmises that the *Trotula* is actually the work of three separate writers who were influenced by Greco-Roman and Islamicate medicine, through Constantine of Africa's translations. See also G. Bos, 'Ibn al-Jazzār on Women's Diseases and Their Treatment', *Medical History* 37 (1993), 296–312. The magnet, or lodestone, was thought to possess the ability to aid the child's delivery by pulling it from the mother. For more on this idea, see N. Harris, 'Loadstones are a Girl's Best Friend: Lapidary Cures, Midwives, and Manuals of Popular Healing in Medieval and Early Modern England', in *The Sacred and the Secular*, ed. Bowers and Keyser, pp. 189–225. The *Trotula* was allegedly the work of Trota of Salerno, an eleventh- or twelfth-century figure who was rumoured to be the first female professor of medicine.

36 J. Evans, *Magical Jewels of the Middle Ages and the Renaissance, Particularly in England* (London, 1921), p. 112.

37 J. Carney, ed., *Regimen na sláinte: Regimen sanitatis Magnini Mediolanensis* (Baile Átha Cliath: Oifig an tSoláthair) (Dublin, 1942), pp. 202, 212.

These texts offered no explanation for the purpose and intent of this procedure. Yet coral's long-credited efficacy against bleeding and Pliny, Dioscorides and Damigeron's recognition of it as an effective apotropaic amulet, presumably for both mother and child, gave its medieval obstetric use some validity. Constantine's suggestion that coral eased pains in the stomach, could staunch the flow of blood from the matrix (i.e., womb or uterus) and remedied convulsions further expanded coral's medical connection to childbirth. Convulsions before, during or after labour were a recognised risk for birthing mothers (a condition now known as eclampsia) and were thought at the time to be caused by the combined cessation of the menstrual flux (presumably during the months of pregnancy) and vapours rising from the uterus.[38] Infants were also considered to be at frequent risk of convulsions following birth and through the first few years of life – hence the expression 'Children's Disease'.[39] Since convulsions were associated with the uterus within the Hippocratic corpus, both mother and child were thought to be especially susceptible to the condition during the process of labour.[40]

Another indication that this obstetric use of coral was at least partially intended to ward off the risk of convulsions, indicative of modern eclampsia, is the *Trotula*'s reference to 'physical remedies whose power is obscure', perhaps an allusion to the belief that convulsions required a cure drawn from an occult property (early modern texts often noted that coral possessed occult properties).[41] Childbirth iconography from a fifteenth-century Florentine birthing tray by Bartholomeo di Fruosino offers evidence for the practical

38 Hippocratic teachings considered the cessation of menstrual flux to be a cause of epilepsy in women, while suggesting that healthy menses was preventative. The development of ideas linking epilepsy and eclampsia can be traced to Paul of Aegina, a seventh-century Byzantine physician. Temkin, *Falling Sickness*, pp. 29, 23, 195. Eclampsia is derived from Greek and means, in its basic sense, 'brightness'. Various authors have credited the use of the term to Bossier de Sauvages, an eighteenth-century French physician, who, in turn, attributed it to Hippocrates in *Coan Prognoses*. In fact, while the word does appear in some manuscript versions of *Coan Prognoses* (*CP* 214), it is in reference to eye disorders, a 'brightness' that prevents the pupil from dilating. I am indebted to Helen King for this explanation of the use of the term within the Hippocratic corpus. See H. King, *Hippocrates Now: The 'Father of Medicine' in the Internet Age* (London, 2020). Eclampsia came into common usage in connection with the obstetric disorder only in the latter half of the nineteenth century, as physicians sought to define it as a symptom of a condition separate from epilepsy and to develop effective treatments for their patients. Today eclampsia is a rare but serious complication of pre-eclampsia that results in seizures during pregnancy. See L. Ghulmiyyah and S. Baha, 'Maternal Mortality from Preeclampsia/Eclampsia', *Seminars in Perinatology* 36 (2012), 56–9. My thanks to Monica Green for her help and insights into this topic.

39 During the Middle Ages, Salernitan physicians referred to it as 'pedicon', from the Greek 'paidion', and categorized it as an infectious disease. Temkin, *Falling Sickness*, pp. 29, 115–16.

40 Temkin suggests that the Hippocratic corpus drew parallels between epilepsy and 'hysterical attacks'. Ibid., pp. 29, 32, 50, 122.

41 Green, *Trotula*, p. 82.

implementation of these theories.[42] The reverse of the tray includes an image of a child with a branch of red coral around his neck. The inscription on the tray reads 'May God give health to every woman who gives birth ... may the child be born without fatigue or danger' ('FACCIA IDDIO SANA OGNI DONNA CHFFIGLIA EPADRI LORO...RO... ERNATO SIA SANZA NOIA ORICHDIA ISONO UNBANBOLIN CHESULI').[43] Images of children wearing branched coral amulets or beaded coral necklaces are found commonly in the iconography (portraits, woodcuts and statues, for example) of medieval and early modern Italy, Germany, Holland and England, including depictions of Madonna and Child.[44]

Mendicants, teaching texts and the early popularisation of the use of coral

Mendicant friars and other clerical authors also influenced the medieval development and spread of ideas about the medical and protective uses of coral. In the thirteenth century, members of the Dominican and Franciscan orders, in particular (but not exclusively), authored several separate encyclopaedias, each intended to be a compendium of knowledge about the natural world that could serve as a teaching text for preaching friars. The lapidaries embedded within these texts are written in a utilitarian format that proved to be useful reference guides for preachers, health practitioners and general readers alike. The earliest of these works, *De finibus rerum naturalium* by Arnoldus Saxo, a cleric in lower orders, is primarily a shortened version of the late eleventh-century Latin hexameter lapidary entitled *De lapidibus* written by Marbode of Rennes that, for its part, had largely copied the properties of coral found in Damigeron.[45] However, Arnold additionally included

[42] I am grateful to Rudolph Bell for his suggestion that the iconography of birthing trays might provide important insights into the obstetric use of coral in Renaissance Italy.

[43] A. Bayer, ed., *Art and Love in Renaissance Italy* (New Haven, 2008), p. 152. For more on birthing trays and other objects unique to the birth culture of Renaissance Italy, see J. M. Musacchio, *The Art and Ritual of Childbirth in Renaissance Italy* (New Haven, 1999) and C. de Carli, *I deschi da parto: e la pittura del primo Rinascimento toscano* (Torino, 1997).

[44] Harris, 'Lapidary Medicine', p. 191.

[45] The most significant post-classical lapidary is the late eleventh-century prose composition entitled *Liber lapidum seu de gemmis*, or *De lapidibus*, written by Marbode, bishop of Rennes. Composed in Latin hexameter and addressing the physical appearance and healing properties of sixty stones, this work circulated widely throughout Western Europe in its original format as well as in a number of vernacular translations (including French, Provençal, Italian, Spanish, Irish, Danish and Hebrew). The fact that *De lapidibus* was written in verse form likely facilitated its oral circulation, which further added to its popularity even beyond its wide manuscript dissemination. Arnold drew upon some source material that he does not name; at other times, he gives his source as 'Dyascorides'. The content Marbode attributes to Dioscorides does not, however, appear in *De materia medica*. John Riddle suggests that this material appearing in Marbode is actually an extended version of Damigeron, now lost, which the authors of each mendicant encyclopaedia thereafter erroneously attributed to Dioscorides. See Riddle, *Marbode*, pp. 12–15.

a broader summation of the medicinal uses of coral as found in Constantine's *Liber de gradibus*. Here, coral is credited with efficacy against convulsions ('epylenciam') and 'any type' of 'fluxus sanguinis'.[46] The expansiveness of this last attribute is perhaps meant as a summation of the various types of bleeding, including menstruation and dysentery or bowel issues, for which Constantine had used the single term 'fluxus sanguinis'. It might also refer to the fact that Constantine suggested that coral-based remedies prescribed for one type of bloody flux were similarly useful for others.

Franciscan author Bartholomaeus Anglicus included a lapidary within his encyclopaedia, *De proprietatibus rerum*, which cites the authority of Isidore of Seville, Marbode and 'Dyascorides', as well as medical authors such as Constantine and Avicenna. Providing a thorough description of the origin and physical appearance of white and red coral, Bartholomew offered an abbreviated account of its medicinal properties, stating simply that the red variety is effective against 'fluxus sanguinis' and convulsions ('epilepsia').[47] The lapidary in Dominican friar Thomas of Cantimpré's encyclopaedia, *Liber de natura rerum*, provided a single medical attribute for coral: effectiveness against the build-up of phlegm.[48] While Thomas did not directly specify coral's use against convulsions, Hippocratic tradition held that epileptiform activity arose from an abundance of phlegm in the brain, and so perhaps the link was to be understood.[49] Thomas also provided a novel explanation for why coral was effective against demons, suggesting that its branched shape often resembled the form of a cross, thereby revealing a new manifest virtue.[50] The idea that convulsions were the result of a demon entering the patient's body was a long-held popular belief in the ancient world, one that many Christian theologians adopted, starting in the third century.[51] Although Thomas did not identify coral as a remedy against any

46 'Valet contra quemlibet fluxum sanguinis et epylenciam ...' Arnoldus Saxo, *Die Enzyklopädie des Arnoldus Saxo: Zum ersten Mal nach einem Erfurter Codex*, ed. E. Stange, Beilage zum Jahresbericht des Königlichen Gymnasiums, 3 vols. (Erfurt, 1905–7) III, 71. I am indebted to Richard S. Williams for his valuable insights into the medieval transmission of classical medical ideas in mendicant texts. For more on the works of Arnoldus Saxo see among others, I. Draelants, 'Une mise au point sur les œuvres d'Arnoldus Saxo 1ère partie', *Bulletin de philosophie médiévale* 34 (1992), pp. 163–80.

47 Oxford, Bodleian Library, MS Ashmole 1474, fol. 8r; *De proprietatibus rerum* xvi.33 (Frankfurt, 1561), p. 732; *On the Properties of Things. John Trevisa's Translation of* Bartholomaeus De proprietatibus rerum. *A Critical Text*, ed. M. C. Seymour et al., 3 vols. (Oxford, 1975–88), II, 842–3, § xxxii; sources listed in M. C. Seymour et al., *Bartholomaeus Anglicus and his Encyclopaedia* (Farnham, 1992), p. 176 (under 842–3).

48 'Valet et contra corrosivum flegma'. For a printed edition of the Latin text, see T. de Cantimpré, *Thomas Cantimpratensis, Liber de Natura Rerum*, ed. H. Boese (Berlin, 1973), p. 359. Thomas also summarized Damigeron's claims about coral's usefulness in resisting lightning and tempests.

49 Temkin, *Falling Sickness*, p. 4.

50 'Demonibus terribilis est, et hoc forte quia frequenter modum crucis habet ramorum eius distentio'. Cantimpré, *Liber de Natura Rerum*, p. 359.

51 Temkin, *Falling Sickness*, pp. 91–2.

ailment specific to children, then, he did recommend its virtues against two perceived causes of convulsions: phlegm and demons.

Vincent of Beauvais, Dominican author of another popular and widely disseminated mendicant encyclopaedia, *Speculum majus*, included an extensive lapidary within one of its three parts, *Speculum naturale*.[52] Two chapters of Book VIII are devoted to the physical and medicinal properties of coral. The first contains traditional descriptions and therapeutic virtues found within the works by Pliny, 'Dioscorides',[53] Isidore, Marbode, Arnold and Thomas. Mirroring Arnold's phrasing, Vincent affirmed coral's effectiveness against any type of 'fluxus sanguinis' and convulsions. The second chapter begins with an extensive list of medicinal applications of coral attributed to Avicenna, including the assertions that it vehemently restrains 'fluxus sanguinis' and spitting up blood, cleanses sores, comforts the bowels and spleen, washes the eyes, relieves heart palpitations, effectively treats stomach illnesses and relieves pain when directly suspended over the stomach.[54] This last property is cited as the reason why coral is hung around the necks of children ('Et ideo collis puerorum appenditur').[55]

Additionally, Vincent credited Avicenna with the statement that coral is useful in filling up holes in weak teeth ('impleantur ex eo concauitates infirmorum dentium'), removing them by the root and, if hung about the necks of children (presumably as a teether), is most comforting when rubbed against the gums ('est summus in confortatione gingiuarum').[56]

52 Vincent of Beauvais, *Speculum naturale*, in *Speculum quadruplex sive, Speculum maius, naturale, doctrinale, morale, historiale*, 4 vols. (Douai, 1624), I, 493–552; two chapters on coral, 522–3.

53 See n. 44.

54 'dolorem stomachi remouet, ac prohibit super os eius directe suspensus'. Ibid. Avicenna did include coral in the *Canon of Medicine*, citing its astringent properties and usefulness in stopping haemorrhaging, cleaning the eyes, removing scars, heart palpitations, swellings of the spleen and intestinal ulcers. However, early modern editions of the Latin translation emphasize the usefulness of red coral for stomach pain (citing Galen). See Ibn Sina, *Canon of Medicine* (New Delhi, 1998), pp. 96–7. For coral in an early modern edition of the Latin translation available to Vincent, which includes applications for stomach pain, convulsions and its use for children, see Avicenna, *Liber canonis* II.2.cxxiv (Venice, 1517; reprint, Hildesheim, 1964), fol. 101r.

55 Vincent of Beauvais, *Speculum naturale*, p. 523.

56 Ibid. Dental and periodontal applications of coral appear in early modern Latin editions of the *Canon*, such as those editions printed in Venice in 1517 and Basel in 1556. Mentions of coral being used to fill dental caries and to remove teeth are also present in the *Thesaurus pauperum* by Petrus Hispanus, who later became Pope John XXI (1215–77). To remove a decayed tooth the text directs, 'Put the pouder of redde Coral in the hole of thy tothe and it wyl faul out by the rote.' Additionally, it recommends that 'The pouder of corall being layd theron also is mooste pryncypall in comfortyng the gumes.' A printed marginal notation in the text attributes this last statement to Avicenna. Pope John XXI, *The Treasury of Healthe* (London, 1553). *Thesaurus pauperum* or *Treasury of the Poor* was translated into English by Humfrey Lloyd, who added a few materials of his own and published it under the title *Treasury of Health*. At least seven editions of the *Treasury of Health* appeared in English print, 1550 (two variant editions), 1553, 1556, 1558, 1570 and 1585. I am grateful to Herbert C. Edwards, DDS, MAGD, for generously sharing his insights into premodern dental techniques and theories.

Revisiting statements about the medicinal properties of coral earlier attributed to Arnold, Vincent added a qualification that coral should be worn around the neck to preserve against convulsions.[57] He concludes his thoughts on the uses of coral by repeating the claim that branches of coral in the shape of a cross are effective against demons, erroneously attributing the idea to Arnold rather than Thomas.[58]

Another thirteenth-century text authored by the renowned Dominican academic, natural philosopher, bishop and saint Albertus Magnus sought to combine utility with a comprehensive investigation of the specific nature and properties of gemstones, minerals and metals. Albert's entry on coral ('corallus') in *Mineralia* draws upon Pliny, Dioscorides, Damigeron, Constantine and his mendicant counterparts, suggesting that coral was useful against any sort of bleeding and, if worn around the neck, was effective against convulsions, the action of menstruation, storms, lightning and hail.[59] In a chapter dedicated to providing a philosophical justification for the orthodoxy and effectiveness of ligatures and suspensions, Albert repeated Constantine's assertion that suspending coral directly over the stomach soothed pain in that location, though Albert attributed the statement to both Galen and Avicenna.[60]

The inclusion of therapeutic properties attributed to coral within mendicant encyclopaedias and mineralogical studies is significant: not only did it facilitate the transmission of these ideas to large audiences across Europe via preaching friars, but it also ensured that it was included in mendicants' purported training of midwives and their spread of ideas about paediatric medicine.[61]

---

57 'Coralius est qui collo suspensus epileptici casum eius prohibit'. Beauvais, *Speculum naturale*, pp. 523

58 Ibid.

59 'valet contra quemlibet fluxum sanguenis'. Albertus Magnus, *De mineralibus et rebus metallicis libri quinque* (Coloniæ, 1569), p. 130.

60 Magnus, *Mineralia*, Book II, tractate iii, chapter 6. John Riddle suggests that Albert's statement here attributing this partly to Galen comes from Qusṭā ibn Lūqā [Costa Ben Luca], 'Galen: Lapis corallius multum valet ad passiones stomacho, si super stomache suspensus fuerit vel in collo patientis.' I cannot find this statement in the modern corpus of Galen's works, nor was Riddle able to locate it. Riddle, *Marbode*, p. 110. Wyckoff suggests that Albert's sources for this chapter include Qusṭā ibn Lūqā (whom Albert refers to as 'Constabulence'), Arnold of Saxony and the *Lapidary of Aristotle*. Wyckoff, *Book of Minerals*, pp. 151, 277–8. As previously noted, the Latin translation of the *Canon* lists the treatment of stomach pain as a medical attribute of coral, citing Galen as the source.

61 Peter Biller's studies on birth control and childbirth in the Middle Ages argue that friars – and Dominicans in particular – were highly effective in popularizing ideas about obstetric and paediatric medicine: they not only showed specific interest in the work of midwives, but also took an active intellectual and practical role in their education and training. See P. Biller, 'Childbirth in the Middle Ages', *History Today* 36 (1986), 42–9 (p. 46) and P. Biller, 'Birth-Control in the West in the Thirteenth and Early Fourteenth Centuries', *Past and Present* 94 (1982), 3–26. Monica Green urges caution, however, noting that these texts may be 'merely "armchair gynecology"' rather than evidence of actual teaching practice. M. H. Green, 'Women's Medical Practice and

Paediatric and obstetric use of coral in early modern popular print

The advent of print technology in the fifteenth century and the consequent development of a print market revolutionised methods of constructing and circulating medical knowledge in early modern Europe.[62] Among the many social and cultural changes brought about by this development, the growing availability of cheaply printed texts dramatically altered the methods by which ideas about the paediatric uses of coral circulated. Reflecting a changing dynamic aimed at a mass market with the specific goal of turning a profit, early modern print lapidaries, pharmacopoeias and medical treatises often took the form of easy-to-read practical advice manuals designed to meet a growing demand for direct access to medical information.[63]

Health Care in Medieval Europe', *Signs* 14 (1989), 434–73 (p. 460). Angela Montford's recent works on the medical activities of friars likewise make no mention of midwifery. A. Montford, *Health, Sickness, Medicine and the Friars in the Thirteenth and Fourteenth Centuries* (London, 2017) and '"Brothers Who Have Studied Medicine": Dominican Friars in Thirteenth-Century Paris', *Social History of Medicine* 24 (2011), 535–53.

62 The most widely circulating classical and medieval lapidaries did not generate equal market demand in the various vernacular print cultures across Europe. Several enormously influential scholarly works of the classical and medieval periods were available only in Latin manuscript form in England until the seventeenth or eighteenth centuries, and many of those were not published in English until well into the twentieth. While interest in these texts and their authors remained, their availability in printed form was entirely dependent on consumer demand across Europe and, thus, on the ability of a printer to turn a profit. The reality of early modern print culture was such that a popular advice manual by a native celebrity physician who incorporated the work of a renowned classical or medieval healer often sold far better than an edition of the original text itself. For more on the early modern print marketplace, printed advice manuals and popular medical literature in England, see M. E. Fissell, 'Popular Medical Writing', in *Oxford History of Popular Print Culture, vol 1: Cheap Print in Britain and Ireland to 1660*, ed. J. Raymond (Oxford, 2011), pp. 418–31; E. L. Furdell, *Publishing and Medicine in Early Modern England* (Rochester NY, 2002); and P. Slack, 'Mirrors of Health and Treasure of Poor Men: The Uses of the Vernacular Medical Literature of Tudor England', in *Health, Medicine and Mortality in the Sixteenth Century*, ed. C. Webster (Cambridge, 1979), pp. 237–74.

63 Rudolph Bell's inquiry into the use of popular advice manuals in sixteenth-century Italy evidences the great range of printed medical advice books published during this period. It furthermore demonstrates the value of such texts in providing insight into early modern attitudes towards sexual activity, conception, childbirth and parenting. See R. M. Bell, *How to Do It: Guides to Good Living for Renaissance Italians* (Chicago, 1999). See also S. Cavallo and T. Storey, *Healthy Living in Late Renaissance Italy* (Oxford, 2013). On the desire for practical medical information in England, see P. M. Jones, 'Information and Science', in *Fifteenth-Century Attitudes: Perceptions of Society in Late Medieval England*, ed. R. Horrox (Cambridge, 1994), pp. 97–111 (p. 100). See also L. Astbury, '"Ordering the Infant": Caring for Newborns in Early Modern England', in *Conserving Health in Early Modern Culture: Bodies and Environments in Italy and England*, ed. S. Cavallo and T. Storey (Manchester, 2017), pp. 80–103.

In this way, print manuals on the popular practices of 'physick', surgery, midwifery and the domestic arts transmitted ancient and medieval ideas about the prophylactic and therapeutic properties of coral to early modern audiences.[64] Printed dispensatories and pharmacopoeias likewise provided readers with instructions for producing and administering new complex 'chymical' formulations based on the methods proposed by Paracelsus and his followers.[65] Since the publication of printed texts was driven by local popular demand, vernacular print created language-specific medical cultures that varied greatly from one geographic and linguistic area to another. Medical consumers in any one country or city were guided by those authors whose work made it into popular print in their own unique marketplace. Therefore, my study narrows at this point to examine the social, cultural, intellectual and economic forces that supported the popular use of coral for paediatric disease and childbirth within the medical marketplace of early modern England.

Among the earliest medical books printed in England was John Trevisa's 1495 English translation of Bartholomaeus Anglicus' *De proprietatibus rerum*, which brought into wider circulation traditional ideas about the applications of coral and bolstered the credibility of its use among parents and practitioners. New texts incorporated these ideas as well, such as the first book in English on paediatric medicine: *The Boke of Children written by the physician Thomas Phayer*. First published in 1544, the work was embedded, at least initially, within a larger compendium that included Phayer's translations of a regimen of health and a plague treatise; at least seven editions followed over the next half century.[66] This text provided sixteenth-century physicians and parents with coral-based remedies for dysentery, eye complaints, vomiting, pestilence, teething and convulsions. On the topic of the 'falling evil' – which he explains to his readers is called 'epilepsia … in the greke tonge' – Phayer writes that although young children are often afflicted with the disease,

64 For a useful explanation of the differences between the terms 'medicine' and 'physic' in late medieval and early modern England, see H. Cook, 'Physick and Natural History in Seventeenth-Century England', in *Revolution and Continuity: Essays in the History of Philosophy of Early Modern Science*, ed. P. Barker and R. Ariew (Washington, 1991), pp. 63–80.

65 Paracelsus, whose real name was Philip Theophrastus Aureolus Bombast von Hohenheim (1493–1541), was a Swiss German alchemist, surgeon and theologian, whom some scholars dismiss as a charlatan and others hail as the father of modern medicine. Paracelsus's conceptualisation of medicine dismissed Galenic theories that focused on balancing humours through purging, bloodletting and diet, in favour of using alchemy to utilise the 'virtues' of natural substances by incorporating them into chemical remedies. See P. Ball, *The Devil's Doctor: Paracelsus and the World of Renaissance Magic and Science* (New York, 2006), p. 164. The popularity of these new ideas increased the use of lapidary medicine in the sixteenth century and beyond.

66 J. Goeurot, *The regiment of life, whereunto is added a treatise of the pestilence, with the boke of children, newly corrected and enlarged by T. Phayre* (London, 1550). Extant editions from 1544, 1550, 1553, 1560, 1567, 1578 and 1596 demonstrate the popularity of Phayer's ideas among early modern English readers.

the threat lessens around the age of seven.[67] He offers the following guidance to protect children from the falling evil:

> I fynde that manye thynges have a natural vertue against ye falling evill, not of any qualitye elementall, but by a singuler propertye, or rather an influence of heaven, whiche almyghtye god hathe geven unto thynges here in earth, as be these and other. Saphires, smaragdes, redde coral, piony ...[68]

With this advice, Phayer lent both his authority and his encouragement to employ coral amulets to combat or even prevent convulsions in children. When Reginald Scot's *Discoverie of Witchcraft* was first published in 1584, at least six different editions of *The Boke of Children* had already appeared in English print over the previous forty years.

On the subject of teething, Phayer explained that the process began at about seven months and, although teething is a natural process, it often came with 'sondry diseases and pains' such as swelling in the gums and jaws, 'unquieted' crying, fevers, cramps, palsies, fluxes and other infirmities. To remedy these issues, Phayer recommended the use of red coral amulets:

> redde coralle in lyke maner, hanged about the necke, wher upon the chylde shuld oftentimes labour his gummes, and many other lyke, whyche I leave out at this time, to avoide tediousnes, onely content to declare this of coral, that by consent of al authours, it resisteth the force of lyghtenyng, helpeth the chyldren of the fallynge evyll, and is verye good to be made in pouder, & dronken agaynst al maner of bleeding of the nose or fundament.[69]

Phayer's suggestion that a child might use coral amulets to 'labour his gummes' is a reference to coral teething sticks, a popular and useful accessory for sixteenth- and seventeenth-century children. Surviving records show that in 1548, four years after the first edition of Phayer's text had appeared, a child by the name of Frances Cavendish was bought 'a coral for her teeth' costing 7d., a sum that represents a little less than the daily wage for a skilled labourer in this period.[70] Other records note that a coral teething piece

67 Febrile seizures occur in young children, usually aged between six months and five years, and are triggered by fevers. They may accompany colds and other common childhood diseases and involve the uncontrollable shaking of arms and legs; sometimes they include the loss of consciousness. The National Institute of Neurological Orders and Stroke notes that a prolonged history of this type of seizure can carry the added risk of developing epilepsy later in life. https://www.ninds.nih.gov/Disorders/Patient-Caregiver-Education/Fact-Sheets/Febrile-Seizures-Fact-Sheet.

68 While sapphires and 'smaragdus' certainly appear in lapidary sources in this regard, red coral and peony had been consistently recommended as cures for convulsions since at least the sixth century. Goeurot, *Regiment of life*, pp. 154–5.

69 'Fundament' refers to the anus. Norri, *Dictionary*, p. 449.

70 S. Levey, 'References to Dress in the Earliest Account Book of Bess Hardwick', *Costume* 34 (2000), 13–24 (p. 16).

was stolen from the house of an Essex yeoman in 1576, suggesting that ownership was not limited to the wealthy or upper classes.[71] The smooth, hard surface of polished coral would have provided teething children with a benign surface to work their gums; a study of coral teethers from this period reveals that they do, in fact, show signs of wear and use.[72]

The popular use of red coral teethers, amulets and beaded necklaces is further evidenced in a variety of English portraits from this period. A portrait of John Dunch and his nurse Elizabeth Field (c. 1588) features a gold-set coral 'teething stick' and whistle suspended from the child's neck on a matching red ribbon (figure 10.1). Gold or silver ornaments, such as teething pieces, rattles and whistles, could be seen as high-status ornaments meant to indicate the social position of the wearer and are frequently observed in English portraits of infants and toddlers after the 1550s.[73] It is important to note that the dress and presentation of the children in these portraits were both planned and deliberate in their communication with the viewer. In each of these images, the use of coral was not only chosen to be part of the visual message: the eye of the viewer is often directed towards its significance.

A 1596 portrait of Barbara Gamage with her two sons and four daughters, by Marcus Gheeraerts the Younger, for example, shows her youngest child, a boy, wearing a red coral beaded bracelet and holding a teether made from a branch of red coral suspended from a ribbon around his neck. This image, which shows children of various ages, demonstrates a trend that can be observed from images of other Tudor children: red coral amulets or jewellery appear only on infants and toddlers, ages that might actively be experiencing the health effects of teething. A study of Tudor children, their clothing and accessories, based on early modern images, revealed that just under one quarter of babies and 11 per cent of toddlers in the images surveyed were pictured with a simple teething piece or one that was combined with a rattle (figure 10.2). The presence of coral teethers was equally represented among male and female children.[74]

While Thomas Phayer focused on treating illnesses in children, other writers emphasised the ways in which coral could cure the ills of women, especially childbearing women. In 1651, for example, English physician Nicholas Culpeper authored a popular advice manual directed towards a female audience entitled *A Directory for Midwives*. It became an instant success and served as the definitive guide to obstetric and paediatric medicine in England for more than a century.[75] Culpeper employed various lapidary remedies in this text, including the use of emeralds, eagle-stones, lodestones and red coral. For women

71 F. Emmison, *Elizabethan Life: Disorder, mainly from Essex Sessions and Assize Records* vol. 1 (Chemsford, 1970), pp. 56, 262.

72 J. Huggest and N. Mikhaila, ed., *The Tudor Child: Clothing and Culture 1485–1625* (Lightwater, 2013), p. 28.

73 Ibid.

74 Ibid.

75 N. Culpeper, *A Directory for Midwives: Or, a Guide for Women* (London, 1651). By far the most popular manual on childbirth sold in early modern England, *A Directory for Midwives* was first

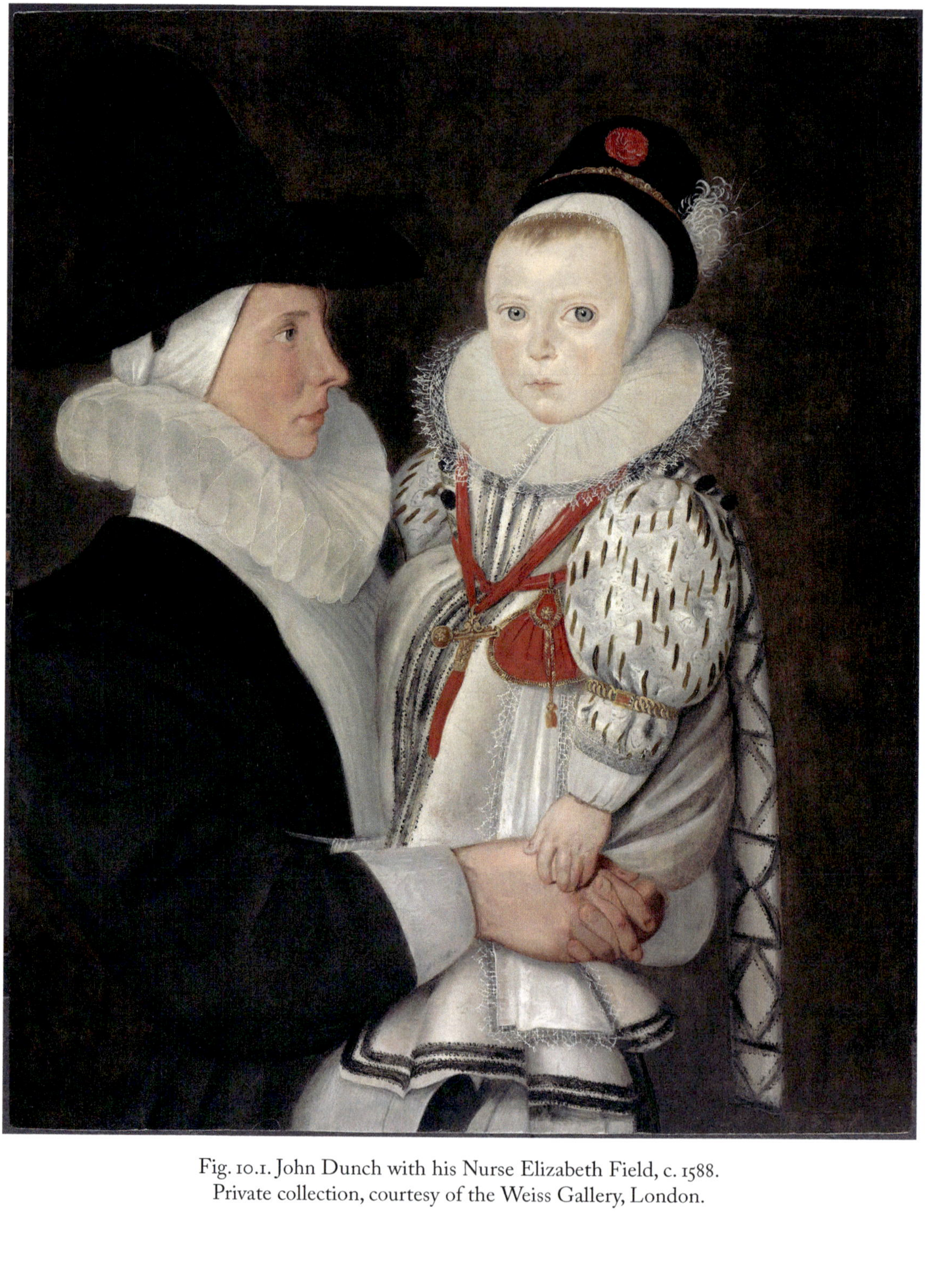

Fig. 10.1. John Dunch with his Nurse Elizabeth Field, c. 1588.
Private collection, courtesy of the Weiss Gallery, London.

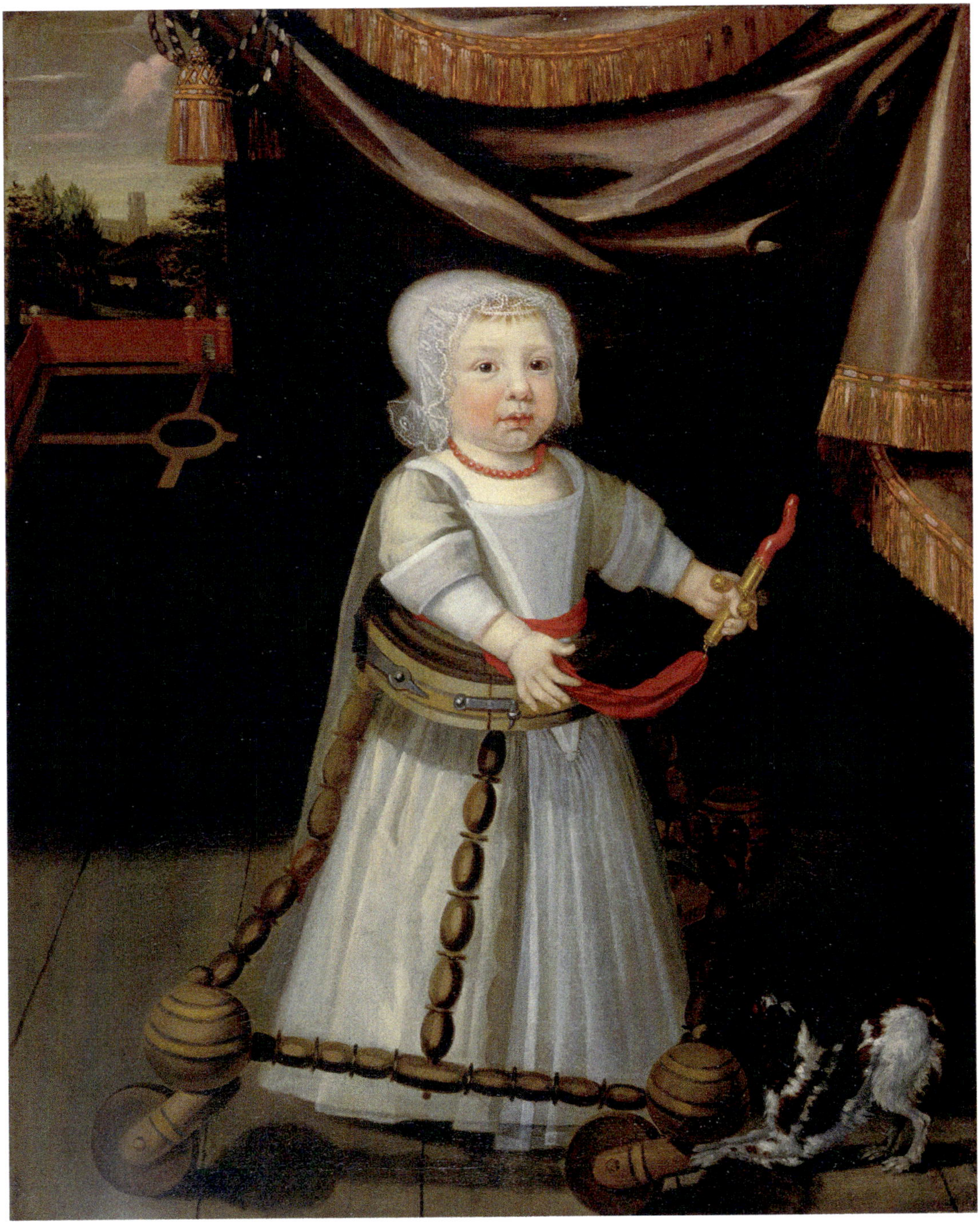

Fig. 10.2. Portrait of a Boy with a Coral Rattle by an unknown painter. English school, c. 1650–60. Norfolk Museums Service (Norwich Castle Museum and Art Gallery).

with 'overflowing' menses, he suggested that a variety of herbs and red coral be boiled and added to 'your ordinary drink'; he likewise recommended the use of dittany, betony, pennyroyal and coral, should a woman's waters break before the child was due.[76] His advice for pharmaceutical aids to ease childbirth included 'A piece of coral hung near the said place', echoing advice found in the *Trotula* and other medieval medical treatises compiled centuries earlier.

Beginning with its 1662 edition, which appeared eight years after Culpeper's death, *A Directory for Midwives* incorporated the work of Daniel Sennert, a renowned German physician, chemist and faculty member at the University of Wittenberg. Sennert was a proponent of chemical medicines and his recommendations on the topics of obstetric and paediatric care incorporated a variety of chemical techniques and formulations, including new discussions about the use of coral for illnesses in children. To prevent a miscarriage, the text suggests ingesting a powder of magistery of coral, pearl, ivory, mastic, kermes and *Manus Christi* with an egg. To reduce the 'flux of blood' after childbirth, it provides a recipe for an electuary made of roses, tormentil, quinces, bole and coral added to a syrup of currants and coral. To explain convulsions in children, this updated version of Culpepper's work offered a variety of causes, including 'the bad humours that twitch the membranes of the brain, as in Meazles and small Pox'. The following remedy was suggested to ward off infantile convulsions at birth:

> *Give this Pouder to prevent it, to a child as soon as it is born. Take* male Piony roots gathered in the decrease of the Moon a scruple, Magistery of Coral half a scruple, with Leaf-gold make a Pouder. *Or, Take* Piony roots a dram, Piony seeds, Mistleto of the Oak, Elkes hoof, Mans skull,[77] Amber, each a scruple; Musk two grains, make a Pouder.[78]

Here we see the culmination of ancient mineralogy, Byzantine remedies, mendicant ideas and early modern medical chemistry that sought to produce cures by separating the pure and impure parts of a substance to extract and distil its therapeutic virtues. The 'magistery of coral' included in these formulas, for example, is the solid precipitate remaining after ground coral had been dissolved in vinegar or another natural acid in order to isolate its vital essence. The gold leaf is a contribution from Paracelsus, who advocated for the

---

published in 1651, followed by at least sixteen subsequent editions in 1652, 1656, 1662, 1668, 1671, 1671, 1675, 1676, 1684 and 1700.

[76] Culpeper, *Directory for Midwives*, pp. 100, 169–70.

[77] Ancient sources often cite human bones as an effective cure for convulsions. Temkin, *Falling Sickness*, p. 13.

[78] N. Culpeper, *A Directory for Midwives* (London, 1662), pp. 244–5, italics in the original. Theophilus Garencieres attributes the idea that children should be given coral immediately following birth to Arnaldus de Villa Nova. T. Garencieres, *Thw* [sic] *admirable virtues, and wonderful effects of the true and genuine tincture of coral* (London, 1676), p. 7.

use of coral and/or gold leaf dissolved in wine to treat convulsions.[79] This revised version of *A Directory for Midwives* also listed coral-based paediatric cures for scabs, ulcers and 'frights in the sleep', all of which it cautioned were causes of convulsions. Hanging coral about children's necks, on the basis of its 'occult property', was also suggested, not only for convulsions, but also for a variety of issues such as vomiting and the 'flux of the belly'.[80]

Apothecary inventories from this period not only substantiate the general acceptance and widespread use red coral as a popular therapeutic, but also provide an estimate of the relative price and affordability for London consumers seeking to either purchase or self-formulate the coral-based cures recommended in popular advice manuals and pharmacopoeias. The inventories of apothecary wholesaler Estwick and Coningsby, for example, specify different grades of coral (fine, coarse, middle, worst) and colours (red or white), of which red was thought to possess superior medicinal qualities.[81] An inventory from October 1661 lists fourteen pounds of red coral priced at 14d. per pound; one pound of white coral appears at the slightly lower price of 12d. Five and three-quarters pounds of 'fine' coral are significantly more expensive, at 2s. 8d. per pound. One ounce of magistery of coral, considered to be the 'vital essence' with one hundred times the healing virtue, is listed for 3s. The final entry shows just over a hundredweight of coral, with a total value of £1 15s.[82] While the prices of coral found in other Estwick and Coningsby inventories fluctuated by month and year, the relative value difference between the various

79 Coral figures prominently in Paracelsian cures for the Falling Sickness and a condition that Paracelsus describes as convulsions in women caused by conditions of the womb. Throughout his writings, Paracelsus is clear that the healing virtues of coral are entirely natural and derived from God. T. von Hohenheim, called Paracelsus, *The Diseases That Deprive Man of His Reason, Such as St Vitus' Dance, Falling Sickness, Melancholy, and Insanity, and Their Correct Treatment*, trans. G. Zilboorg in *Four Treatises of Theophrastus Von Hohenheim Called Paracelsus*, ed. H. Sigerist (Baltimore, 1941), pp. 127–207. A significant section of Paracelsus's *Herbarius* discusses the therapeutic properties of coral, including that they 'are good for women giving birth so that they lie-in well disposed and are delivered [of a child] in good health … [and] take away convulsions and justify nature so that a person does not lapse into the falling sickness … [and] take epilepsy … away from the young'. It further 'quiets all bleeding in whatever way it occurs in the body'. B. T. Moran, 'The "Herbarius" of Paracelsus', *Pharmacy in History* 35 (1993), 99–127 (p. 122). On Paracelsus's use of gold and coral for convulsions, see E. E. DuBruck, 'Theophrastus Bombastus von Hohenheim, Called Paracelsus: Highways and Byways of a Wandering Physician (1493–1541)', *Fifteenth Century Studies* 25 (2000): 1–10 (p. 5).

80 Culpeper, *A Directory for Midwives*, pp. 253–6. A copy of the 1682 edition of this text bears the following inscription, presumably from a midwife, '*Mary Hillyer, her book God give her grace there unto look, not to look, but to understand, care is better than house and land. July 2, 1790*', demonstrating not only the popularity of Culpeper's ideas but also the lengthy circulation of his work.

81 These notations are drawn from an analysis of The National Archives of the UK (TNA): Public Record Office (PRO) C 104/130, the inventories of the apothecary wholesale business Estwick and Coningsby (1661–85). My thanks to Patrick Wallis at the London School of Economics for his help in initially locating these apothecary inventories in TNA and for his willingness to share some of his own research on the topic.

82 A hundredweight, abbreviated as cwt, is equal to 112 pounds.

colours, grades and forms of coral remained constant. The quantities of coral on hand in any one inventory indicate the existence of a significant supply of and demand for pharmaceutical coral, especially considering that the amounts required to formulate most cures suggested in manuals of popular healing are measured in the much smaller grains, scruples and drams.[83]

Following the economic success of Culpeper's *A Directory for Midwives*, which dominated the midwifery book market for at least half a century, numerous other manuals dedicated to obstetric medicine and the training of midwives appeared in English popular print during the seventeenth century.[84] The majority of these texts drew heavily upon information and instructions originally found in Culpeper and show how ideas about the obstetric applications of coral became increasingly popularised. One such imitator, a 1671 practical advice manual entitled *The Midwives Book, or, The Whole Art of Midwifery Discovered*, was attributed to a 'Mrs. Jane Sharp', an English woman credited with practising midwifery for thirty years and purportedly being the first female author of such a text in England. Sharp offered a number of recipes containing coral to aid several female maladies, including stomach 'looseness' during labour, 'rage of the womb' (i.e., hysteria), 'long ulcers in the neck of the womb' and risk of miscarriage, as well as remedies to address vomiting, sleeplessness and over-leanness in children.[85] Sharp specified that red coral was most effective in countering the risk of miscarriage and hysteria. Here, it is the woman's obstetrical health, rather than the child's, that takes centre-stage with respect to the medicinal value of coral.[86]

Two other popular advice manuals written in seventeenth-century England by the physician John Pechey, by contrast, detail how and why red coral was useful to prevent convulsions in children. In his 1695 work entitled *The Store-house of Physical Practice*, Pechey called convulsions in children *Epilepsia puerorum*, which he defined as convulsions that occurred soon after birth or during teething:

> We must endeavour to prevent these Convulsions in Children and Infants, or to cure them, when they are come; for if the former Children of the same Parents have been

[83] In the troy apothecary weight system, 1 pound = 12 ounces = 96 drams = 288 scruples = 5,760 troy grains. For an important study of the supply and consumption of drugs in the medical marketplace of early modern England, see L. H. Curth, ed., *From Physick to Pharmacology: Five Hundred Years of British Drug Retailing* (Aldershot, 2006).

[84] This success is judged in terms of editions sold as well as the multitude of comments made by authors of competing midwives' manuals, who alternatively acknowledge or belittle the success of Culpeper's text.

[85] J. Sharp, *The Midwives Book: Or the Whole Art of Midwifery Discovered* (London, 1671), pp. 248–50, 325–6, 279–80, 224, 400, 411, 414. Sharp's book was republished in 1674, 1724 and 1725.

[86] Numerous well-known midwifery manuals of the era contain frequent references to – and thus provide evidence of the ongoing importance of – coral for gynaecological and/or obstetric conditions. Among others, see, N. Fonteyn, *The Womans Doctour* (London, 1652), T. Chamberlayne, *The Compleat Midwifes Practice* (London, 1656) and J. Pechey, *The Compleat Midwife's Practice Enlarged* (London, 1698).

> subject to Convulsive Fits, this Disease ought to be prevented by the early use of Remedies, in such as are born after. To this end it is customary to give to new-born Babes, as soon as they begin to breath, some Medicine proper for Convulsions ...[87]

Pechey advised that infants be given twice daily spoonfuls of 'the waters of Black Cherries and Rue, each one ounce and an half, of Langiuses, Epileptick water, one ounce, of Syrup of Coral, six drams, of prepared Pearl fifteen grains; mingle them in the Viol'. In another book published about the same time, Pechey recommended that coral be applied both internally and externally to combat convulsions, nightmares, falling sickness and teething pains in young children. On the topic of nightmares and night fears in children, which Hippocratic theory held could provoke epilepsy and lapidaries suggested coral could prevent, Pechey endorsed a diet-based cure combined with several pharmaceuticals, including coral and peony. He also described the external application of coral:

> Nurses in *England* hang it about Children's Necks, to promote Cutting of the Teeth; for, by reason it is soft and cold, Children love to have their Gums rub'd with it; and so the Eruption of the Teeth is render'd more easie.[88]

An English painting by an unknown artist dated to the mid-seventeenth century, entitled *Portrait of a Boy with a Coral Rattle*, provides iconographic evidence that substantiates Pechey's claim (see figure 10.2). The portrait shows an upper-class child wearing a short strand of red coral beads of a type that is commonly depicted in Continental portraits of children found in Italy, Germany and the Netherlands from the thirteenth through the eighteenth centuries. The toddler is shown holding a golden rattle with a large branch of red coral protruding from the end, presumably for use as a teething stick. The child holds the rattle, which is tied to his waist by a thick red sash, towards the viewer, as if to call attention to its significance.

The arrangement of the portrait is obviously meant to show a well-cared-for child surrounded by common articles of daily life, such as a wheeled, wooden walker to help support his legs as he learns to walk, a pet dog to amuse and guard him, a coral necklace to protect him from danger and childhood illnesses as well as a rattle with its practical coral teething stick. Pechey explains that the hard, cool nature of the coral was thought to be an ideal medium for such an item and it allowed children to sooth their gums during the teething process. A manuscript that appears to be the work of a practical lapidary who ran a jewellery business in London during the second half of the seventeenth century prices

[87] J. Pechey, *The Store-House of Physical Practice Being a General Treatise of the Causes and Signs of All Diseases Afflicting Human Bodies: Together with the Shortest, Plainest and Safest Way of Curing Them, By Method, Medicine and Diet: To Which is Added, For the Benefit of Young Practicers, Several Choice Forms of Medicines Used By the London Physicians* (London, 1695), p. 9.

[88] J. Pechey, *The Compleat Herbal of Physical Plants Containing All Such English and Foreign Herbs, Shrubs and Trees as are Used in Physick and Surgery* (London, 1694), p. 247.

branches of coral at 10d., at a time when the average daily wage of a skilled labourer was close to two shillings a day.[89]

The 1696 edition of the *Pharmacopoiea Londinensis* lists twenty-four separate preparations of coral, including Salt of Coral, Liquor of Corals, Magistery of Coral, Oil of Coral, Syrup of Coral, Essence of Corals and Tincture of Coral.[90] For each, the *Pharmacopoeia* provided readers with detailed instructions of how to grind, mix, distil and calcine coral to produce medicine using chemical methodologies. Coral is credited with the ability to cure all manner of conditions and diseases: megrim (i.e., migraine), vertigo, Falling Sickness, apoplexy, convulsions, scurvy, gout, consumptions, fevers, fluxes 'of all sorts', the whites,[91] terms (menstruation problems), gonorrhoea, spitting of blood, distempers of the head, diarrhoea, 'dysenteria', the stone, frights in children, impurities of the blood, madness, melancholy and pestilential fevers.[92] Oil of Coral and Tincture of Coral are likewise recommended for Falling Sickness. The use of coral as an aid to childbirth is no longer mentioned here, however. Instead, in accordance with trends beginning in late seventeenth-century popular advice manuals, the emphasis has shifted to coral's use in curing various venereal diseases.[93]

89 K. Coman, 'Wages and Prices in England, 1261–1701', *Journal of Political Economy* 2 (1893), 92–4 (p. 93). For the manuscript, see London, British Library, Sloane MS 2539, fol. 44r. Seventeenth-century English authors reported that coral was imported from Tunis and Spain. The lapidary notes in his journal that coral branches were effective remedies against the Falling Sickness and that their expense was largely due to the labour spent polishing them smooth with sand and oil.

90 The Latin version of this text, together with two English-language versions authored by Nicholas Culpeper and William Salmon, appeared in at least forty print editions between 1618 and 1696. Harris, 'Lapidary Medicine', 111. The original Latin text of the *Pharmacopoeia Londinensis* appeared at least seventeen press-run editions in 1618, 1627, 1632, 1639, 1650, 1651, 1655, 1662, 1668, 1677, 1678, 1689 and 1699. Two variant editions of the Latin text were printed in 1618, 1655, 1668 and 1677. Popular demand for a more accessible English version of the same work motivated Nicholas Culpeper to offer a translation in 1649; subsequent press-run editions appeared in 1650, 1651, 1653, 1654, 1655, 1659, 1661, 1667, 1669, 1672, 1675, 1679, 1683 and 1695. Two variant editions of Culpeper's text were printed in the years 1649 and 1654. Print editions of yet another English-language version, this one authored by William Salmon, appeared in 1678, 1682, 1685, 1691 and 1696. Two variant press-run editions of Salmon's text were printed in 1691. For a history of the *Pharmacopoeia Londinensis*'s influence into the nineteenth century, with particular focus on the Culpeper translation, see C. J. Fowler, *Pharmacopoeia Londinensis 1618 and Its Descendants* (London, 2018). For more on press-run editions and early modern audiences see A. B. Farmer and Z. Lesser, 'What Is Print Popularity? A Map of the Elizabethan Book Trade', in *The Elizabethan Top Ten: Material Readings in Early Modern Culture*, ed. J. Daybell and A Smith (London, 2016), pp. 19–54.

91 Whitish discharge from the genitals sometimes used to refer to gonorrhoea.

92 W. Salmon, *Pharmacopoeia Londinensis, or, The New London Dispensatory* (London, 1696), pp. 422–28.

93 For more on venereal disease in this period see K. Siena, *Venereal Disease, Hospitals and the Urban Poor: London's 'Foul Wards,' 1600–1800* (Rochester, 2004).

Conclusion

Just three years later, the 1699 edition of the *Pharmacopoeia Londinensis* lists few 'stones' among the indexed 'materia medica' and mentions of the therapeutic applications of coral are entirely absent.[94] This omission signalled the decline in popularity of coral-based pharmaceuticals that occurred in eighteenth-century England. New understandings of obstetric conditions like pre-eclampsia and eclampsia, and the development of drugs and techniques in the eighteenth and nineteenth centuries, replaced traditional Galenic remedies and chemical formulations, bringing hope and relief to expectant mothers. The use of red coral amulets and teething necklaces for children, however, did continue throughout the nineteenth century, although evidence suggests that the theories behind their medicinal uses and properties were well lost by then on contemporary consumers and heathcare practitioners. In his 1855 edition of Pliny's *Natural History*, John Bostock, Fellow of the Royal College of Surgeons, commented that coral hung about the necks of children was 'a practice still retained, though the original intention of it has been lost sight of'.[95] Photographs of Queen Elizabeth II as an infant and toddler often show her wearing a beaded coral necklace, resembling those seen on portraits of early modern English children, but it may well have been just an ornament by this point. The demise of the use of coral in children's medicine corresponds with the rise of modern antipyretic therapy and the production of the stable, palatable fever- and pain-reducing drug marketed as 'Aspirin' at the turn of the twentieth century.[96] The power to reduce the fevers that frequently appear in infancy and during teething, paired with the effective means to treat or vaccinate against common childhood illnesses, means that few modern observers have witnessed a child experiencing febrile convulsions. Modern parents have no need for medicinal amulets or healing stones, which even some premodern sources suggest probably worked in a mind–body sense, providing peace of mind to those who employed them. In the end, the history of medicine teaches us that medical ideas and popular healthcare practices are often the result of cultural trends that find intellectual affirmation in society and are not always those which yield measurable results by modern scientific standards.

94 *Pharmacopoeiæ Collegii Regalis Londini* (London, 1699). 'Corallina' remains listed, but was recognized as a plant and separate from coral. While some later editions, such as the 1720 edition credited to Nicholas Culpeper, continued to suggest coral's efficacy for menstrual bleeding and venereal disease in women and 'Falling Sickness or Convulsions' in children, the 1699 edition reflects the waning popularity of many lapidary cures, including the pharmaceutical uses of coral, in the eighteenth and nineteenth centuries.

95 Pliny, *Natural History*, ed. J. Bostock (London, 1855), 32.11. Bostock's statement appears in note 6.

96 For the development of modern antipyretics, see P. A. Mackowiak, 'Brief History of Antipyretic Therapy', *Clinical Infectious Diseases*, 31 (2000), S154–6.

PART III

Studying, Analysing and Interpreting

11

Leprosy in Medieval Europe: An Immunological and Syndemic Approach

FABIAN CRESPO[1]

> Amongst all infirmities, the disease of leprosy may be considered the most loathsome, and those who are smitten with it ought at all times, and in all places, as well as in their conduct as in their dress, to bear themselves as more to be despised and as more humble than all other men.[2]

Leprosy deeply impacted on the lives of medieval European populations, even though its prevalence declined after the thirteenth century.[3] Social attitudes and responses to the disease varied in time and space, making its history and the reason for its decline

[1] I thank Lori Jones and Nükhet Varlık for inviting me to participate in this volume, for their inmense help with the editing process and especially for their patience and support. I also thank Charlotte Roberts and Keith Manchester for reviewing an early draft of this chapter; their comments significantly helped me to improve the text and ideas. Many others' work on leprosy in medieval Europe has been a great inspiration for me. I further thank Jacob White and Haleigh Mitchell for their help in collecting the experimental data presented in this chapter. Finally, I thank Ann Carmichael and Monica Green for their constant support and assistance in helping me to understand diseases in the past, especially in medieval Europe.

[2] This quote (c. 1335–49) comes from the leprosarium at St Albans and corresponds to the first injuction of a book of rules drawn up for the guidance of its inmates. Cited in S. N. Brody, *The Disease of the Soul: Leprosy in Medieval Literature* (Ithaca NY, 1974), p. 78.

[3] The most common and current biomedical terminology is Hansen's disease and the term leprosy is no longer used in most contemporary populations. During the twentieth century, many researchers advocated for removing the term from medical literature; a personal view on that issue recently appeared in P. Deps and A. Cruz, 'Why We Should Stop Using the Word Leprosy', *The Lancet Infectious Diseases* 20 (2020), 75–8. Yet there are still debates about whether Hansen's disease is the proper terminology, since 'Hansen's disease substitutes a word representing misconceptions with a term that honours a man guilty of abusing a patient by unethical experimentation. The neutral term mycobacterial neurodermatosis would be a better choice.' C. R. Butlin and D. N. Lockwood, 'Why We Should Stop Using the Word Leprosy', *The Lancet Infectious Diseases* 20 (2020), 900–1. The debate over the disease's biomedical terminology, as well as the use of 'leper', is not yet over. However, given this chapter's historical approach, I do use the historical terms 'leprosy' or 'leper' where appropriate, especially since they better support the hypothesis that an individual's immune competence is a biosocial process or construct, rather than simply a biological one. From an immunological perspective, stigmatization (past and present) could have played a significant role in the rise and/or decline of endemic leprosy in medieval Europe.

difficult to reconstruct or explain with any certainty. One hypothesis for this decline is cross immunity between the biologically related pathogens responsible for leprosy and tuberculosis; that is, cases of leprosy may have diminished due to the increasing prevalence of tuberculosis. However, without ruling out some partial impact of tuberculosis, other environmental, social and biological factors should also be considered when examining changes in the prevalence of leprosy. This chapter explores how different biosocial factors affected – either increased or decreased – an individual's capacity to mount a proper immunological response against leprosy, in order to explain changes in its prevalence in medieval Europe. In particular, the chapter uses a syndemic approach to consider how a set of different biosocial factors could have worked together, synergistically (or counter-synergistically), to affect an individual's capacity to fight leprosy.

This chapter does not offer a complete historical and bioarchaeological review of leprosy in medieval Europe. Instead, it uses historical and bioarchaeological evidence to explore how larger bioecological environments and social structures converged to produce infected or uninfected spaces. This, in turn, reveals that complex and heterogeneous immunological landscapes marked the disease's prevalence. The syndemics approach helps to expand the 'immunity' concept by replacing it with 'immune competence'. It also generates a new dialogue among and between disciplines such as immunology, bioarchaeology and history to reconstruct potential interactions between them. It equally helps to identify mortality burden contributions of chronic infectious diseases and biosocial factors in past populations.

Hansen's disease is an infectious disease caused by *Mycobacterium leprae*, which commonly generates a chronic infection primarily affecting nerves and skin.[4] It is one of humankind's most disabling and deforming infectious diseases.[5] With regard to host immune responses, it can show a broad spectrum of clinical signs and symptoms: patients with tuberculoid leprosy express an extensive cell-mediated immune response (high resistance) and thus have few severe or long-lasting effects, while patients with lepromatous leprosy experience a significantly reduced cell-mediated or innate response (low resistance) and thus can be severely affected.[6] However, in reality a continuous spectrum exists between these polar states.[7]

4 Until 2008, *Mycobacterium leprae* was the only known microbial pathogen that causes Hansen's disease. More recently, a unique form of diffuse lepromatous leprosy was identified in Mexico: *Mycobacterium lepromatosis*. X. Y. Han et al., 'The Leprosy Agents *Mycobacterium lepromatosis* and *Mycobacterium leprae* in Mexico', *International Journal of Dermatology* 51 (2012), 952–9.

5 H. C. Covey, 'People with Leprosy (Hansen's disease) during the Middle Ages', *The Social Science Journal* 38 (2001), 315–21.

6 G. Kapplan, 'Cytokine Regulation of Disease Progression in Leprosy and TB', *Immunobiology* 191 (1994), 564–8.

7 D. S. Ridley and W. H. Jopling, 'Classification of Leprosy According to Immunity', *International Journal of Leprosy* 31 (1966), 255–73.

While significant progress has been made over the past century in both preventing and treating this disease, global incidence remains high.[8] The highest numbers of new cases of Hansen's disease today are found in South America (primarily Brazil), Central and East Africa (primarily the Democratic Republic of the Congo and Ethiopia) and South-East Asia (primarily India).[9] Since this chronic infection was both common and endemic in the European high Middle Ages, yet is largely absent from there now, it offers an interesting and challenging case study from a historical, social and epidemiological perspective.

Palaeogenetic studies provide evidence of the presence of specific pathogens in human remains, help in the reconstruction of their phylogenetic trees, suggest their geographical distribution and signal genetic changes potentially associated with pathogenic virulence. Yet pathogen palaeogenetics cannot reveal host (i.e., human) biology and the complex interaction between host and pathogen. Investigating both sides of the equation is the only way to fully grasp (or get closer to) the evolution of any infectious disease in human history. Moreover, from the host perspective, it is an oversimplification – or mistake – to think that host biology can be reduced to host genetics. This chapter thus proposes that host immune responses have both a biological *and* a social dimension. When revisiting leprosy's prevalence or decline in medieval Europe, taking an immunological approach is crucial because host immune responses significantly dictate the infection's progress and clinical features.[10] In this chapter, the concept of immune competence (IC) represents the capacity of an individual to generate an appropriate immune response that involves innate and/or acquired mechanisms. Further, and crucial for this chapter's main argument, the IC of individual people is influenced not only by biological factors but also by the environmental and social factors that influence their lives.[11]

This chapter will review biological, archaeological and historical evidence to discuss five interrelated issues. First, whether the pathogen *Mycobacterium leprae* changed its virulence over the course of the Middle Ages. Second, whether bioarchaeology can explore changes in immune competence in the human host during the Middle Ages. Third, using my own unpublished experimental data, whether other *Mycobacterial* species might have shaped human host immune competence. Fourth, whether social attitudes towards leprosy in medieval Europe generated heterogeneous social landscapes. Finally, how heterogeneous social landscapes could have generated equally heterogeneous immunological landscapes

8 World Health Organization, 'Global Leprosy Update, 2018: Moving toward a Leprosy-Free World', *Weekly Epidemiological Record* 94 (2019), 389–412.

9 See the World Health Organization's interactive leprosy map at https://apps.who.int/neglected_diseases/ ntddata/leprosy/leprosy.html. Last accessed 9 March 2020.

10 R. L. Modlin, 'The Innate Immune Response in Leprosy', *Current Opinion in Immunology* 22 (2010), 48–54; I. Nath, C. Saini and V. L. Valluri, 'Immunology of Leprosy and Diagnostic Challenges', *Clinics in Dermatology* 33 (2015), 90–8; Ridley and Jopling, 'Classification of Leprosy', 255–73.

11 F. A. Crespo and M. B. Lawrenz, 'Heterogeneous Immunological Landscape and Medieval Plague: An Invitation to a New Dialogue between Historians and Immunologists', *The Medieval Globe* 1 (2014), 229–57.

that ultimately could help us to present a *syndemics* approach/model to explain leprosy prevalence in medieval Europe.

Did *Mycobacterium leprae*'s virulence change during the Middle Ages?

The genome of *M. leprae* is one of the smallest in the *Mycobacterium* family.[12] It has undergone significant reductive evolution, whereby approximately 40 per cent of its genes were inactivated or became pseudogenes over time.[13] Interestingly, this massive gene decay or reduction took place in those bacterial lineages that adapted to a specific host (or hosts).[14] The evolution of Hansen's disease bacteria appears to have taken place in at least two stages: the initial period occurred around twenty million years ago – when hypothetically the last bacterial common ancestor underwent a massive reductive genetic evolution (or change) to become adapted to a new ecological niche – and a second stage (genetically speaking) that has taken place over the past ten million years. It is only in the last 100,000 years that *M. leprae* appears to have infected humans or human ancestors.[15]

These hypothetical phylogenetic historical reconstructions are based on comparative analyses using modern bacterial genomes. In the decade since 2008, different studies on ancient *M. leprae* genomes have generated crucial information about the pathogen's recent genetic evolution, drawn especially from medieval European samples.[16] Verena Schuenemann and colleagues, for example, compared ancient bacterial genomes recovered from medieval human skeletal samples in the United Kingdom, Sweden and Denmark with contemporary bacterial genomes representing diverse geographical origins. Their main conclusion, based on bacterial genetics, is that ancient and modern genomes show remarkable similarities (high genetic conservation) over the last 1,000 years; this, in turn, suggests that leprosy's post-medieval decline in Europe was *not* due to decreased bacterial genetic virulence.[17] Tom Mendum and colleagues studied the remains of two individuals excavated from tenth- to twelfth-century burial sites in a leprosarium cemetery at St

12 A genome is an organism's complete set of DNA, including all of its genes. Each genome contains all the genetic information needed to build and maintain that organism. For more information see the web page from the National Center for Biotechnology Information – NIH: https://www.ncbi.nlm.nih.gov/genome/.

13 S. T. Cole et al., 'Massive Gene Decay in the Leprosy Bacillus', *Nature* 409 (2001), 1007–11; X. Y. Han and F. J. Silva, 'On the Age of Leprosy', *PLoS Neglected Tropical Diseases* 8 (2014), e2544.

14 L. Gómez-Valero et al., 'Reconstructing the Ancestor of Mycobacterium leprae: The Dynamics of Gene Loss and Genome Reduction', *Genome Research* 17 (2007), 1178–85.

15 Han and Silva, 'On the Age of Leprosy', e2544.

16 For a comprehensive review of all *M. leprae* ancient genomes (including lipid biomarkers) recovered and published up to 2018, see H. D. Donoghue et al., 'The Distribution and Origins of Ancient Leprosy', in *Hansen's disease: The Forgotten and Neglected Disease*, ed. W. Ribòn (London, 2019), pp. 7–36 (pp. 12–14).

17 V. J. Schuenemann et al., 'Genome-wide Comparison of Medieval and Modern Mycobacterium leprae', *Science* 341 (2013), 179–83.

Mary Magdalen, Winchester, United Kingdom.[18] They argue that genetic differences from contemporary genomes are unlikely to encode phenotypic or functional changes.[19] More recently, Verena Schuenemann and colleagues further demonstrate *M. leprae*'s complex and high genetic diversity in medieval Europe, but note that it is still not clear whether all genetic branches differ in virulence.[20] Taken together, these studies suggest that virulence and transmissibility probably did not differ between genetic branches, or at least not enough to have a significant short-term effect. Another study exploring ancient genomes in skeletons from the St Jorgen leprosarium cemetery in Odense, Denmark showed bone lesions associated with lepromatous leprosy. Surprisingly, this study revealed the presence of many different genetic strains within a remote locality over just a few hundred years. Yet, in agreement with previous studies, no differences were identified in these medieval bacterial genomes that could suggest a change in virulence or function.[21]

To date, most ancient DNA information retrieved from skeletal remains suggests that, from a genetic perspective, changes in pathogen virulence cannot explain leprosy's decline or any change in its prevalence in medieval Europe. Instead, correlating genomic data with the presence of palaeopathological evidence for leprosy unveils a complex scenario that suggests, as expected for Hansen's disease, the necessity to consider the immune competence of each individual to explain the biological differences observed in various studies.[22] The problem is that detecting immune competence using skeletal remains presents a challenging immunological reconstruction.

Can bioarchaeology inform us about host changes in immune competence during the Middle Ages?

Immune competence (IC), which encompasses but is not limited to immunity, represents the capacity of an individual to generate an appropriate immune response involving innate and/or acquired mechanisms.[23] Just as we refer to the fitness of an individual,

18 Bioarchaeological analysis and reconstruction by S. Roffey and K. Tucker, 'A Contextual Study of the Medieval Hospital and Cemetery of St Mary Magdalen, Winchester, England', *International Journal of Paleopathology* 4 (2012), 170–80.

19 T. A. Mendum et al., '*Mycobacterium leprae* Genomes from a British Medieval Leprosy Hospital: Towards Understanding an Ancient Epidemic', *BMC Genomics* 15 (2014), 270.

20 This study included four whole genomes of *M. leprae* taken from individuals with leprosy in Italy, Hungary, Czech Republic and United Kingdom. V. J. Schuenemann et al., 'Ancient Genomes Reveal a High Diversity of Mycobacterium leprae in Medieval Europe', *PLoS Pathogens* 14 (2018), e1006997.

21 B. Krause-Kyora et al., 'Ancient DNA Study Reveals HLA Susceptibility Locus for Leprosy in Medieval Europeans', *Nature Communications* 9, no. 1569 (2018).

22 S. A. Inskip et al., 'Osteological, Biomolecular and Geochemical Examination of an Early Anglo-Saxon Case of Lepromatous Leprosy', *PLoS One* 10 (2015), e0124282; Mendum et al., '*Mycobacterium leprae* Genomes', 270.

23 Crespo and Lawrenz, 'Heterogeneous Immunological Landscape', 229–57.

the term 'immunological fitness' is useful when understanding and reconstructing IC. From a biological perspective, 'fitness' implies the capacity of an organism to survive and reproduce and, when exposed to a no-self or foreign entity (i.e., a microbial pathogen), to mount an appropriate immunological response. The ability to do so is crucial for an individual's fitness.

However, it is a mistake to understand or describe 'immunological fitness' only as a biological concept. During their lifetimes, humans are immersed in specific environments and social networks that could impact on their IC. These environments can be highly heterogeneous, even within the same populations, towns and families. During the Middle Ages, why (and how) some individuals infected with deadly diseases survived without modern antibiotics and modern medical treatments is unknown.[24] It is thus necessary to reconcile historical and scientific information to answer such questions, including bioarchaeological studies that can provide crucial information when reconstructing IC in past populations.

Following Vilhelm Møller-Christensen's initial osteological work on leprosy, Stephen Ell attempted to reconstruct the epidemiology of leprosy in Scandinavia.[25] One of his main considerations was the necessity to include 'the social, religious, and legal situations of leprosy patients in order to correct for any biases that may vitiate the statistical data'.[26] In his comparative analysis of skeletons from three Danish cemeteries, Jesper Boldsen found different prevalence of bone lesions associated with leprosy (lesions associated with lepromatous leprosy) across two cemeteries commonly associated with the leprosy hospitals of St Jørgen in Odense and St Jörgen in Malmö and one rural cemetery in Tirup.[27] He suggested that the differential inclusion of individuals with leprosy in lepers' institutions makes it very difficult to study the true prevalence and spread of the disease in medieval Europe.[28] Importantly, Boldsen warned that the specificity and sensitivity of leprosy-re-

24 It could be argued that being exposed continuously to 'dirty' environments, people's immune systems became strong and resistant to different pathogen invasions, suggesting that relative virulence changed across regions/locations influenced by different 'microbial pathogenic environments'.

25 V. Moller-Christensen, 'Location and Excavation of the First Danish Leper Graveyard from the Middle Ages: St. Jørgeb's Farm, Næstved', *Bulletin of the History of Medicine* 27 (1953), 112–23.

26 S. R. Ell, 'Reconstructing the Epidemiology of Medieval Leprosy: Preliminary Efforts with Regard to Scandinavia', *Perspectives in Biology and Medicine* 31 (1988), 496–506.

27 J. Boldsen's comparative analysis of skeletons from these three Danish cemeteries involved complex statistical analysis and not all the lesions included were specific to leprosy. Further, Boldsen and Mollerup hypothesised that the skeletal lesions of leprosy in medieval Europe were probably different from skeletal lesions in modern-day people. J. L. Boldsen and L. Mollerup, 'Outside St. Jørgen: Leprosy in the Medieval Danish City of Odense', *American Journal of Physical Anthropology* 130 (2006), 344–51.

28 J. L. Boldsen, 'Epidemiological Approach to the Paleopathological Diagnosis of Leprosy', *American Journal of Physical Anthropology* 115 (2001), 380–7; J. L. Boldsen, 'Leprosy and Mortality in the Medieval Danish Village of Tirup', *American Journal of Physical Anthropology* 126 (2015), 159–68; Boldsen and Mollerup, 'Outside St. Jorgen', 344–51.

lated osteological alterations probably have changed over the centuries, due to changing host and bacteria co-evolution.[29]

There is no dispute that the skeletal data show a complex landscape when considering the impact of leprosy on past populations. The first problem is that data on modern Hansen's disease show that only around 5 per cent of patients exhibit skeletal signs of the disease.[30] Furthermore, most skeletal markers or lesions (bilateral and symmetrical) are found in persons suffering from lepromatous leprosy (LL); in tuberculoid leprosy (TL) patients, such markers can be minimal and are usually unilateral.[31] In the case of TL, where an extensive cell-mediated immune response is present, many skeletons may not show any chronic bone changes at all.[32] Clearly, a skeleton showing no visible signs of leprosy could have been a person suffering the infection but who died before developing bone lesions; this suggests that skeletal remains with signs of leprosy or Hansen's disease infection must have had a long-lasting chronic infection.[33]

It is also important to consider that other factors – such as living conditions and diet – may have affected the extent of skeletal involvement in leprosy, as well as the individual's IC.[34] As noted above, IC will determine the clinical progress of Hansen's disease and probably will also determine the immunopathological lesions (i.e., due to a long and chronic inflammatory process) that will determine, in part, whether skeletal lesions will develop. Consequently, it is crucial to recognise that a complex interaction exists between those factors that simultaneously influence both the progress of skeletal lesions in leprosy and overall IC. The emerging question here is, can we reconstruct the overall IC of an individual just using skeletal markers? Currently, I am attempting such an osteo-immunological reconstruction in various skeletal samples using and integrating different skeletal markers where inflammation is observed. This also involves incorporating ancient proteomic

29 Boldsen, 'Epidemiological Approach', 380–7.

30 D. Resnick and D. Niwayama, 'Osteomyelitis, Septic Arthritis, and Soft Tissue Infection: Organisms', in *Diagnosis of Bone and Joint Disorders*, ed. D. Resnick (Edinburgh, 1995), pp. 2448–558.

31 V. M. J. Matos, 'O diagnóstico retrospectivo da lepra: complementaridade clínica e paleopatóligica no arquivo médico do Hospital-Colónia Rovisco Pais (Século XX, Tocha, Portugal) e na colecção de esqueletos da leprosaria medieval de St. Jorgen's (Odense, Dinamarca) [The Retrospective Diagnosis of Leprosy: Clinical and Paleopathological Complementarities in the Medical Files from the Rovisco Pais Hospital-Colony (20th Century, Tocha, Portugal) and in the Skeletal Collection from the Medieval Leprosarium of St Jorgen's (Odense, Denmark)]' (unpublished Ph.D. dissertation, Universidade de Coimbra, 2009).

32 C. A. Roberts, 'The Bioarchaeology of Leprosy and Tuberculosis: A Comparative Study of Perceptions, Stigma, Diagnosis, and Treatment', in *Social Bioarchaeology*, ed. L. Meskell, R. A. Joyce, S. C. Agarwal and B. A. Glencross (Chichester, 2011), pp. 252–81.

33 C. A. Roberts, *Leprosy: Past and Present* (Gainsville, 2020), pp. 127–31.

34 C. A. Roberts, 'The Antiquity of Leprosy in Britain: The Skeletal Evidence', in *The Past and Present of Leprosy: Archaeological, Historical, Palaeopathological and Clinical Approaches*, ed. C. A. Roberts, M. Lewis and K. Manchester (Oxford, 2002), pp. 213–22.

analysis to identify the expression of different immune proteins, and ultimately testing a palaeopathological reconstruction of IC using modern experimental osteo-immunological protocols. Such complex immunological reconstruction using ancient skeletal samples was recently introduced as the skeletal inflammatory index or SINDEX.[35] I propose that the future integration of SINDEX and osteological markers of inflammation indicative of leprosy-related lesions can help to reconstruct IC in individuals who experienced chronic leprosy or Hansen's disease, in past populations.

Given that most skeletal markers for leprosy are generally found in LL patients, a second question emerges: should we predict a higher IC for individuals with TL? Unfortunately, most of the skeletal evidence is absent for this disease state. Consequently, when studying skeletal remains it is important to carefully explore immunological differences between TL and LL. However, as Alicia Wilbur and colleagues note, more problems arise, since many studies do not distinguish between these two disease states.[36] Moreover, a complex and heterogeneous landscape emerges when contemporary epidemiological data show significant variation among populations for LL/TL ratios in the occurrence of leprosy.[37] Again, recognising and distinguishing between LL and TL (especially in palaeopathological analysis) could be crucial for assessing the immunological status of each individual. Interestingly, it has been suggested that in the late Middle Ages, leprosy did not disappear but instead shifted to a higher frequency of TL, mostly undetectable in skeletal analysis.[38]

Did other mycobacterial species train the host innate immune system?

It has been recognised that innate and acquired immune responses work in concert and protect us from infection through a complex, multilayered network of cooperation; the two responses are commonly associated with different cell components and mechanisms.[39] The old idea that innate cellular mediated responses lack memory has been reconsidered.[40] In recent years, it has been proposed that the term 'trained immunity' should be used to

35 The osteological, molecular, experimental description and reconstruction of this skeletal index (SINDEX) is beyond the scope of this chapter. For comprehensive information on the theoretical and methodological approach for SINDEX, see F. A. Crespo, 'Reconstructing Immune Competence in Skeletal Samples', in *Theoretical Approaches in Bioarchaeology*, ed. C. M. Cheverko, J. R. Prince-Buitenhuys and M. Hubbe (New York, 2021), pp. 76–92.

36 A. K. Wilbur, J. E. Buikstra and C. M. Stojanowski, 'Mycobacterial Disease in North America: An Epidemiological Test of Chaussinand's Cross-Immunity Hypothesis', in Roberts, Lewis and Manchester, *The Past and Present of Leprosy*, pp. 247–58.

37 J. M. Hunter and M. O. Thomas, 'Hypothesis of Leprosy, Tuberculosis and Urbanization in Africa', *Social Science & Medicine* 19 (1984), 27–57.

38 Roberts, 'The Bioarchaeology of Leprosy and Tuberculosis', pp. 252–81.

39 D. Danilova, 'Evolution of the Human Immune System', in *Handbook of Human Molecular Evolution*, vol. 1, ed. D. Cooper and H. Kehrer-Sawatzki (Chichester, 2008), pp. 1068–74.

40 J. Quintin et al., 'Innate Immune Memory: Towards a Better Understanding of Host Defense Mechanisms', *Current Opinion in Immunolology* 29 (2014), 1–7.

describe enhanced innate host defence, while mounting evidence is showing that innate memory can be found in mammals.[41]

This 'trained immunity' against reinfection can be applied to the same or different pathogens. Most species within the *Mycobacteriaceae* family share many antigens and therefore it can be expected that there would be a complex pattern of immunological interaction between concomitant infections or casual exposure to different mycobacterial species.[42] Revisiting the cross-immunity tuberculosis–leprosy hypothesis has shown that, in some regions, the prevalence of leprosy was inversely correlated with the prevalence of tuberculosis (TB), caused by *Mycobacterium tuberculosis*.[43] These observations support earlier work on the hypothesis, although some epidemiologists have challenged the conclusions.[44]

It has been proposed as well that other mycobacterial species, such as *Mycobacterium bovis*, which is most commonly found in cattle and related animals, played a role in priming our immune system. In sub-Roman and Anglo-Saxon England, for example, especially in isolated village-oriented communities, TB likely was primarily of the gastrointestinal form due to *M. bovis* infection.[45] Indeed, before milk pasteurisation, *M. bovis* was likely a major source of tuberculosis infection worldwide.[46]

Following that line of thought, one cannot rule out that exposure to different environmental species of mycobacteria (i.e., the saprophytic and generally non-pathogenic *Mycobacterium smegmatis*) also may have played a role in the evolution of immune responses

41 M. G. Netea, 'Training Innate Immunity: The Changing Concept of Immunological Memory in Innate Host Defence', *European Journal of Clinical Investigation* 43 (2013), 881–4; M. G. Netea, J. Quintin and J. W. van der Meer, 'Trained Immunity: A Memory for Innate Host Defense', *Cell Host Microbe* 9 (2011), 355–61.

42 Antigens can be defined as molecules (commonly present in bacteria and other non-self particles or organisms) that contain distinct sites or epitopes that are recognised and interact with various components of the immune system. See more detailed information in *Encyclopedia of Analytical Science*: https://www.sciencedirect.com/topics/medicine-and-dentistry/antigen). P. Fine, 'Leprosy and Tuberculosis – an Epidemiological Comparison', *Tubercle* 65 (1984), 137–53.

43 F. A. Crespo, J. White and C. A. Roberts, 'Revisiting the Tuberculosis and Leprosy Cross-Immunity Hypothesis: Expanding the Dialogue between Immunology and Paleopathology', *International Journal of Paleopathology* 26 (2019), 37–47.

44 R. Chaussinand, 'Tuberculosis and Leprosy: Mutually Antagonistic Diseases', *Leprosy Review* 24 (1953), 90–4; K. Manchester, 'Tuberculosis and Leprosy: Evidence for Interaction of Disease', in *Human Paleopathology: Current Syntheses and Future Options*, ed. D. C. Ortner and A. C. Aufderheide (Washington, 1991), pp. 23–5. For challengers, see T. Lietman, T. Porco and S. Blower, 'Leprosy and Tuberculosis: The Epidemiological Consequences of Cross-Immunity', *American Journal of Public Health* 87 (1997), 1923–7; Wilbur, Buikstra and Stojanowski, 'Mycobacterial Disease in North America', pp. 247–58.

45 Manchester, 'Tuberculosis and Leprosy', pp. 23–5.

46 R. M. Smith et al., '*Mycobacterium bovis* Infection, United Kingdom' *Emerging Infectious Diseases* 10 (2004), 539–41.

Fig. 11.1. Case study: Are different mycobacterial species training our innate immune system? Fabian Crespo.

Chronic exposure to other mycobacteria species, including different environmental mycobacteria (EM), could have played a role on and training human immune responses. EM (atypical or nontuberculous bacteria) exhibit a great variation in growth rates and virulence.[1] Most EM are not obligate pathogens and their interaction with humans is transient, but still, this interaction involves the release of potent immunomodulatory proteins, and such proteins were detected in *Mycobacterium. smegmatis*[2] where chronic exposure to EM can result in systemic tolerance, and ultimate influencing the protective efficacy of TB vaccines such as BCG.[3] Therefore, a more comprehensive approach should be considered when studying the cross-immunity and potential interaction of *Mycobacterium leprae* and other mycobacterial species and expanding experimental *in vitro* protocols can help to understand the complex interaction of EM and human immune system.

Experimental question: Is it possible that early *in vitro* exposure of human immune cells (PBMCs) to different mycobacterial species (*Mycobacterium. tuberculosis* or *Mycobacterium bovis* or *M. smegmatis*) causes an immunological shift affecting the expression of key pro-inflammatory proteins (such as TNFα and IFNγ) when same cells are re-exposed to *M. leprae*?

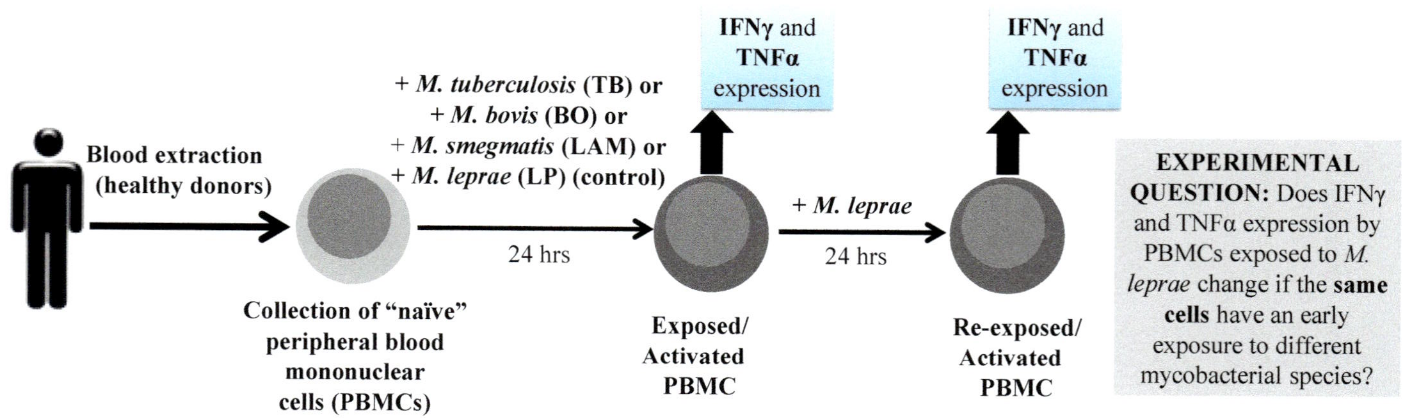

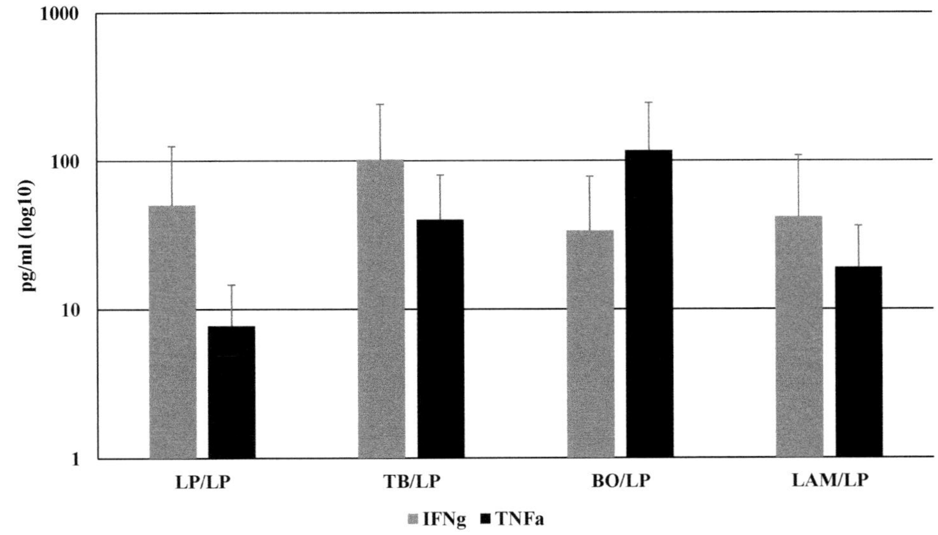

IFNγ (grey columns) and **TNFα** (black columns) expression (pg/ml) from 21 individuals* corresponding to the second day of culture. **LP/LP** represents cells exposed to *M. leprae* lysate (day1 – 24 hrs.) and re-exposed to *M. leprae* lysate (day 2 – 24 hrs.); **TB/LP** represents cells exposed to *M. tuberculosis* lysate (day 1- 24 hrs.) and re-exposed to *M. leprae* lysate (day 2 – 24hrs.); **BO/LP** represents cells exposed to *M. bovis* lysate (day 1 – 24 hrs.) and re-exposed to *M. leprae* lysate (day 2 – 24hrs.); and **LAM/LP** represents cells exposed to lipoarabinomannan (from *M. smegmatis*) (day 1 – 24 hrs.) and re-exposed to *M. leprae* lysate (day 2 – 24hrs.); (*) n= 15 for LP/LP and TB/LP; n=6 for BO/LP and LAM/LP

Experimental results: *In vitro* exposure to different mycobacterial species affects the expression of inflammatory proteins when same cells are re-exposed to antigens from *M. leprae* (when compared to control: *M. leprae* both days). Interestingly, there is an increased TNFα when cells are pre-exposed to all mycobacterial species.

These experimental results support the potential priming or "training" of the innate immune response by other mycobacterial species before exposure to *M. leprae*.

1 T. P. Primm, C. A. Lucero and J. O. Falkinham, 'Health Impacts of Environmental Mycobacteria', *Clinical Microbiology Reviews* 17 (2004), 98–106.

2 J. S. Tyagi and D. Sharma, '*Mycobacterium smegmatis* and Tuberculosis', *Trends in Microbiology* 10 (2002), 68–9; K. A. Sweeney et al., 'A Recombinant *Mycobacterium smegmatis* Induces Potent Bactericidal Immunity against Mycobacterium Tuberculosis', *Nature Medicine* 17 (2011), 1261–8.

3 D. N. Price, D. F. Kusewitt, C. A. Lino et al., 'Oral Tolerance to Environmental Mycobacteria Interferes with Intradermal, but Not Pulmonary, Immunization against Tuberculosis', *PLoS Pathogens* 12.5 (2016): doi 10.1371/journal.ppat.1005614.

against different mycobacterial species, probably acting as 'natural vaccines'.[47] Environmental mycobacteria (EM), atypical or nontuberculous bacteria exhibit great variation in growth rates and virulence.[48] It has been shown, for example, that some of the proteins of *M. smegmatis* can modify mammalian host immune response.[49] Notably, this mycobacterial species has been isolated from diseased animals, most frequently from cattle.[50]

To study the impact of different mycobacterial species on immune responses, we collected *in vitro* experimental data to test if the pre-exposure of naïve human immune cells (cell culture of peripheral blood mononuclear cells) to other mycobacterial species (*M. tuberculosis*, *M. bovis* and *M. smegmatis*) could generate a shift in the immune response that might, in turn, affect response to *M. leprae* (see the case study in figure 11.1).[51]

Leprosy and social attitudes in medieval Europe: a heterogeneous social landscape?

To better understand the social landscape of leprosy in the Middle Ages, it is necessary to examine historical scholarship rather than solely rely on what palaeopathological study of skeletons reveals. These two fields of study on leprosy are beginning to interact more closely now, but have traditionally worked in isolation or, in some cases, drawn only marginally from each other's conclusions, given the very different questions they asked, the different methodologies they used and the different mindsets with which they approached their subjects.

47 J. L. Stanford and C. A. Stanford, 'Leprosy: A Correctable Model of Immunological Perturbation', in *Past and Present of Leprosy*, ed. Roberts, Lewis and Manchester, pp. 25–38; Wilbur, Buikstra and Stojanowski, 'Mycobacterial Disease in North America', pp. 247–58.

48 T. P. Primm, C. A. Lucero and J. O. Falkinham, 'Health Impacts of Environmental Mycobacteria', *Clinical Microbiology Reviews* 17 (2004), 98–106.

49 J. S. Tyagi and D. Sharma, '*Mycobacterium smegmatis* and Tuberculosis', *Trends in Microbiology* 10 (2002), 68–9; K. A. Sweeney et al., 'A Recombinant *Mycobacterium smegmatis* Induces Potent Bactericidal Immunity against Mycobacterium Tuberculosis', *Nature Medicine* 17 (2011), 1261–8.

50 H. Bercovier and V. Vincent, 'Mycobacterial Infections in Domestic and Wild Animals Due to *Mycobacterium marinum, M. fortuitum, M. chelonae, M. porcinum, M. farcinogenes, M. smegmatis, M. scrofulaceum, M. xenopi, M. kansasii, M. simiae* and *M. genavense*', *Revue scientifique et technique* 20 (2001), 265–90.

51 This preliminary experimental work was conducted in Fabian Crespo's lab at the University of Louisville with the assistance and collaboration of Jacob White and Haleigh Mitchell. The primary references for this case study are T. P. Primm, C. A. Lucero and J. O. Falkinham, 'Health Impacts of Environmental Mycobacteria', *Clinical Microbiology Reviews* 17 (2004), 98–106; Tyagi and Sharma, '*Mycobacterium smegmatis*', 68–9; Sweeney et al., 'Recombinant *Mycobacterium smegmatis*', 1261–68; D. N. Price et al., 'Oral Tolerance to Environmental Mycobacteria Interferes with Intradermal, but Not Pulmonary, Immunization against Tuberculosis', *PLoS Pathogens* 12 (2016), e1005614.

Leprosy was not the only affliction associated with perversion and impurity, but early historical scholarship on the disease insisted that its conception as a 'moral disease' was particularly intense and deeply rooted during the Middle Ages.[52] Saul Brody, for example, insisted that medieval leprosy was associated first and foremost with sin and corruption. He did acknowledge that 'the leper was by turn the object of vilification and of sympathy', whereby a physician simultaneously could describe that the disease was a sign that God had chosen to grant someone's soul salvation while including in the diagnosis that the patient was morally corrupt. In the end, however, Brody argued that when balancing all social attitudes to leprosy, the disease was mostly considered a stigma.[53] Peter Richards joined Brody and argued that medieval attitudes towards lepers were uniform and contained heavy moral associations.[54] More than a decade later, Richards wrote that 'Separation of lepers in the Middle Ages was essentially a requirement of church law', although he later added a recognition that 'attitudes differed in time and place'.[55]

The term or category, *lepra*, in fact had a dual history, stemming from both biblical and medical traditions; this makes it rather challenging to parse out its exact meaning in any given context, since the etymology of the term *lepra* can have different origins or meanings.[56] Another problem or limitation when working with leprosy in the past, specifically in the Middle Ages, is determining what disease described in different medieval documents actually was leprosy. As Brody noted, without a precise clinical description there can be no standardised report by which to compare all medieval depictions.[57]

Taking heterogeneous social and clinical landscapes into consideration makes it clearer that different *social* responses to disease may have ultimately affected immunological phenotypes or overall IC, thereby generating in turn heterogeneous immunological landscapes among individuals or populations. The fact that leprosy in medieval documents did not always refer to the same infectious disease (Hansen's disease, as we know it today), or that most cases cannot be confidently associated with the same pathogenic experience, could also partially explain different immunological landscapes. This makes it more difficult to present a simple and linear rise and decline of leprosy in medieval Europe, or of attitudes towards it. Diagnosis of leprosy during the Middle Ages also depended on available information and its interpretation, which differed across geographic regions.[58]

The case of the diagnosis of Jean de Bierville, a Master of Arts in the diocese of Rheims, shows how, in some cases, doctors of that time – in this case the Masters-Regent in the

52 Brody, *Disease of the Soul*, pp. 60–1

53 Ibid.

54 P. Richards, *The Medieval Leper and His Northern Heirs* (Cambridge, 1977), pp. 70–1.

55 Richards, *Medieval Leper*, p. 60.

56 For a detailed etymology of the word *lepra*, see L. Demaitre, *Leprosy in Pre-Modern Medicine: A Malady of the Whole Body* (Baltimore, 2007), p. 92.

57 Brody, *Disease of the Soul*, pp. 60–1.

58 K. Manchester and C. A. Roberts, 'The Palaeopathology of Leprosy in Britain: A Review', *World Archaeology* 21 (1989), 265–72.

Faculty of Medicine in Paris – were addressing a clinical condition rather than generating condemnation: 'the said Jean ought not to be disturbed, bothered or disquieted by anyone; nor should his company be feared on account of contagious disease'.[59] As Luke Demaitre points out, perhaps the real reason why Bierville looked for medical attention and diagnosis was that he wanted help after being suspected and reported by some people as having the disease.[60]

François-Olivier Touati's work on leprosy in the 1990s might be considered a paradigm shifter.[61] He noted that medieval leprosy and its history provide a unique opportunity to study the interplay of scientific and intellectual elaboration of the notion of contagion. By the early modern era, a skewed perception of the disease had emerged, predicated on a polarising equation between leprosy and contagion: lepers and rejection, leper houses and segregation. Most physicians embraced this misleading, unified monolithic perception, as Touati clearly expressed:

> Unfortunately, the greater part of local erudition and scholarly publications arose in such circumstances: reflecting the current wisdom, they prejudged what the Middle Ages should have been by embracing one directed interpretation of the sources. The indolent repetition of 'facts' without confirming their foundation in the historical record, the usual attempts of physicians (but not historians) to write history without any basic methodology in historical research beyond a commitment to their own a priori judgements …//… Medieval culture – conceived in terms of monolithic unity enduring for more than one thousand years, and supposedly uniform from the North Sea to the Mediterranean – was under the primary influence of the Bible and its Levitical prescriptions of 'Unclean! Unclean! You will stay out of the camp!'[62]

Touati used three examples to show misunderstandings (lost in translation?) that were used to create the leprosy paradigm that insisted on uniform rejection of the leper. One of these is illustrated in the story of Josaphat meeting a leper and a disabled person at the gate of his castle (figure 11.2). The common interpretation of the image was 'A guard at the gate of a city prohibits the leper's approach', but in fact a translation of the text in the original manuscript reads exactly the opposite: Josaphat (not a guard) is welcoming both the impaired person and the leper.[63]

Touati notes that the first medical text to suggest that lepers were segregated – the *Breviarium practicae* of circa 1494 – actually appeared after the disease was long in decline. He also suggests further that (perhaps) Guy de Chauliac, in the wake of the

[59] Demaitre, *Leprosy in Pre-Modern Medicine*, p. 75.

[60] Demaitre, *Leprosy in Pre-Modern Medicine*, p. 76.

[61] F. O. Touati, 'Contagion and Leprosy: Myth, Ideas and Evolution in Medieval Minds and Societies', in *Contagion: Perspectives from Pre-Modern Societies*, ed. L. I. Conrad and D. Wujastyk (London, 1999), pp. 179–201.

[62] Ibid., pp. 182–3.

[63] Ibid., p. 184.

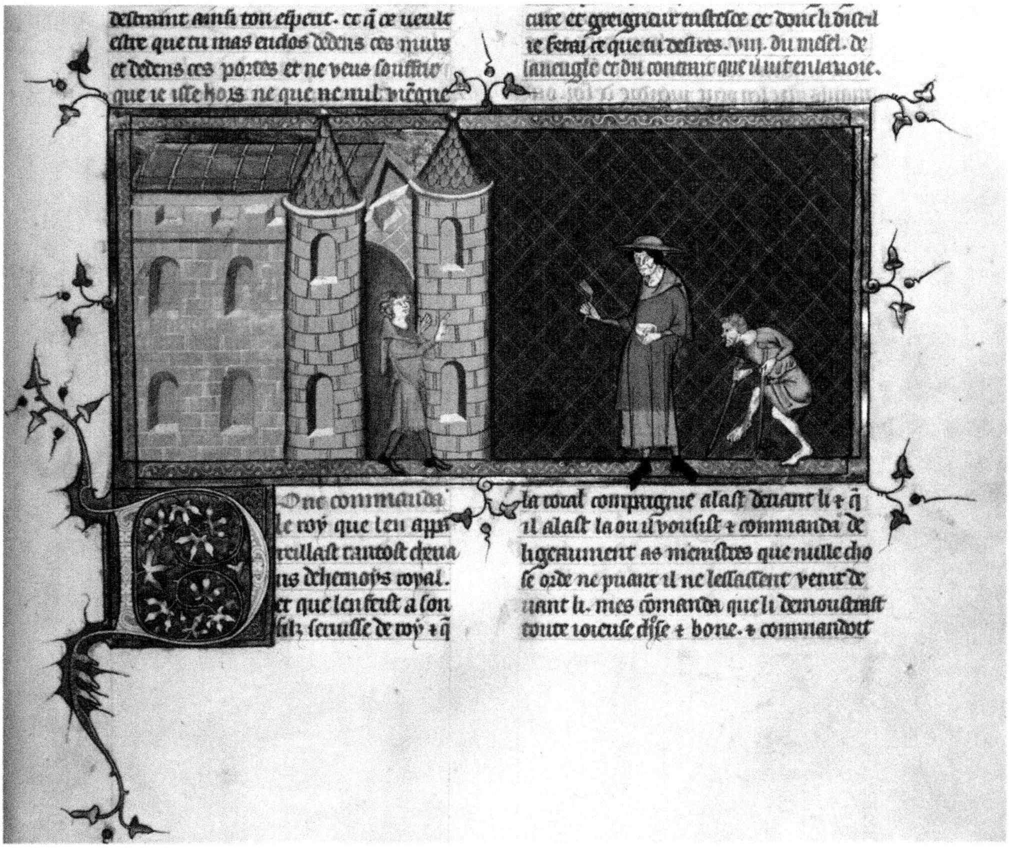

Fig. 11.2. *Josaphat Meets a Leper and a Cripple at the Gate of Jerusalem* (or *Two Lepers Begging*), detail from Vincent Beauvais, *Le miroir historial*, Paris, Bibliothèque de l'Arsenal, MS 5080, fol. 373. Bridgeman Art Library, New York. Reproduced with permission.

mid-fourteenth-century Black Death, had imposed a new contagion paradigm by suggesting that the main cause of plague was corrupted air and contact with lepers. Taken at face value in later centuries, these accounts then imposed an 'anachronistic view of contagion of leprosy to the entire course of the Middle Ages'.[64] Touati further addressed incorrect perceptions of leprosy and lepers tied to the origins of leper houses. He linked the creation of such specific communities with the 'revolution of charity' in the eleventh century, whereby 'leprosy offered [donors] a positive opportunity for redemption and sanctification'.[65]

At the beginning of the twenty-first century, other scholars joined Touati in challenging or revisiting monolithic interpretations that described lepers as constantly stigmatised and

64 Ibid., p. 198.

65 Ibid., p. 199.

expelled from their communities.[66] Carole Rawcliffe argues that the image of the excluded medieval leper was mostly constructed by early microbiologists and colonial administrators in the nineteenth century to justify their own campaigns for mandatory segregation:

> The powerful image of ostracism, forcible detention and rampant fear of contagion fostered by an increasingly influential and vociferous medical lobby soon seized the imagination of poets and novelists on both sides of the Channel. The results still permeate the pages of scholarly as well as popular studies of Hansen's disease, which inevitably present the leper as a marginal figure, shunned throughout the ages by his or her fellow man.[67]

Leprosaria, leprosy hospitals or leper houses are now also known to have had different functional or social interpretations, thus adding more support to the idea that heterogeneous social landscapes existed for medieval leprosy in Europe. Touati argues that leprosaria could be seen as monastic institutions, serving as sites for conversion into religious life.[68] Simon Roffey's archaeological research suggests that the status and organisation of these institutions varied across time and space. However, unlike monastic institutions, there was no regular plan or predefined layout for leprosy hospitals.[69] This organisational heterogeneity probably impacted on diet, sanitation, treatment and the daily lives of those who lived in these institutions. Overall, scholars agree that institutional differences can be observed during the peak prevalence of leprosy in Medieval Europe, while regional differences in attitudes towards people are also evident.[70] In Western Europe, variant religious responses (Christian, Jewish and Muslim) also added complexity, underscoring the fact that social attitudes were not monolithic. In the case of Muslims, for example, lepers were segregated, but less harshly viewed when compared with some Christian attitudes.[71] Likewise, while not ruling out the establishment of leprosaria, Elma Brenner noted that Jewish charitable practices were more commonly associated with private care in the home.[72]

Bruno Tabuteau has noticed a change between the twelfth and thirteenth centuries, when people with leprosy were commonly found in an open brotherhood (not in a 'prison

[66] Demaitre, *Leprosy in Pre-Modern Medicine*; C. Rawcliffe, *Leprosy in Medieval England* (Woodbridge, 2006); Roberts, 'Antiquity of Leprosy in Britain', pp. 213–22.

[67] Rawcliffe, *Leprosy in Medieval England*, p. 5.

[68] F. O. Touati, *Maladie et société au Moyen Âge. La lèpre, les lépreux et les léproseries dans la province ecclésiastique de Sens jusqu'au milieu du XIVe siècle* (Brussels, 1998).

[69] S. Roffey, 'Medieval Leper Hospitals in England: An Archaeological Perspective', *Medieval Archaeology* 56 (2012), 203–33.

[70] E. Brenner, 'Recent Perspectives on Leprosy in Medieval Western Europe', *History Compass* 8 (2010), 388–406; Demaitre, *Leprosy in Pre-Modern Medicine*; Rawcliffe, *Leprosy in Medieval England*; Roberts, 'Bioarchaeology of Leprosy and Tuberculosis', pp. 252–81.

[71] M. W. Dols, 'Leprosy in Medieval Arabic Medicine', *Journal of the History of Medicine and Allied Sciences* 34 (1979), 314–33.

[72] Brenner, 'Recent Perspectives on Leprosy', p. 394.

or sepulchral world'), and the fourteenth through sixteenth centuries, when most people with leprosy were probably relocated outside the city in communities sitting at the junction of the rural and urban worlds.[73] Writing of the transition, Tabuteau states:

> This change excluded people with leprosy from the house and marginalized those that retained the right to enter it. Their homeless and wandering peers were caught up in the rising pauperism, exciting fears and reaction to 'the impure' and 'the stranger'.[74]

Clearly, historical scholarship on leprosy has evolved, reflecting the difficulties of trying to grasp the full picture of the disease – or diseases – in medieval Europe. Perhaps the most significant conclusion is that leprosy did not have a uniform clinical and social existence, either during the Middle Ages or across Europe.

Recent bioarchaeological studies are also showing that, in some regions, segregating those with leprosy is a more recent social response than previously thought.[75] Even within the same region, complex societal changes can affect the social perception of an infectious disease whose related pathogen may not have changed at all.[76] In India, for example, one of the three areas in today's world with the highest rate of 'new cases', such social and institutional disparities, in time and space, must have a significant impact on disease progress, on overall health and, ultimately, on the IC of people with leprosy.[77]

One factor that may have influenced a change in social responses towards lepers (in receipt of charity) was the Fourth Lateran Council's (1215) promulgation of the idea of 'holy poor' that included individuals diagnosed with leprosy (especially those residing in leprosaria). These individuals, while suffering in life, were headed for salvation and thus offered an important focus for prayers and charity. In this light, founding or endowing leper institutions were deemed to be good investments.[78]

Elma Brenner has noted that much evidence for the status of medieval lepers remains ambiguous. Considering the complex and changing dynamics of medieval societies, there were in fact multiple and heterogeneous social responses across time and space.[79] Moreover, she insists that the two notions attributed to lepers – punishment or salvation – were

73 B. Tabuteau, 'Historical Research Developments on Leprosy in France and Western Europe', in *The Medieval Hospital and Medical Practice*, ed. B. S. Bowers (Aldershot, 2007), pp. 41–55.

74 Tabuteau, 'Historical Research Developments', p. 44.

75 B. J. Baker and K. L. Bolhofner, 'Biological and Social Implications of a Medieval Burial from Cyprus for Understanding Leprosy in the Past', *International Journal of Paleopathology* 4 (2014), 17–24.

76 G. Robbins Schug, 'Begotten of Corruption? Bioarchaeology and "Othering" of Leprosy in South Asia', *International Journal of Paleopathology* 15 (2016), 1–9.

77 For global Hansen's disease information, see WHO web page: https://www.who.int/publications/i/item/who-wer9536, last updated 4 September 2020.

78 J. Magilton, 'Leprosy, Lepers and Their Hospitals', in *Lepers Outside the Gate: Excavations at the Cemetery of the Hospital of St. James and St. Mary Magdalene, Chichester, 1986–87 and 1993*, ed. J. Magilton, F. Lee and A. Boylston (Chichester, 2008), pp. 9–21.

79 Brenner, 'Recent Perspectives', pp. 388–406.

not actually irreconcilable, since the leprous could have been viewed simultaneously as 'sinners who had been singled out to be redeemed'.[80]

Here again, then, it becomes clear that if medieval perceptions of and social responses towards leprosy were neither monolithic nor uniform, we cannot expect there to have been a homogeneous impact of heterogeneous social factors on IC.[81] Therefore, we must embrace the existence of heterogeneous immunological landscapes when exploring the complex process associated with leprosy prevalence and decline in medieval Europe.

Heterogeneous social landscapes generate equally heterogeneous immunological landscapes: building a syndemics approach for leprosy in medieval Europe

At its simplest level, syndemic refers to the interaction of two or more epidemics, with that interaction exacerbating the burden and clinical outcome of one or both diseases in a population.[82] Biological synergism also exists among co-dwelling diseases (i.e., pathogens). A more comprehensive definition of syndemic, however, embraces the additional impact of social and environmental conditions on the health of individuals and populations.[83] Emily Mendenhall has noted that the syndemic (or syndemics) concept has three core features: (a) clustering of two or more diseases within a population; (b) the biological, social and psychological interaction of those diseases; and (c) the large-scale social forces that precipitate the clustering of such diseases.[84] In essence, syndemics highlight the adverse interactions of diseases exacerbated by environmental and social factors, where differential disease outcomes emerge under conditions of health inequality caused by poverty, stress and stigmatisation, among other factors.[85]

In her study of plague in Renaissance Florence, Ann Carmichael ingeniously pointed out that plague did not simply displace other infections; instead, she described a situation in which 'a plague was many plagues', meaning that other infections coexisted or co-occurred alongside plague outbreaks in medieval Europe.[86] Clearly, plague was a devastating

80 Brenner, 'Recent Perspectives', p. 393.

81 These include social factors that likely included different economic, dietary and sanitary approaches or responses.

82 Synergistically interacting epidemics (CDC: https://www.cdc.gov/nchhstp/programintegration/definitions.htm, last accessed 11 June 2020). See also M. Singer and S. Clair, 'Syndemics and Public Health: Reconceptualizing Disease in Bio-Social Context', *Medical Anthropology Quarterly* 17 (2003), 423–41.

83 Singer and Clair, 'Syndemics and Public Health', p. 423–41.

84 E. Mendenhall, 'Syndemics: A New Path for Global Health Research', *The Lancet* 389 (2017), 889–91.

85 M. Singer et al., 'Syndemics and the Biosocial Conception of Health', *The Lancet* 389 (2017), 941–50.

86 A. G. Carmichael, *Plague and the Poor in Renaissance Florence* (Cambridge, 1986), p. 14.

infection in medieval and early modern Europe, yet clinical descriptions without specific reference to buboes could also have reflected a mixture of epidemic infections. As Carmichael wrote,

> unmixed, pure bubonic plague was an unlikely occurrence ... Herding poorer people into isolation hospitals was not characteristic of plague provisions in the fourteenth century. Isolation of plague sufferers and their contacts may have had more profound effects on the differential mortality rates of rich and poor than it did on the spread of plague. Truly contact-born infections were more likely to spread within the miserable populations of a lazaretto.[87]

Consequently, it is important to consider that more than one infectious disease was undermining the health and challenging the IC of medieval European populations. Moreover, when studying a long-lasting chronic infectious disease such as Hansen's disease, exposure to other infectious diseases during the individual's lifetime might have played a significant role in depressing the host immune system and, in the end, influencing the clinical progress and outcome of Hansen's disease. For example, Helen Donoghue and colleagues state that impairment in the cell-mediated immune response found in LL, commonly identified in archaeological remains, could, when coupled with social factors, lead to a reactivation of latent TB and perhaps induce a speedier death. This, in turn, could lead to a decline in the number of individuals *living* with leprosy.[88] Concurrent infections is syndemics at its simplest level.

Without ruling out disease interaction, it is possible to develop an even more comprehensive syndemics model for medieval leprosy, wherein the changing prevalence of infection by *M. leprae* was not significantly influenced by changes in pathogen virulence but, rather, by changes in the host's biology. Here, fluctuations in IC are determined more, or as much, by a person's biological and socio-ecological contexts. Merrill Singer and colleagues already expanded the 'syndemic lexicon' among modern populations to include the concept of countersyndemics – whereby one biological, behavioural or social condition provides a protective benefit against other disease interactions – and unintended countersyndemics – whereby efforts to treat one disease improve the elimination of another.[89] Consequently, building a syndemics approach to understand the prevalence of fluctuations of leprosy in medieval Europe must consider an emerging discipline: ecological immunology. This discipline studies the human immune system in its own ecological and social context.[90] Ecological immunology expands our understanding of how the immune system

87 Ibid., p. 18.

88 H. D. Donoghue et al., 'Co-Infection of *Mycobacterium tuberculosis* and *Mycobacterium leprae* in Human Archaeological Samples: A Possible Explanation for the Historical Decline of Leprosy', *Proceedings of the Royal Society B: Biological Sciences* 272 (2005), 389–94.

89 Singer, 'Syndemics', pp. 941–50.

90 S. S. French, M. C. Moore and G. E. Demas, 'Ecological Immunology: The Organism in Context', *Integrative and Comparative Biology* 49 (2009), 246–53; T. W. McDade, 'The Ecologies of

works, by demonstrating how multiple ecological and social factors can affect innate or acquired immune responses. Such an immunological approach requires a careful reconstruction of the lifetime of each individual or population, since all social and ecological contexts, past and present, shape an individual's IC.[91]

Inflammatory responses involve cellular mechanisms that play a significant role in the clinical progress of Hansen's disease.[92] Long-lasting systemic inflammation is shaped by more than one factor, though, and can be associated with a homeostatic imbalance affecting the function and regulation of the immune system.[93] Along with pathogens, any disruption to an individual's systemic homeostasis can trigger an immunological response; repeated experiences of acute or chronic stress, for example, can induce changes in the inflammatory processes.[94] Clearly, medieval leprosy is an excellent model with which to consider a complex multidimensional process wherein biosocial factors experienced during a person's lifetime can shape their immunological phenotype, ultimately determining if the individual will mount, or not, an appropriate immunological response to infection.

Christos Lynteris argues that Singer's syndemics approach clearly 'de-medicalises' epidemics and opens up the field for a new anthropological approach.[95] Moreover, Lynteris adds a crucial phenomenological dimension for epidemics:

> What syndemic theory and other, less overarching, processual approaches to epidemics seem to neglect is a crucial phenomenological dimension of outbreaks: that these are, more often than not, experienced by their victims as ruptures in social, political and economic life; that they are experienced not as long-term processes but as short-term catastrophic events, which are often attributed not to a multiplicity of causes, but to a single or unilateral cause.[96]

I propose that leprosy in medieval Europe should be reconstructed using both approaches: a syndemic approach that also considers that many people with leprosy experienced their diagnosis as a relatively short-term catastrophic event and wherein each event (in time and space) should not be always associated with the same 'single or unilateral cause'. Leprosy

---

the Human Immune Function', *Annual Review of Anthropology* 34 (2005), 495–21.

91 T. W. McDade, 'Life History, Maintenance, and the Early Origins of Immune Function', *American Journal of Human Biology* 17 (2005), 81–94; T. W. McDade, 'Early Environments and the Ecology of Inflammation', *Proceedings of the National Academy of Sciences* 109 (2012), 17281–8.

92 Modlin, 'Innate Immune Response', pp. 48–54.

93 P. H. Black, 'The Inflammatory Response Is an Integral Part of the Stress Response: Implications for Atherosclerosis, Insulin Resistance, Type II Diabetes and Metabolic Syndrome X', *Brain, Behavior, and Immunity* 17 (2003), 350–64.

94 P. H. Black and A. S. Berman, 'Stress and Inflammation', in *Cytokines: Stress and Immunity*, ed. N. P. Plotnikoff, R. E. Faith, A. J. Murgo and R. A. Good (Orlando, 1999), pp. 115–32; Black, 'The Inflammatory Response', pp. 350–64.

95 C. Lynteris, 'Introduction: The Time of Epidemics', *The Cambridge Journal of Anthropology* 32 (2014), 24–5.

96 Ibid., p. 25.

in medieval Europe was not an isolated regional phenomenon that took place within a homogeneous social and environmental landscape. The installation and development of large-scale institutional care in the form of leprosaria, for example, show us that the status and organisation of such institutions varied in time and space, including social attitudes and responses.[97] So too did the status, perception, care and health status of the people residing in these institutions vary across time and space.

Considered a neglected tropical disease (NTD),[98] Hansen's disease today is used as an example for the *new syndemics theoretical approach*, wherein patients could have been incubating *M. leprae* that reactivated or manifested the disease only when a second infection decreased their immunity.[99] The syndemics concept has been revamped and expanded in the last decades but is primarily applied only to contemporary populations or case studies. I propose that it is necessary to apply and expand syndemics theoretical approaches to past populations and their infectious diseases and epidemics. I therefore argue for a multifactorial model to approach and study changes in leprosy prevalence in medieval Europe, whereby multiple factors influenced, directly or indirectly, overall IC in individuals and populations (figure 11.3). As previously noted for medieval plague, homogeneous or uniform changes did not exist in time and space for IC in all medieval European populations.[100] This model thus should be conceptualised in a syndemic framework that can highlight the complex interaction of biological, social and environmental factors that synergistically (syndemic or countersyndemic) could have influenced leprosy prevalence. It is important to recognise that other syndemic approaches can be proposed for leprosy's decline or changes in its prevalence, such as lack of exposure to the pathogen or other factors that do not directly affect the host's IC. However, differential exposure alone cannot explain overall changes in leprosy prevalence.

Conclusion

Our modern COVID-19 pandemic is showing us that physical distance, wearing masks and improved hygiene (including avoiding exposure) play important roles in keeping overall infection rates as low as possible. Nevertheless, changes in an individual person's biosocial context that impact on IC (stress, herd immunity, therapeutically immune activation, passive immunity by donor antibodies or active immunity by exposure or vaccines)

97 Demaitre, *Leprosy in Pre-Modern Medicine*; Rawcliffe, *Leprosy in Medieval England*; Roberts, 'Bioarchaeology of Leprosy and Tuberculosis'; Roffey, 'Medieval Leper Hospitals'.

98 1042 WHO https://www.who.int/neglected_diseases/diseases/en/, last accessed 20 June 2020). NTD are a diverse group of communicable diseases that prevail in tropical and subtropical conditions in 149 countries, where populations living in poverty, without adequate sanitation and in close contact with infectious vectors and domestic animals and livestock are worst affected.

99 M. Singer and N. Bulled, 'Interlocked Infections: The Health Burdens of Syndemics of Neglected Tropical Diseases', *Annals of Anthropological Practice* 36 (2012), 328–45.

100 Crespo and Lawrenz, 'Heterogeneous Immunological Landscape', pp. 229–57.

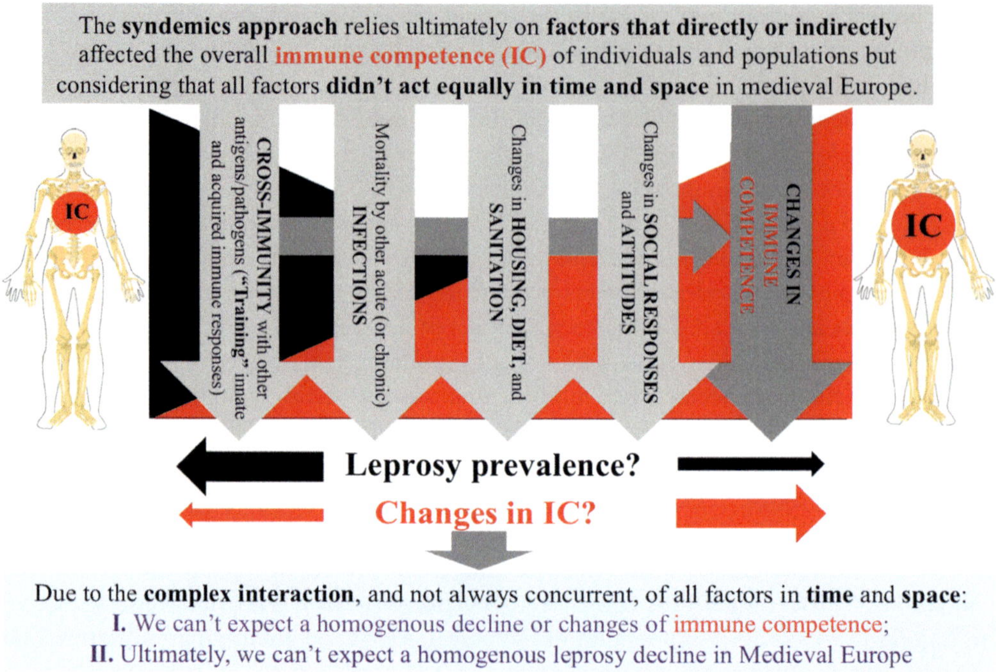

Fig. 11.3. Diagram that summarises the syndemic rationale for the decline of leprosy. Fabian Crespo.

will ultimately determine the fate and co-evolution of the SARS-CoV-2 pathogen and humans.[101] The COVID-19 pandemic is also showing intersectionality generally as a set of biological, social and environmental factors that come together to generate disease.[102] This chapter is being finalised while we are still trying to understand the global health and epidemiological crisis generated by COVID-19. It is clear that a syndemic approach is being utilised to explain heterogeneous landscapes for infection, spread, clinical outcomes and differential mortality. A growing literature is exploring the COVID-19 pandemic (news, blogs and peer-reviewed articles) using the 'syndemics of COVID-19' model to show how pre-existing conditions, social groups or social inequalities can help to explain differential outcomes or mortality.[103] Clearly, the COVID-19 pandemic is teaching us a

[101] These changes in immune competence include natural/biological processes (e.g., stress, herd immunity) or medically acquired processes (therapeutically immune activation, passive immunity by donor antibodies or active immunity by exposure or vaccines).

[102] For example: age/gender/ethnicity/genetics/immune system or diet/living conditions/ occupations/behaviour/stigma and marginalization.

[103] C. Herrick, 'Syndemics of Covid-19 and Pre-Existing Conditions', *Somatosphere* 30 March 2021, http://Somatosphere.Net/2020/Syndemics-of-Covid-19-and-Pre-Existing Conditions.html; T. A. Kenny, 'The Coronavirus Doesn't Exist in Isolation – It Feeds on Other Diseases, Crises', *The Conversation*, 25 May 2021, https://theconversation.com/the-coronavirus-doesnt-

lesson: understanding immunological susceptibility, disease progress and differential mortality requires us to conduct complex multidisciplinary studies. The same lessons can also be applied to the past.

Numerous authors have explored already how ecological and social factors (co-infections, diet and social attitudes, among other factors) could help to explain the prevalence and decline of leprosy in medieval Europe.[104] Keith Manchester has also proposed a potential and direct link between some of these factors and the immune system (immunocompromised individuals).[105] I propose that using a syndemics approach, it is time to explore past epidemics and pandemics by unravelling broader social, historical and ecological contexts and ultimately understanding how they affected host biology and people's capacity to mount a lasting and successful immune response. Medieval Hansen's disease or medieval leprosy offers a unique opportunity to expand such a complex immunological and syndemic approach. As long as heterogeneous social and ecological landscapes existed in past populations, we cannot rule out their impact on immune responses and the role they played in generating heterogeneous immunological landscapes. After all, these heterogeneous landscapes had a significant effect on disease prevalence and mortality burdens.

exist-in-isolation-it-feeds-on-other-diseases-crises-135664; T. Poteat et al., 'Understanding Covid-19 Risks and Vulnerabilities among Black Communities in America: The Lethal Force of Syndemics', *Annals of Epidemiology* 47 (2020), 1–3.

104 Donoghue et al., 'Co-Infection'; Ell, 'Reconstructing the Epidemiology'; Manchester, 'Tuberculosis and Leprosy'; Rawcliffe, *Leprosy in Medieval England*; Roberts, 'Antiquity of Leprosy'; Roffey, 'Medieval Leper Hospitals'; Touati, 'Contagion and Leprosy'; A. S. Wilson, K. Manchester and N. Lynnerup, 'Mycobacterial Cross-Immunity: A Possible Factor in the Medieval Decline of Leprosy', *American Journal of Physical Anthropology* 153 (2014), 274.

105 Personal communication, 7 July 2019.

12

Past Plagues: On the Synergies of Genetic and Historical Interpretations of Infectious Disease

HENDRIK POINAR[1]

There are no facts, only interpretations of facts.[2]

Introduction

Lester Little's brilliant and prescient 2011 review article 'Plague Historians in Lab Coats' ends with the first draft genome of the ancient pathogen *Yersinia pestis*, the causative agent of plague, being reconstructed from ancient DNA (aDNA).[3] The pathogen was found in the teeth of human remains discovered in a mid-fourteenth-century burial site in East Smithfield, London.[4] In the article, Little addressed the emerging gap between historians, who had occupied the retrospective plague space for decades, and geneticists all too eager to claim this space as their own. With modern techniques paving the way for ancient pathogen detection, geneticists felt well placed to bring the years-long debates

1 I humbly dedicate this chapter to the intrepid historian Ann G. Carmichael, who has generously enlightened me on various aspects of plague (and other) history, to think critically about plague reservoirs and the over-interpretations that come from singular records, whether archival or DNA. I am proud to say that I, in turn, have taught her the meaning of ascertainment bias. This chapter would not have come to fruition without the tremendous help of Debi Poinar, Nükhet Varlık and Lori Jones, whose endless suggestions, edits and positive feedback were both much needed and welcomed. I present here data collected, analysed and interpreted by three of my phenomenal students, Katherine Eaton, Maddie Tapson and Ravneet K. Sidhu, as well as collaborators without whom I would be a much lesser scientist: Eddie Holmes, Ann Carmichael, Nükhet Varlık, Sharon DeWitte, Dan Salkeld, Luis Barriero, Rebecca Redfern, Sebastian Duchene, Leo Featherstone, Gino Fornaciari, Brian Golding and Timothy Newfield. This work has been funded by the Social Sciences and Humanities Research Council of Canada and the Canadian Institute for Advanced Research (CIFAR). Opinions and errors herein are entirely my own.

2 F. Nietzsche, *The Will to Power*, paragraph 481, trans. W. Kaufmann and R. J. Hollingdale (New York, 1967).

3 Importantly, the 'ancient' in aDNA does not necessarily mean the genome was drafted using the remains of an individual who died in antiquity or any specific historical period. In fact, aDNA has been applied to genomes drafted from the twentieth century.

4 L. K. Little, 'Plague Historians in Lab Coats', *Past and Present* 213 (2011), 267–90 (pp. 270–1). For the East Smithfield research, see K. I. Bos et al., 'A Draft Genome of *Yersinia pestis* from Victims of the Black Death', *Nature* 478 (2011), 506–10.

about the causative agents, origins, timing of the emergence and disappearances of past plagues to a close.[5]

Seen in hindsight, Little's chronicling of the discovery of the aetiological agents of historical plague outbreaks is rather like a brisk walk – nothing like the frenetic pace of new discoveries today. His paper echoes back to the early days of germ theory and microbial identity, which were synonymous for disease at the time. In 1873, the Norwegian physician Gerhard Armauer Hansen discovered the leprosy bacillus. Subsequent discoveries, including those by Robert Koch and Louis Pasteur, not only informed thinking about modern disease but also were often applied retrospectively to the past with no evidence to either support or refute such applications.[6] It was not until more recent palaeopathology and aDNA work enabled definitive proof of the presence (but not the absence) of some particular pathogens that somewhat less tenuous retrospective histories could be offered.

Although the advent of new scientific methodologies has enabled positive identification of pathogens responsible for infectious disease that have long been visible in bone (e.g., leprosy and tuberculosis) or presumed present (e.g., plague) and have been instrumental in rendering the once-invisible (e.g., salmonella and Hepatitis B virus (HBV)) perceptible, they nevertheless still require appropriate context to be useful and meaningful in the broader scholarship. In short, while these scientific techniques revealed new facts, they also generated additional challenges with interpretation. One must be cautious with the presumed power of a DNA sequence. In much the same way that a single historical document or object can offer only a snapshot of a particular moment or place in time and cannot nor should not readily be extrapolated, an aDNA sequence without proper context derived from additional historical, biochemical, archaeological and other evidence likewise remains anecdotal.[7]

Out of the old and into the new

While many historians were quick to jump on the early plague aDNA results as vindication of their retrospective diagnoses, I can attest that much controversy still existed in the

5 For retrospective diagnosis wars among historians, see, among others O. J. Benedictow, *What Disease Was Plague? On the Controversy over the Microbiological Identity of Plague Epidemics of the Past* (Leiden, 2010) and *The Black Death, 1346–1353: The Complete History* (Woodbridge, 2004); G. Twigg, *The Black Death: A Biological Reappraisal* (London, 1984); S. Scott and C. J. Duncan, *Return of the Black Death: The World's Greatest Serial Killer* (Chichester, 2004) and *Biology of Plagues: Evidence from Historical Populations* (Cambridge, 2001); S. K. Cohn, 'The Black Death: End of a Paradigm', *The American Historical Review* 107 (2002), 703–38 and *The Black Death Transformed: Disease and Culture in Early Renaissance Europe* (London, 2002).

6 S. Kitasato, 'The Bacillus of Bubonic Plague', *The Lancet* 144 (1894), 452.

7 S. Duchêne et al., 'The Recovery, Interpretation and Use of Ancient Pathogen Genomes', *Current Biology* 30 (2020), R1215–31.

scientific fields involved in the discovery of these results.[8] Until the first ancient pathogen genome was literally 'captured' in 2011 (see later), aDNA analyses relied almost exclusively on the use of Polymerase Chain Reaction (PCR). This technique enables identification of the pathogen by targeting and copying a tiny portion of a single gene so that it may be visible (denoting a positive presence) and/or sequenced (revealing the actual order of bases and thus far more discriminatory than a simple positive PCR). For the bulk of early aDNA *Y. pestis* work, scientists used the plasminogen activator gene (*pla*), which is found commonly (although not always) in one of the bacterium's three plasmids (extra chromosomal circular genomes). Plasmids are often found in multiple copies per bacterium and thus should, in theory, be more easily detected than chromosomal genes. Even so, the amplification (or increase in the number of copies) of the PCR target represents less than 0.0002% of the entire genome of the plague bacillus. It is thus useful only in the positive placement of plague in an individual at a site, but cannot speak to its evolutionary history or relatedness to other, existing strains.

Little was correct to highlight inconsistencies in the early identifications of *Y. pestis* aDNA, since PCR is extremely sensitive to minute amounts of DNA contamination, the sources of which can be difficult to identify. The early results, often showing remarkably high positivity rates, could not be replicated, an essential criterion that underpins the scientific method and was essential for the burgeoning field of palaeogenetics. This was due, in part, to the fact that preservation of aDNA is volatile and its presence in one sample does not and cannot guarantee its presence in another. Even samples taken from the same burial setting – or even the same individual – can contain completely different DNA content and thus generate separate negative or positive results regarding the pathogen of interest. It is not surprising that the methodology gave inconsistent findings in the first decade of looking for *Y. pestis* in ancient remains. This, in turn, often led to misinterpretations or over-interpretation of results.

Evolutionary biologist Tom Gilbert has addressed the important issue of negative scientific findings.[9] His article outlining his inability to reproduce earlier work was groundbreaking in and of itself, since far too few scientific journals publish negative results. In fact, my own first attempts to find plague in samples from East Smithfield, sent to me in 2003 by my collaborator Sharon DeWitte and using methods similar to those published previously by others, were also consistently negative. Yet, samples taken from the same site and sent to me in 2008, five years later, were the ones that – using novel methodologies (see later) – ultimately yielded the data that formed the basis of the first ancient genome paper.[10] I did not publish the negative results, but wish that I had. As such, Gilbert's paper

8 See, for example, D. Raoult et al., 'Molecular Identification by "Suicide PCR" of *Yersinia pestis*', *Proceedings of the National Academy of Sciences* 97 (2000), 12800–3; A. Cooper and H. N. Poinar, 'Ancient DNA: Do It Right or Not at All', *Science* 289 (2000), 1139.

9 M. T. P. Gilbert et al., 'Absence of *Yersinia pestis*-Specific DNA in Human Teeth from Five European Excavations of Putative Plague Victims', *Microbiology* 150 (2004), 341–54.

10 Bos et al., 'Draft Genome'.

was key in keeping vigilance in the field, while also highlighting the significance of PCR negatives (absence of evidence). For all the recent success of the field, one must remember that most samples have overwhelmingly yielded negative results.

Rather like the much discussed 'Big Bang' (polytomy) that gave rise to the four main branches of *Y. pestis* shortly before the Black Death, the 2011 conclusion of Little's review sits at its own polytomy, that of the emergence of the field of genomics of ancient infectious disease.[11] In the decade since the publication of Little's article and at the time of this writing, 240 ancient microbial genomes have been reconstructed (and published) from diverse infectious agents of human victims. By far the most prevalent of these have been *Yersinia pestis* (plague), with 135 draft genomes representing 56 per cent of the total.[12]

11 The culminant study identifying the so-called 'Big Bang' is Y. Cui et al., 'Historical Variations in Mutation Rate in an Epidemic Pathogen, *Yersinia pestis*', *Proceedings of the National Academy of Sciences* 110 (2013), 577–82. I discuss subsequent work on this below. For studies leading to the discovery of the polytomy, see G. Morelli et al., '*Yersinia pestis* Genome Sequencing Identifies Patterns of Global Phylogenetic Diversity', *Nature Genetics* 42 (2010), 1140–3 (p. 1142–3); M. Achtman et al., 'Microevolution and History of the Plague Bacillus, *Yersinia pestis*', *Proceedings of the National Academy of Sciences* 101 (2004), 17837–42; J. Parkhill et al., 'Genome Sequence of *Yersinia pestis*, the Causative Agent of Plague', *Nature* 413 (2001), 523–7; M. Achtman et al., '*Yersinia pestis*, the Cause of Plague, Is a Recently Emerged Clone of *Yersinia pseudotuberculosis*', *Proceedings of the National Academy of Sciences* 96 (1999), 14043–8.

12 See, for example, A. Seguin-Orlando et al., 'No Particular Genomic Features Underpin the Dramatic Economic Consequences of 17th Century Plague Epidemics in Italy', *iScience* 24 (2021), 102383; M. Guellil et al., 'A Genomic and Historical Synthesis of Plague in 18th Century Eurasia', *Proceedings of the National Academy of Sciences* 117 (2020), 28328–35; I. Morozova et al., 'New Ancient Eastern European *Yersinia pestis* Genomes Illuminate the Dispersal of Plague in Europe', *Philosophical Transactions of the Royal Society B Biological Sciences* 375 (2020), 20190569; M. A. Spyrou et al., 'Phylogeography of the Second Plague Pandemic Revealed through Analysis of Historical *Yersinia pestis* Genomes', *Nature Communications* 10 (2019), 4470; J. Susat et al., '*Yersinia pestis* Strains from Latvia Show Depletion of the *pla* Virulence Gene at the End of the Second Plague Pandemic', *Scientific Reports* 10 (2020), 14628; M. Keller et al., 'Ancient *Yersinia pestis* Genomes from across Western Europe Reveal Early Diversification during the First Pandemic (541–750)', *Proceedings of the National Academy of Sciences* 116 (2019), 12363–72; P. B. Damgaard et al., '137 Ancient Human Genomes from across the Eurasian Steppes', *Nature* 557 (2018), 369–74; A. Namouchi et al., 'Integrative Approach Using *Yersinia pestis* Genomes to Revisit the Historical Landscape of Plague during the Medieval Period', *Proceedings of the National Academy of Sciences* 115 (2018), E11790–7; M. A. Spyrou et al., 'Analysis of 3800-year-old *Yersinia pestis* Genomes Suggests Bronze Age Origin for Bubonic Plague', *Nature Communications* 9 (2018), 2234; A. A. Valtueña et al., 'The Stone Age Plague and Its Persistence in Eurasia', *Current Biology* 27 (2017), 3683–91; Bos et al., 'Draft Genome'; M. Feldman et al., 'A High-Coverage *Yersinia pestis* Genome from a Sixth-Century Justinianic Plague Victim', *Molecular Biology and Evolution* 33 (2016), 2911–23; M. A. Spyrou et al., 'Historical *Y. pestis* Genomes Reveal the European Black Death as the Source of Ancient and Modern Plague Pandemics', *Cell Host Microbe* 19 (2016), 874–81; K. I. Bos et al., 'Eighteenth Century *Yersinia pestis* Genomes Reveal the Long-Term Persistence of an Historical Plague Focus', *Elife* 5 (2016), e12994; S. Rasmussen et al., 'Early Divergent Strains of *Yersinia pestis* in Eurasia 5,000 Years Ago', *Cell* 163 (2015), 571–82; D. M. Wagner et al., '*Yersinia pestis* and the Plague of Justinian 541–543 AD:

Success has also been achieved with *Mycobacterium leprae* (leprosy, twenty-two genomes), *Mycobacterium tuberculosis* (tuberculosis, six genomes), *Salmonella enterica* (salmonella, thirteen genomes), *Variola virus* (smallpox, fourteen genomes), *Influenza* virus (influenza, twenty-one genomes), *Helicobacter pylori* (Helicobacter pylori infection, one genome), *Treponema pallidum* (syphilis, eight genomes), *Hepatitis* B virus (HepB or HBV, seventeen genomes), *Measles morbillivirus* (measles, six genomes) and *Human Immunodeficiency Virus* 1 (HIV-1, ten genomes), among others.

The explosion in data acquisition over the decade since 2011 has been possible because of the development of new methods for the retrieval of DNA from ancient samples, notably the advent of – and oddly labelled – next generation sequencing (NGS) (what will the ensuing change be called, if this one is already labelled 'next'?). NGS was the catalyst to the genomics revolution because it allowed for the miniaturisation and parallelisation of sequencing reactions. To offer a comparison, in 2005, the most commonly used sequencing machine (ABI 3730) produced 356 sequences (each of those sequences – termed a read – is between 300 and 700 base pairs in length), while in 2006 the first NGS instrument (454 GS FLX) produced one million reads, each between 100 and 200 base pairs in length. As prices dropped, it increasingly became cost-effective for researchers to evaluate greater numbers of samples. Today, the latest iterations (e.g., NOVAseq, Illumina) produce over one *billion* reads, at a cost of about ten cents per one million bases; this represents a cost savings of nine orders of magnitude in less than fifteen years. We might say that we are in the midst of a genomics revolution merely via the explosion of cheaply available sequencing data.

More importantly, however, the real benefit of NGS methodology over PCR for aDNA is that it can sequence nearly everything within a sample, in an unbiased way. It can also sequence molecules at the edge of their bioinformatic utility, molecules that are about twenty-four base pairs in length, which is about half the size of the smallest, useful PCR fragments. Further, whereas PCR required preliminary insight, or a best guess, as to the underlying cause of a given epidemic so that a pathogen could be targeted specifically, next generation and high-throughput (NGS/HTS) required no insight at all. It also had the advantage of producing millions of reads per sample, thereby allowing the total spectrum of DNA present in a sample to be retrieved (i.e., human, fungal, bacterial, viral and environmental). This could, in theory, then be linked to known pathogens in contemporary databases via various computational analyses. In other words, with NGS/HTS scientists could let the analyses tell them what infectious agents were in their samples rather than having to search or target something in particular. This ability to unearth the unrecognised or otherwise invisible has dramatically increased the number and range of pathogens found and identified in historical remains.[13]

A Genomic Analysis', *Lancet Infectious Diseases* 14 (2014), 319–26; P. Skoglund et al., 'Genomic Diversity and Admixture Differs for Stone-Age Scandinavian Foragers and Farmers', *Science* 344 (2014), 747–50.

13 Duchêne et al., 'Recovery, Interpretation and Use'.

As the study of aDNA progressed from PCR to NGS/HTS methodologies, it also became possible, for the first time, to acquire enough genetic material (DNA) from a sample to reconstruct a draft genome, as was the case for *Y. pestis*.[14] Here, it is important to note that a draft genome is not a complete genome. Very few modern genomes are actually complete or, in genome parlance, closed, because they are limited by the length of reads produced by NGS/HTS methodologies and the repetitive nature of most genomes. This is more so the case for ancient genomes, whose reads are exceptionally short due to the degraded nature of the extracted DNA. An incomplete or draft genome is problematic for retrospective analyses for several reasons. First, it means that the strain isolated from an ancient epidemic may lack some of its phylogenetically informative changes (or SNPs – see later). These changes are of critical importance for describing the strain's relationship to other strains (its position on a phylogenetic tree). Second, a draft genome may lack truly novel gene content, or the correct order of its genes, which could be responsible for altering a pathogen's virulence, transmission or other phenotype.

Even with all this new genomic data, most retrospective aDNA work on infectious disease still lacked the significant and necessary contextual information that historians could (and would) have contributed, such as: the context for the disease's emergence (from trade and communication to politics, agriculture and environmental variability); how the individual(s) may have contracted the disease; how they understood their condition; or how they lived and perhaps died with or of their disease. They also had little to add to historical questions related to larger epidemics or pandemics: how pathogens erupted and (were) moved across space and through time. This is partly an artefact of the way in which a DNA sequence from a particular pathogen was purposed in earlier studies. Most PCR-based work sought simply to identify the presence of a pathogen in a set of remains in order to confirm the existence of an infectious disease in a specific location at an approximate point in time. While interesting in and of themselves, such findings were usually void of any real contextual information regarding the sample; of course, this did not always keep scientists from speculating on the historical implications of their findings, often relying on outdated historical sources and narratives to do so.[15] Hence they performed as what Little aptly called 'plague historians in lab coats'.

Fast-forward ten years from Little's review, and we are now in the midst of an ancient infectious disease genomics revolution. Numerous recent reviews highlight significant progress in the field. This chapter, however, focuses specifically on insights drawn from recent sequencing efforts of both modern and ancient *Y. pestis* genomes to explore the

[14] Bos et al., 'Draft Genome'.

[15] See, for example, R. Barbieri, '*Yersinia pestis*: The Natural History of Plague', *Clinical Microbiology Reviews* 34 (2021), e00044–19; B. Bramanti et al., 'Assessing the Origins of the European Plagues following the Black Death: A Synthesis of Genomic, Historical and Ecological Information', *Proceedings of the National Academy of Sciences* 118 (2021), e2101940118; M. Drancourt and D. Raoult, 'Molecular History of Plague', *Clinical Microbiology and Infection* 22 (2016), 911–15.

limitations of existing scientific data and to demonstrate how our desire to interpret aDNA results has outpaced the limitations of said data. To help place this in context, I begin by briefly describing the current limitations of aDNA work, where potential biases and over-interpretations may pose problems. Then I explore what we can – and, importantly, cannot – say from the current state of the field for plague genomes specifically. In doing so, I hope to highlight the critical importance of interdisciplinary collaboration to study past pandemics.[16]

Limitations of aDNA work

There are very real limitations concerning access to and interpretations of aDNA data. While by no means offering an exhaustive exploration of these themes, I describe here some of the major points that should be of interest to non-specialists.[17]

Most obviously, not everyone has access to the human (or animal) remains that may be relevant to the timeline of a particular infectious disease's history. Access is not, and never has been, a democratic process. Rather, it often is driven by colonial legacies (collections in museums sitting outside their original burial locations), funding decisions and/or politics. The ethics of storing and working on these remains is just beginning to be addressed, following well-established protocols that are already in place for indigenous remains in North America – the Native American Graves Protection and Repatriation Act. Similar protocols will play out across the field in due time.

The greatest limitation of the work, scientifically speaking, is molecular taphonomy – meaning how organisms' DNA and proteins decay and vanish or become preserved and thus detectable. Many centuries-old human remains do not contain DNA, neither of the host itself nor of any infection pathogen.[18] Once an organism dies, the post-mortem degradation of nucleic acids (DNA and RNA) is swift – within hours – with internal, commensal bacteria being responsible for the bulk of that loss. The molecules that do survive do so in an environmentally controlled fashion where fewer interactions with environmental contaminants, namely exogenous bacteria and fungi as well as water and other factors, are ultimately responsible for long-term persistence. DNA is more likely to be

16 For examples of a more consilient approach, see Haldon et al., 'History Meets Palaeoscience: Consilience and Collaboration in Studying Past Societal Responses to Environmental Change', *Proceedings of the National Academy of Sciences* 115 (2018), 3210–18; M. H. Green, 'Genetics as a Historicist Discipline', *Perspectives on History* (December 2014), https://www.historians.org/publications-and-directories/perspectives-on-history/december-2014/genetics-as-a-historicist-discipline.

17 For a more comprehensive discussion on the bioarchaeology of plague, see S. DeWitte, 'Misconceptions About the Bioarchaeology of Plague', *Bioarchaeologists Speak Out: Deep Time Perspectives on Contemporary Issues*, ed. J. E. Buikstra (Cham, 2019), pp. 109–31.

18 This is especially true of RNA (ribonucleic acid), which significantly limits access to many viruses (e.g., influenza, HIV, West Nile, yellow fever) whose genomes are based on RNA rather than DNA.

preserved in higher latitudes and altitudinal sites, in sites with colder mean annual temperatures and in cave sites where protection from water is key. Even so, sample variation is so high even within a single site that one cannot simply count on a locale or individual set of remains to repeatedly generate positive DNA results. Such is the frustration of aDNA work. Complicating matters even further, for pathogen detection to be successful, the sampled individual must have died and been buried during the period when they were experiencing high bacteraemia, viraemia or parasitaemia – which is individual, specific and time dependent, and which may not have been the ultimate cause of death. Thus, the very fact that geneticists are able to detect the presence of blood-borne infections in long-dead individuals is remarkable in and of itself.

Despite these limitations, work on detecting pathogen DNA signatures in ancient remains has shifted seismically with the move to NGS/HTS. Little's entire review of the history of plague DNA is based on old PCR technology, whereby, as noted, singular, small sections of a genome or gene are targeted and copied many times, making them accessible (visible) to study. That data is typically used for the simple identification of the pathogen in the remains. However, if enough positions (which is an inordinate amount of work with PCR) on a genome can be typed (to type is to infer the actual base – A, C, G or T – at a position in the genome) they can be used in a simple matrix to describe proximity to or association with a particular branch on the phylogenetic tree.[19] The power of NGS/HTS, by contrast, is that it 'reads' the sequences of *all* DNA in a sample. This is called metagenomics, and although there is a bias towards less-damaged and/or contaminated DNA, some of the biases that exist with PCR are now better managed or pre-empted.[12]

The most recent iteration of the sequencing machines used by aDNA experts today generates a lot of data: between 650 million and 10 billion stretches of DNA that range from 30 to 250 base pairs in length. With prices ranging from about US$5,000 to $20,000 for a single run (which can screen several hundred samples at once), it remains an expensive experiment to conduct, with little guarantee that the results will provide any data on ancient pathogens. Labs must be well funded to do this line of work, thereby limiting which labs can participate and creating monopolies; this further aggravates already existing imbalances in the field. The benefit, however, is that hundreds of samples can be examined at one time, which in theory provides generous sequence diversity, a requirement of finding low-level, preserved DNA reads of a given infectious agent.

Unless there is exceptional preservation and another significant limitation has been met – that of high bacteraemia, viremia or parasitaemia – the data from that single experiment can provide proof of the presence of a pathogen in a given set of remains (like PCR), but it can do little more. Since the DNA of most human remains typically contains far less than 1 per cent of an infecting agent, many of us in the field have had to resort to another method to capture that miniscule proportion of DNA from its background and reconstruct the genomes, using something called targeted or capture-based enrichment.

[19] See Morelli et al., '*Yersinia pestis* Genome Sequencing'.

Like PCR, this can be a biased approach, as it requires the building of a 'bait' set, that is, a set of RNA sequences that mimic the existing diversity of *Y. pestis* as described in contemporary databases. These baits are in essence fishing hooks that capture sequences similar to themselves via hybridisation. Imagine a mirrored image of a written text. When you lay the two texts on top of each other, they match or mirror perfectly. Now imagine altering one of these texts by randomly changing a set of letters, by say 5 per cent, across one page. When laid on top of each other, the pages are still a closer match to each other than they are to other random pages of text from a different source. Thus, you still are able to 'capture' or recognise the original form. However, once more than 25 per cent of the letters on one page have been changed (i.e., a bacterium or virus has diverged significantly from its modern relatives), the two pages are no longer alike enough and the one is no longer useful to capture the other. For targeted DNA capture, 25 per cent nears the maximum divergence (differences in letters) that the current technology can handle and still capture the closest matches in a pool of other unrelated sequences. Beyond that point, the capture is no better at finding its closest relative than any other sequence in the pool; in other words, it is random. But remember, it requires access to the original textual source in the first place. Since baits rely on the diversity in existing databases, truly novel genes still present in ancient pathogen strains, but no longer present in modern ones, will be missed entirely. Deleted genes, however, are readily detectable. Thus, the completeness of modern databases is as important for the design and capture of targets as it is for the post-sequence identification of a pathogen and the construction of its draft genome.

Potential biases and over-interpretations

As is true in any field that studies the past, in ancient genomics the absence of evidence does not imply evidence of absence. Despite best efforts to uncover the true distribution of infectious disease across space and time, sample access, historical contextualisation and preservation – amongst many other issues – create strong biases in the data and thus modify interpretations. These lead to what is called ascertainment biases, that is, a bias in the true representation of a (complete) data set. This bias is often masked in the past for reasons described above and in modern datasets because of sampling artefacts or improperly broad sampling.

Ancient plague studies have the benefit of being slightly less biased than those of other ancient infectious diseases for several reasons. Some archaeological sites can be historically well documented, such as through mass burials with dated historical records to match or funerary inscriptions with suggestive hints. This, in turn, has enabled strategic, almost surgical sampling of many individuals at once, yielding 135 reconstructed genomes stemming from both first and second plague pandemics. Yet even in these best-case scenarios – East Smithfield for example, where individuals are well known to have succumbed during the Black Death – the positivity rate for plague was only 37 per cent of the forty-six teeth sampled and about 6 per cent of fifty-three bones. Complementary historical and archaeological records, including mass or so-called deviant burials as well as textual accounts of contemporary outbreaks, allows for the narrowing or focusing of efforts, thereby increasing likelihoods of aDNA retrieval success. Apart from archival fixed material in museum or hospital pathological collections with clear identification (e.g., influenza, cholera, measles), only two other infectious diseases visible in the archaeological or historical record have been the focus of the ancient human pathogen genomics revolution: tuberculosis (which was once the mainstay of early PCR-based identifications, but also problematic for a host of reasons) and leprosy. Both of these have now been sequenced many times.

In last decade since 2011, genetic research on the pathogen responsible for plague, *Y. pestis*, has contributed significantly to our understanding of its evolutionary history. This is largely, but of course not entirely, due to the many new modern and ancient genomes that have been recently acquired. But genomes offer only one glimpse into the history of this pathogen, requiring essential contextualisation from other disciplines. In the following section I entertain a few of the most significant findings from recent modern and aDNA analyses of plague, highlighting potential limitations of interpretation. It is in these spaces where over-interpretations/analyses of the data have driven narratives that are not always well supported and thus should be considered with caution. Given the pace at which the field is currently moving, there is no doubt that new and exciting data will continue to change and rewrite the existing narratives.

Plague genomics post-2011

On ascertainment bias and seeking origins

One of the early features of the genomic revolution in plague studies was a clear ascertainment bias in the geographic distribution of the samples obtained for sequencing (figure 12.1). Two issues are immediately clear. The first is that sampling is not equally distributed across the entire presumed range of *Y. pestis*. The bulk of contemporary (modern) sequences stem from Asian sources, mostly China, where monitoring and sequencing has been a priority due to high incidence of plague in rodent reservoirs. Until 2013, this led researchers to cite north-western China as the likely origin for the First and Second Plague Pandemics. However, as should have been noted then, most of Africa, the Middle East, the Caucasus and what is today Russia remained unsampled. Any ancient genome placed into the global phylogeny in 2013 would by default have had Chinese-isolated strains sitting basal or ancestral to them, suggesting a Chinese origin. Today, there still remains largely unsampled geographic space, although many newly sequenced strains from Kyrgyzstan, Georgia, Azerbaijan and Armenia are helping to change origins narratives. We require a more evenly distributed sampling from contemporary reservoirs and from more ancient remains prior to proposing alternative source populations – and thus geographic locations – as origin narratives for plague pandemics.

Second, *Y. pestis* found in human remains from both the Late Neolithic Bronze Age (LNBA) and during the First and Second Pandemics are, with a few exceptions, almost

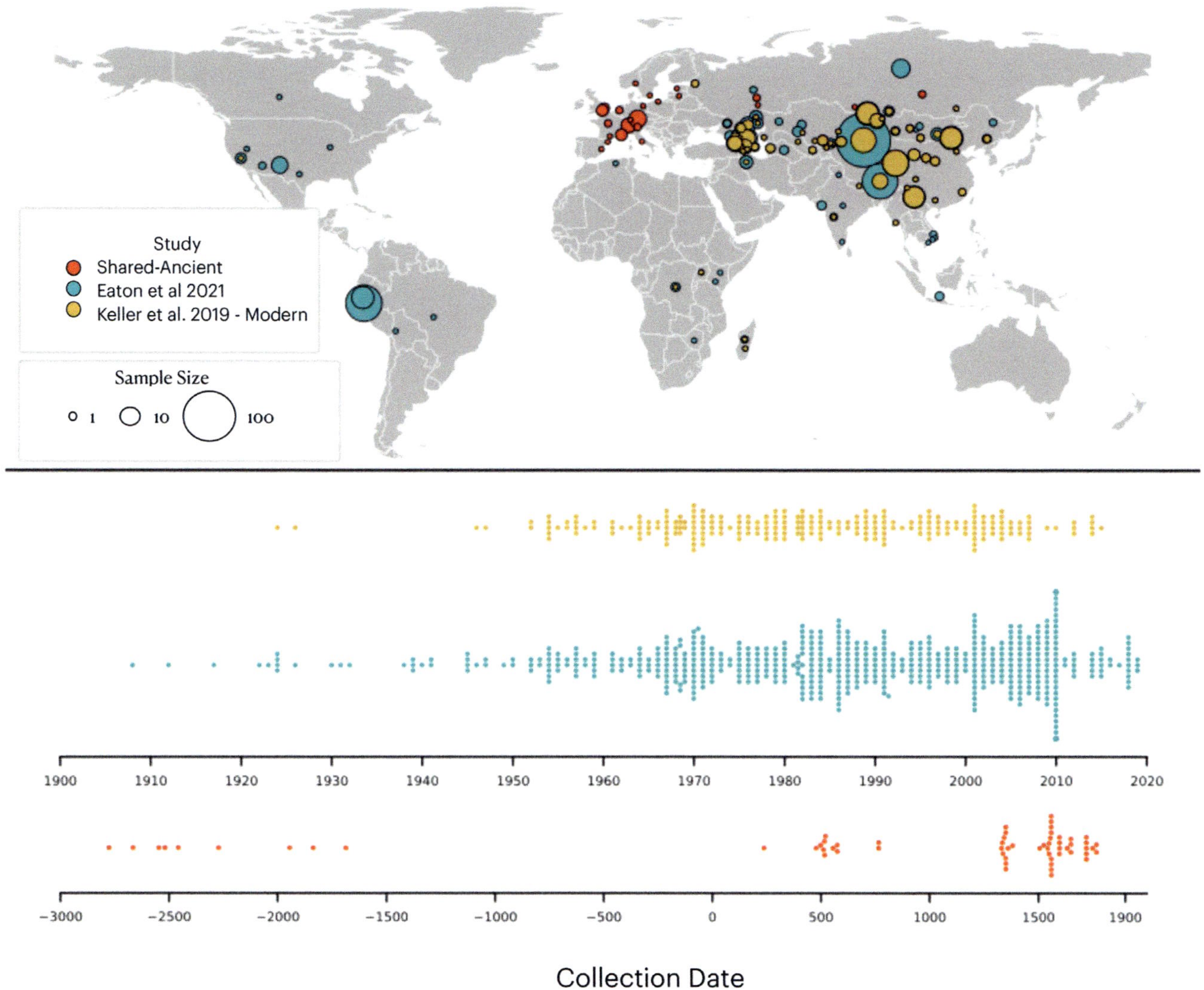

Fig. 12.1. Geographic distribution of *Yersinia pestis* samples from ancient and modern databases. Hendrik Poinar.

entirely from Western and Central Europe.[20] To some extent, the science is able to work alongside historical findings in this region. Elsewhere, this is not often the case. Several recent studies on plague draw on rich historical records from the Middle East and archaeological sites from sub-Saharan Africa for the Second Pandemic, for example, uncovering exciting new possibilities for the history of plague in those regions; but there is, as yet, no ancient *genetic* data to corroborate them.[21] Given the present state of the scientific field, developing origins narratives can seem like a futile effort, since speculative conclusions can be undone as soon as new data – historical, archaeological or genetic – become available. As a case in point, the sequences of related (what we would call 'sister') lineages of non-pandemic strains of *Y. pestis* isolated from European LNBA victims illustrate how little is known of the true geographic distribution of this bacterial pathogen in the past.[22] Before 2015, there was no prior (archaeological, textual or other) evidence to suggest the presence of *Y. pestis* in the LNBA, some 3,000 years prior to the First Pandemic. We simply do not know how long and exactly how widespread reservoirs for pandemic-capable (i.e., flea-adapted *Y. pestis*) plague may have been.

The clonal nature of Yersinia pestis

Since the publication of the first ancient draft genome of *Y. pestis*, there has been an exponential increase in publicly available modern *Y. pestis* genomes. At the time of writing in 2022, there are nearly 1,700 plague genome-sequencing projects in the works, of which some 600 contain well-curated draft genomes and can be used for phylogenetics alongside the 135 ancient genomes.

A comparison of these genomes (each genome is about 4.5 million base pairs long) reveals a very small number of changes between them: in total, only about 4,000 changes (called Single Nucleotide Polymorphisms, SNPs) define the entire *Y. pestis* phylogenetic tree. Compare that with a global phylogeny of *E. coli* or *Vibrio cholerae*, which have some

20 Recent exceptions are Spyrou, 'Phylogeography of the Second Plague Pandemic'; Spyrou, 'The Source of the Black Death'.

21 For an introduction to the historical scholarship on plague in the Middle East, see N. Varlık, 'Plague in the Mediterranean/Islamic World', *ISIS-Current Bibliography*, Special Issue on Pandemics, ed. Stephen P. Weldon and Neeraja Sankaran (2021). For recent studies on the Second Pandemic in the Middle East, see, for example, N. Fancy and M. H. Green, 'Plague and the Fall of Baghdad (1258)', *Medical History* 65 (2021), 157–77; N. Varlık, *Plague and Empire in the Early Modern Mediterranean World: The Ottoman Experience, 1347–1600* (Cambridge, 2015); S. Borsch, *The Black Death in Egypt and England: A Comparative Study* (Austin, 2005). For the possibility of plague in medieval sub-Saharan Africa, see *Afriques* Special Issue 'Sillages de la peste noire en Afrique subsaharienne: une exploration critique du silence', 9 (2018).

22 Some authors have argued that these divergent Bronze Age strains could have been pandemic-like and partially responsible for population decline during the Neolithic period. There is, however, no clear evidence to support this conjecture. See, for example, J. Brooke, 'Thinking Big about the Plague', *Inference* 4 (2018), https://inference-review.com/letter/thinking-big-about-the-plague and S. Rasmussen et al., 'Early Divergent Strains of *Yersinia pestis* in Eurasia 5,000 Years Ago', *Cell* 163 (2015), 571–82.

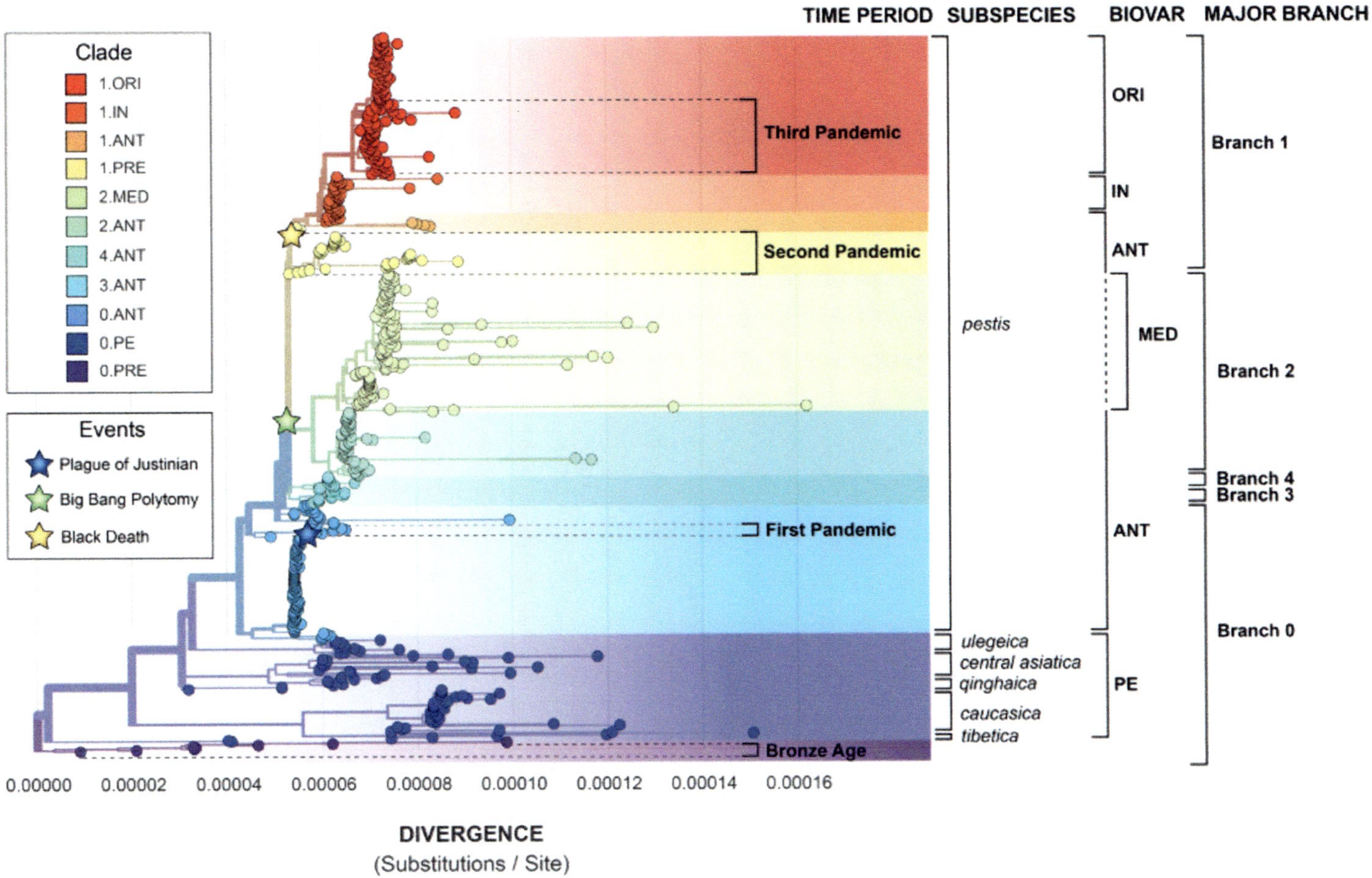

Fig. 12.2. Maximum likelihood tree of both modern and ancient strains with several taxonomic systems that have been used to describe strains of *Yersinia pestis*. Hendrik Poinar.

20,000–30,000 SNP differences describing their respective global phylogenies.[23] For plague, the bulk of that shallow diversity exists within rodent reservoir strains (figure 12.2, branch 0 or the PE biovar) with only a tiny fraction detected in strains associated with plague pandemics (figure 12.2, branch 1.PRE, ANT). This is important, because it means that *Y. pestis*'s evolution is slow; this, in turn, places limitations on what we can say about the relationship (ancestor–descendant) of two or more strains if, on average, they differ by only a few SNPs. If *Y. pestis* changes so little over large swaths of time, then to ascertain the true relationship and movement of strains from one location to another – something that historians and geneticists are especially interested in – one has to sample extremely widely to ensure that strains in neighbouring regions are in fact similar or different (and thus truly descendants of each other). If many sequences, from different locations, are in fact identical or differ only by a single SNP, it is *impossible* to infer direction of import or movement. It also makes diffusion-style maps for the Black Death, such as those promulgated in numerous generalist Black Death publications, completely reliant on historical documents (or old narratives) alone. Genetics cannot easily support these kinds of maps. As an example, early Black Death strains from the UK (East Smithfield), Spain (Barcelona) and Germany (Nabburg) are identical. How many other countries within and outside Western Europe have this identical sequence? With such little diversity, no directionality can be properly inferred from genetic studies. In these cases, we must rely on historical records for insights.

How many plague pandemics were there?

Two, maybe five or eight, but definitely not three.[24] The current three-pandemic narrative is not supported by the genetics and requires reappraisal. Previous historical narratives laid the foundation for the three 'waves' of plague concept, keeping the Second and Third Pandemics as separate and unrelated events. According to twentieth-century scholarship, which still remains influential today, the Second Pandemic started with the Black Death in the mid-fourteenth century and ended – as Europeans claimed – in the early eighteenth century. A clearly defined century-long break was followed by a nineteenth-century emergence in China's Yunnan province that extended until the 1950s. Recent historical scholarship has challenged this out-dated narrative, showing long-term maintenance of plague in the eastern Mediterranean, Caucasus and southern Russia well into the nineteenth century (i.e., the Second Pandemic).[25]

[23] A. M. Devault et al., 'Second-Pandemic Strain of *Vibrio cholerae* from the Philadelphia Cholera Outbreak of 1849', *New England Journal of Medicine* 370 (2014), 334–40; O. Tenaillon et al., 'The Population Genetics of Commensal *Escherichia coli*', *Nature Reviews Microbiology* 8 (2010), 207–17.

[24] This wonderful title was first offered up by Ann Carmichael at a SSHRC-funded conference in Hamilton in 2019.

[25] N. Varlık, 'The Plague That Never Left: Restoring the Second Pandemic to Ottoman and Turkish History in the Time of COVID-19', *New Perspectives on Turkey* 63 (2020), 176–89. Another challenge to the timeline is found in Green, 'Four Black Deaths'.

From a genetics perspective, however, the Second Pandemic strains are directly ancestral to the strains of the modern pandemic (see figure 12.2, 1.PRE and 1.ORI). As such, there is no biological reason to separate them (or to treat them as distinct pandemics). Today, we are still living within the Second Pandemic, as strains descended from it are maintained in plague reservoirs on four continents (Africa, Asia, North and South America) and continue to emerge and spread. This significantly changes the way we should view, think and perhaps write about the legacy of the singular emergence of the Black Death and the earlier polytomy, some 700–800 years ago. Importantly, it also changes the way we should frame the Eurocentric disappearance narrative, ascribing it not to anything singularly unique to Europe at the time, but, rather, most likely to changing reservoir species. So many reservoir species that once existed in European spaces in past centuries may simply no longer exist there; as they disappeared, perhaps so too did plague.[26]

Another out-dated part of the pandemic narrative is the lack of acknowledgement of pandemic-like behaviour for Branch 2, otherwise known as *Medievalis*. This branch contains wide geographic spread throughout Eurasia, stretching from the Caucasus to eastern China; it also has been associated with high-mortality epidemics.[27] As historical plague scholarship extends beyond the bounds of Western Europe, it will be important to consider the role that *Y. pestis*'s other lineages played and how and why we decide to label some branches as pandemics but not others.

Long-term Second Pandemic reservoirs of plague in Europe and the Mediterranean

Related to the point made above about reservoir species, Ann Carmichael postulated in 2014 that marmots in northern Italy may have been an important reservoir for the long-term maintenance of *Y. pestis* during the Second Pandemic.[28] This negates the necessity to infer a human-contagion model of reintroduction of plague from eastern sources for some 500 years. The old narrative that plague came from the East, down the Silk Road, from a distant part of the Central Asian steppes (thousands of kilometres away), remains a common thread in much current work.[29] Recently, palaeoclimatology has been integrated into this old narrative, the cross-Eurasian trek of plague being triggered by climate variability in

26 M. Tapson et al., 'Rodent Reservoirs as a Mechanism for the Persistence and Re-emergence of Plague in Historical Pandemics' (forthcoming).

27 G. A. Eroshenko et al., 'Evolution and Circulation of *Yersinia pestis* in the Northern Caspian and Northern Aral Sea Regions in the 20th–21st Centuries', *Public Library of Science ONE* 16 (2021), e0244615.

28 A. G. Carmichael, 'Plague Persistence in Western Europe: A Hypothesis', *The Medieval Globe* 1 (2014), 157–92.

29 Namouchi et al., 'Integrative Approach'; B. Bramanti et al., 'Plague: A Disease Which Changed the Path of Human Civilization', in *Yersinia pestis: Retrospective and Perspective*, ed. R. Yang and A. Anisimov (Dordrecht, 2016), 1–26; B. V. Schmid et al., 'Climate-Driven Introductions of the Black Death and Successive Plague Reintroductions into Europe', *Proceedings of the National Academy of Sciences* 112 (2015), 3020–5.

the thirteenth or fourteenth centuries.[30] However, here the genetics are very clear. Genome sequences of *Y. pestis* from victims of the Plague of Marseille (1720–22) – now amongst many others from Switzerland, Poland and Lithuania – are descendants of strains very closely related to those isolated from the Black Death victims of East Smithfield. The easiest (or, rather, the most parsimonious) explanation for this is that strains from these early outbreaks of the Second Pandemic made their way into new rodent reservoirs across Europe and the Mediterranean littoral, where they remained, subsequently and repeatedly spilling over into other new, unsuspecting hosts. A GIS analysis of the contemporary rodent distribution mapped on top of known Second Pandemic outbreaks highlights this distinct possibility (figure 12.3). There is no need to infer repeated long-distance dispersal from the East, when available rodent species exist today and most certainly did in the past within the emergence zone.

Deleted genes suggest possible changes to late stages of pandemics

In 2020, Susat et al. reported the deletion of a virulence gene (the plasminogen activator or *pla* gene) from seventeenth-century Second Pandemic plague strains identified in Latvia.[31] The *pla* gene encodes an enzyme that disrupts the host's ability to contain the infection and is an essential virulence factor for flea-borne plague.[32] The authors speculate that this deletion – meaning that the *pla* gene is partially absent from examined strains – could explain the diminution of European plague outbreaks. Interestingly, the gene is also missing in some strains retrieved from later victims of the Justinianic Plague (i.e., the First Pandemic). Furthermore, a recent analysis of multiple plague strains from across both the First and Second Pandemics shows that plasmids from later centuries in either pandemic are also often missing the same gene (figure 12.4, red trend line).[33]

This convergence, or independent loss of the *pla* gene on multiple, separate lineages of *Y. pestis*, is very interesting and suggests possible selection against the gene in later stages of both pandemics. In other words, the gene is deleted (removed) from the plasmid, perhaps to lower its lethality and in turn enable longer survival in the host population. Classic virulence theory posits a delicate balance between the pathogenicity of a microbe (its propensity to kill) and the perpetuation of its population. High virulence can in theory

[30] H. G. Fell et al., 'Volcanism and Global Plague Pandemics: Towards an Interdisciplinary Synthesis', *Journal of Historical Geography* 70 (2020), 36–46; M. H. Green, 'Climate and Disease in Medieval Eurasia', in *Oxford Research Encyclopedia of Asian History* (Oxford, 2018); B. M. S. Campbell, *The Great Transition: Climate, Disease and Society in the Late-Medieval World* (Cambridge, 2016), 463.

[31] Susat et al., '*Yersinia pestis* Strains from Latvia'.

[32] Sebbane et al., '*Yersinia pestis* Plasminogen Activator', *Biomolecules* 10 (2020), 1554.

[33] K. R. Sidhu et al., 'The Depletion of a Plasminogen Activator Locus from Victims of Later Dated Plague Pandemics and Their Implications on Plague's Disappearance' (forthcoming); Susat et al., '*Yersinia pestis* Strains from Latvia'; Keller et al., 'Ancient *Yersinia pestis* Genomes'; Spyrou et al., 'Historical *Y. pestis* Genomes'.

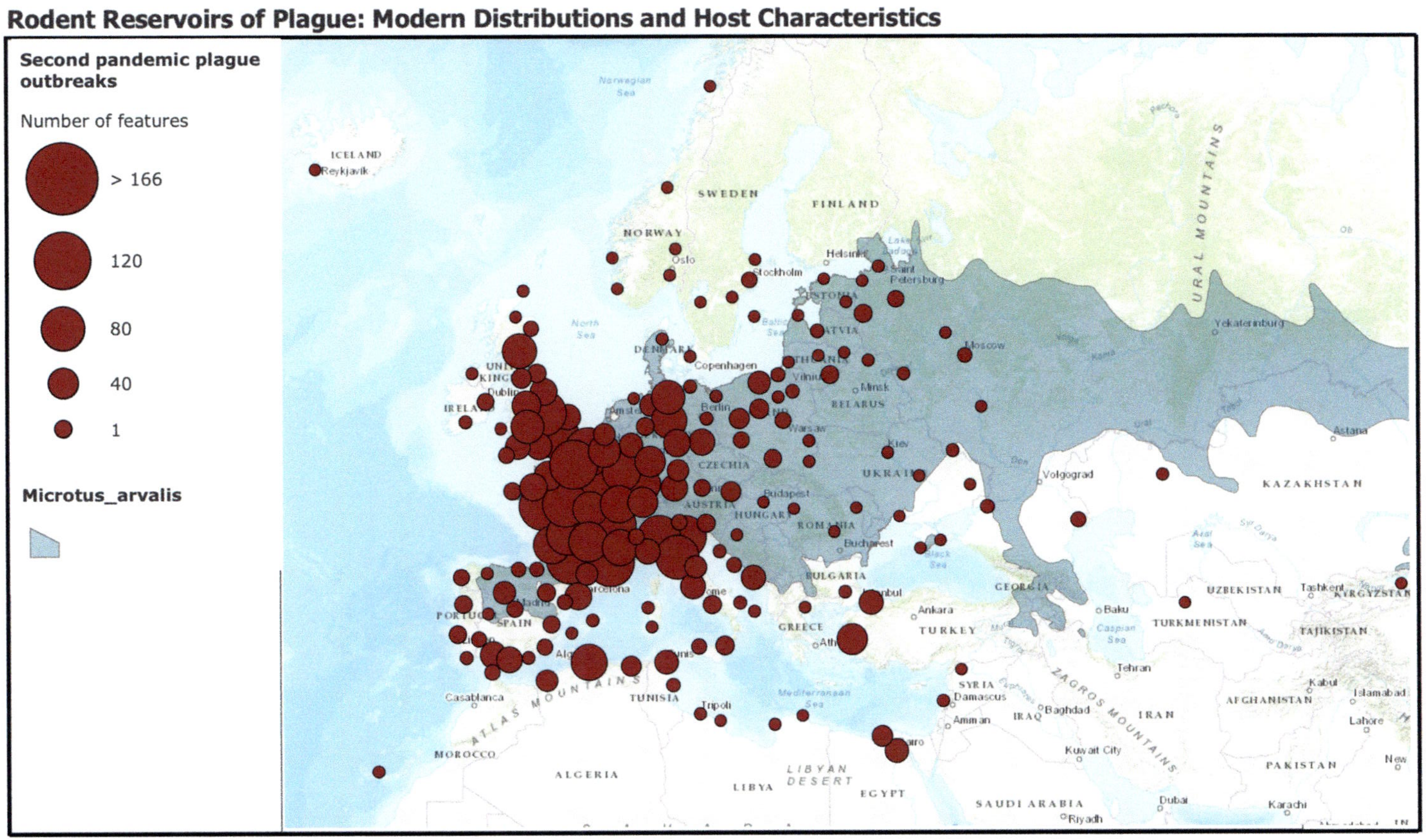

Fig. 12.3. GIS mapped distribution of the rodent species *Microtus arvalis*, known to harbour plague, overlaid onto known outbreaks from the Second Plague Pandemic. Hendrik Poinar.

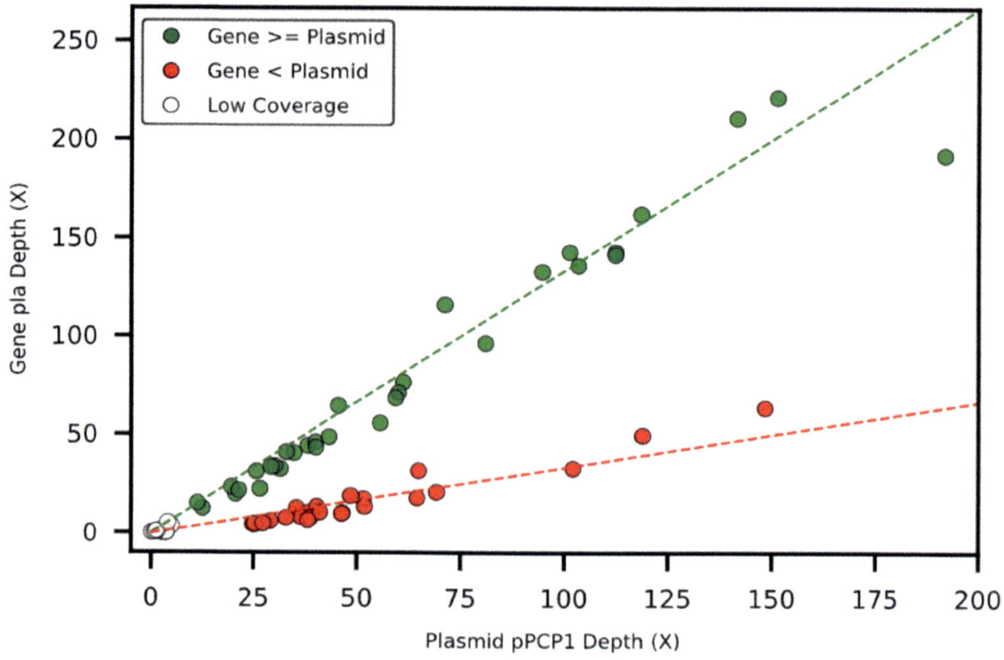

Fig. 12.4. The plasminogen activator (*pla*) gene copy number plotted as a function of the plasmid depth. Hendrik Poinar.

lead to extinction via killing of the host, but low virulence can also lead to extinction, as it is often tied to weaker transmission.[34] Thus, a delicate balance between high and low virulence is key for any pathogen's perpetuation. Perhaps the loss of this gene led to decreased transmission or virulence. However, as this gene is also known to be critical in flea-borne transmission, its deletion could be the result of a change in the host, such as a shift from the commensal black rat to a non-commensal wild species (e.g., *Microtus*, see figure 12.3). Further lab-based biochemical analyses are needed to elucidate the underlying reasons for and implications of this interesting deletion.

The molecular host and clock of Yersinia pestis *are erratic*

One hallmark of what is termed the molecular clock – that is, the rate at which substitutions accumulate over time – of *Y. pestis* is that it is not constant.[35] Rather, across the entire phylogenetic tree, the rate of evolutionary change differs by up to an order of

[34] S. Alizon and Y. Michalakis, 'Adaptive Virulence Evolution: The Good Old Fitness-Based Approach', *Trends in Ecology and Evolution* 30 (2015), 248–54; P. O. Méthot and S. Alizon, 'What Is a Pathogen? Toward a Process View of Host-Parasite Interactions', *Virulence* 5 (2014), 775–85.

[35] See Cui et al., 'Historical Variations'.

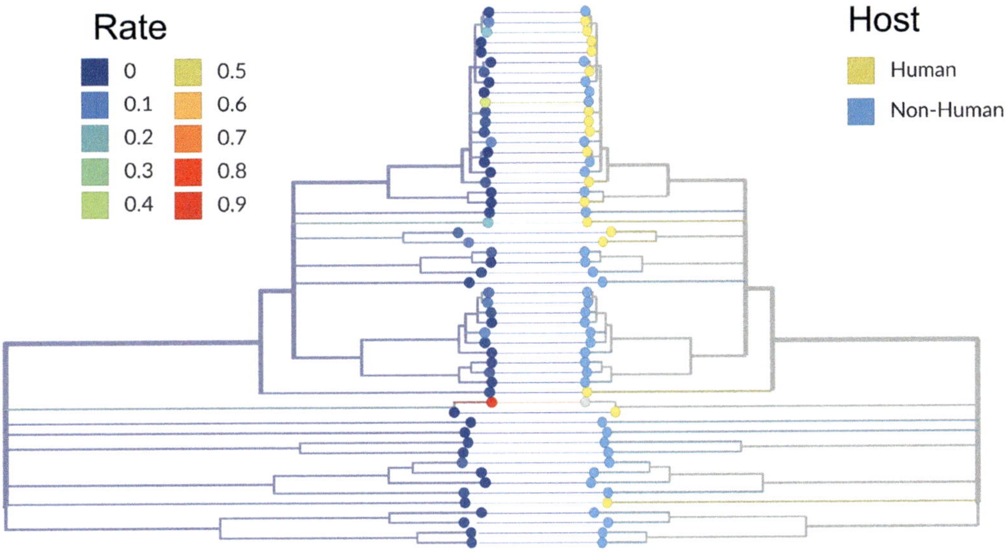

Fig. 12.5. Maximum likelihood tree of Branch 3, highlighting rate variation across the clades as well as the intermixing between both human and non-human hosts. Hendrik Poinar.

magnitude (figure 12.5, Branch 3, left side): sometimes an immense number of changes take place over short periods of time (pandemic phase), while at other times very few changes occur over long periods of stasis (sylvatic phase). Once considered to be one of the slowest-evolving bacteria, similar to *Mycobacterium leprae*, a more thorough statistical analysis across each individual clade (branch) on the phylogenetic tree shows that *Y. pestis*'s mean rate is faster, akin to that of *Mycobacterium tuberculosis*.[36] Why the extensive rate variation? The simplest explanation is likely rationalised by the pathogen's epidemiology. *Y. pestis* is naturally a disease of rodents but is capable of infecting virtually all mammals (figure 12.5, right side). It moves through sylvatic cycles in multiple rodent and flea species, sometimes spilling over into human and non-human hosts and their ectoparasites (i.e., fleas, lice, etc.).[37] Cross-species transfers are known to cause shifts in the rate of substitution, which may account for *Y. pestis*'s tremendous rate variation.

To the plague historian, a calibrated clock with a known number of substitutions expected per year can be used to back-date major bifurcations in the tree, namely polytomies like the

36 K. Eaton et al., 'Plagued by a Cryptic Clock: Insight and Issues from the Global Phylogeny of *Yersinia pestis*', under review at *Communications Biology*.

37 C. G. Zeppelini, A. M. de Almeida and P. Cordeiro-Estrela, 'Zoonoses as Ecological Entities: A Case Review of Plague', *PLOS Neglected Tropical Diseases* 10 (2016), e0004949; K. L. Gage and M. Y. Kosoy, 'Natural History of Plague: Perspectives from More Than a Century of Research', *Annual Review of Entomology* 50 (2005), 505–28.

so-called 'Big Bang', and in turn tie these events to the subsequent movement or associated history of the disease and its progression. Recent analyses suggest that some clades – when separated from the entire global phylogeny – do have a temporal signal.[38] Yet the majority of clades that surround the 'Big Bang' do not have a temporal signal and, as such, they significantly alter any estimate of its timing, which currently contains a wide confidence interval over hundreds of years. To ascertain the timing and emergence of the polytomy will require sequences from multiple remains retrieved from multiple well-described or radiocarbon-dated sites that fall closer to or within the polytomy. The polytomy itself is unlikely to represent a singular event; rather, it would have involved multiple spillovers from multiple reservoirs into different populations of different sizes and different levels of connectivity (i.e., trade routes, ports, etc.). Countless spillovers have undoubtedly occurred in small populations that had limited contact with other peoples, nomadic or otherwise, or with extinct rodent reservoirs. Other spillovers, by contrast, have been responsible for pandemic-scale plague outbreaks. Even among those, though, some ultimately will be 'dead ends', like the First Pandemic, for which no descendants are known.

Genetic diversity versus geographic distance in strains of Yersinia pestis

One way to look at the apportionment of genetic diversity across a geographic landscape is to compare the genetic distance between organisms (or strains) – that is, the differences between each sequence – and the geographic distance that separates them. In many organisms like humans, the further geographically two samples are from one another, the greater genetic distance that separates them. In other words, as related individuals move away from their ancestral homes (origins) and continue to evolve, they become increasingly dissimilar (have greater genetic distance). Single-host pathogens such as *Helicobacter pylori* show a similar trend, one that replicates human migrations.[39] The situation is very different for *Y. pestis*. While strains found in the pestoides (0.PE) branch account for the bulk of the genetic distance measured across *Y. pestis*, that branch accounts for less than 25 per cent of the pathogen's geographic spread (figure 12.6, dark blue circles). Third Pandemic strains (1.ORI), by contrast, account for less than 10 per cent of the genetic distance but 75 per cent of its geographic spread. This says something rather interesting about the epidemiology of plague.

Strains in the 0.PE branch are almost exclusively derived from sylvatic and commensal rodents spread across a fairly vast, currently endemic region of plague. Strains from 1.ORI are almost exclusively human and its spread has been human mediated, with eventual spillover into new wild reservoirs such as prairie dogs in the American south-west.[40] The First and Second Pandemic strains lie somewhere in between, suggesting that, despite the

[38] Eaton et al., 'Plagued by a Cryptic Clock'; Spyrou et al., 'Historical *Y. pestis* Genomes'.

[39] D. Falush et al., 'Traces of Human Migrations in Helicobacter pylori Populations', *Science* 299 (2003), 1582–5.

[40] M. Tapson's work on this is forthcoming.

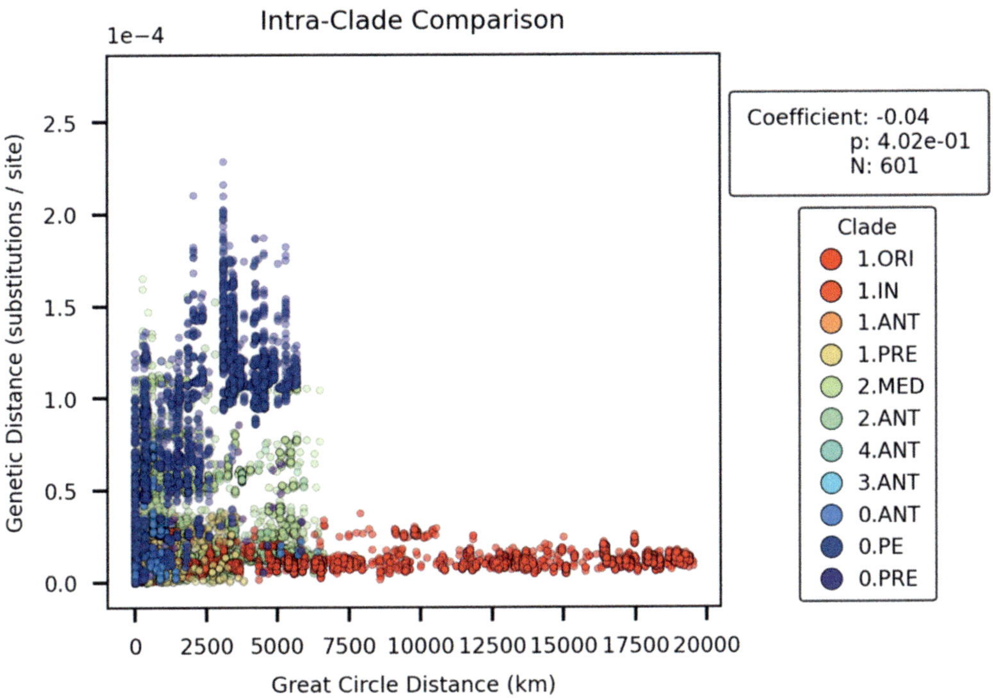

Fig. 12.6. Graph of the genetic distance versus geographic distance for all known strains of *Yersinia pestis*. Hendrik Poinar.

obvious bias that all ancient pandemic strains currently sequenced have been retrieved from human victims, human-mediated dispersal cannot alone explain its genetic distance. Retrospective diagnoses of the Second Pandemic as a human-contagion model are likely prejudiced by the Third Pandemic experience of plague. Perhaps most interestingly is the MED branch, which shows the greatest amount of genetic diversity versus its geographic spread for any single clade, with many isolates stemming from modern human samples. This branch will likely play a pivotal role in future work and re-evaluations of early plague history, including the 'Big Bang'.[41]

Conclusions

Our interpretations of the past are not static, although they are often assumed to be. Rather, they continually change as new data emerges or reinterpretations (analyses) highlight inconsistencies in existing data or historical narratives. It is important for geneticists, archaeologists and historians and all keepers of the past to maintain an open mind to the

[41] See M. H. Green, 'The Four Black Deaths', *American Historical Review* 125 (2020), 1600–31.

ability of aDNA retrieval to rapidly change our understanding of plague's past. Proper consultation with colleagues from many disciplines and the incorporation of multiple lines of evidence, prior to publishing the DNA data in isolation, will likely nuance (even lessen) the importance of any findings. It will also make this line of research less prone to being immediately supplanted by yet another DNA sequence, or even shown to be inaccurate. Occasionally non-specialists over- or misinterpret scientific data. Sometimes historians notice things in the scientific data that the geneticists themselves have missed.[42] Geneticists working in ancient infectious disease should thus rely on the well-informed and strong historical and archaeological frameworks offered by their colleagues in those fields, just as often as historians have followed and updated their own work as new DNA sequences come to light. Without historical contextualisation, geneticists, working in their reductive twenty-first century labs, will not 'solve' anything. Today it is critical that they coexist in a space where mutual interaction and collaboration move the field forward in ways that neither archives nor sequences can possibly do alone.[43]

42 See, for example, the *Contagions* blog post by M. H. Green and B. V. Schmid, 'Plague Dialogues: Monica Green and Boris Schmid on Plague Phylogeny (II)', https://contagions.wordpress.com/2016/06/29/plague-dialogues-monica-green-and-boris-schmid-on-plague-phylogeny-ii/ in which Green outlines her discovery of a misdated sample and the implications this had for genetic understanding of *Y. pestis* Branch 1B.

43 A recently published collaborative article appeared too late for substantive comment here. In this article, *Y. pestis* aDNA data from cemeteries located near Lake Issyk-Kul, Kyrgyzstan are putatively dated to 1338–9. Although suggestive, the clonal nature and very slow substitution rate of plague makes it difficult to claim this as the original emergence event that led to the Black Death. See M. A. Spyrou et al., 'The Source of the Black Death in Fourteenth-Century Central Eurasia', *Nature* 606 (2022), 718–24.

Select Bibliography

This selected bibliography includes the most pertinent references identified by each chapter author. Full details of other cited works are given in the individual chapters.

Albini, G., *Guerra, fame, peste: crisi di mortalità e sistema sanitario nella Lombardia tardomedioevale* (Bologna, 1982).

Arrizabalaga, J., 'Facing the Black Death: Perceptions and Reactions of University Medical Practitioners', in *Practical Medicine from Salerno to the Black Death*, ed. L. García-Ballester, R. French, J. Arrizabalaga and A. Cunningham (Cambridge, 1994), pp. 237–88.

Bergmann, H. and G. Keil, 'Das Münchner Pest-Laßmännchen. Standardisierungstendenzen in der spätmittelalterlichen deutschen Pesttherapie', in *Fachprosa-Studien: Beiträge zur mittelalterlichen Wissenschafts- und Geistesgeschichte*, ed. G. Keil (Berlin, 1982), pp. 318–30.

Black, W., 'Henry of Huntingdon's Lapidary Rediscovered and his *Anglicanus Ortus* Reassembled', *Medieval Studies* 68 (2006), 43–87.

Boldsen, J. L., 'Epidemiological Approach to the Paleopathological Diagnosis of Leprosy', *American Journal of Physical Anthropology* 115 (2001), 380–7.

Boquet, D. and P. Nagy, *Medieval Sensibilities. A History of Emotions in the Middle Ages*, trans. R. Shaw (Cambridge, 2018).

Bos, K. I. et al., 'A Draft Genome of *Yersinia pestis* from Victims of the Black Death', *Nature* 478 (2011), 506–10.

Bos, K. I. et al., 'Eighteenth Century *Yersinia pestis* Genomes Reveal the Long-Term Persistence of an Historical Plague Focus', *Elife* 5 (2016), e12994.

Bouras-Vallianatos P. and B. Zipser, ed., *Brill's Companion to the Reception of Galen* (Leiden, 2019).

Brenner, E., 'Recent Perspectives on Leprosy in Medieval Western Europe', *History Compass* 8 (2010), 388–406.

Brody, S. N., *The Disease of the Soul: Leprosy in Medieval Literature* (Cornell, 1974).

Butler, S. M., *Forensic Medicine and Death Investigation in Medieval England* (New York, 2015).

Caferro, W., *Petrarch's War: Florence and the Black Death in Context* (Cambridge, 2018).

Canalis, R. F. and Ciavolella, M., ed., *Disease and Disability in Medieval and Early Modern Art and Literature* (Turnhout, 2021).

Carmichael, A. G., 'Epidemics and State Medicine in Fifteenth-Century Milan', in *Medicine from the Black Death to the French Disease*, ed. R. French, J. Arrizabalaga, A. Cunningham and L. García-Ballester (Aldershot, 1998), pp. 221–47.

Carmichael, A. G., 'Plague Persistence in Western Europe: A Hypothesis', *The Medieval Globe* 1 (2014), 157–92.

Carmichael, A. G., 'Registering Deaths and Causes of Death in Late Medieval Milan', in *Death in Medieval Europe: Death Scripted and Death Choreographed*, ed. J. Rollo-Koster (London and New York, 2017), pp. 209–36.

Carmichael, A. G., 'Universal and Particular: The Language of Plague, 1348–1350', in *Pestilential Complexities: Understanding Medieval Plague*, ed. Vivian Nutton (London, 2008), pp. 17–52.

Casteen, E., *From She-Wolf to Martyr: The Reign and Disputed Reputation of Johanna I of Naples* (Ithaca, 2015).

Cavallo, S. and T. Storey, *Healthy Living in Late Renaissance Italy* (Oxford, 2013).

Cohn, S. K., *The Cultures of Plague: Medical Thinking at the End of the Renaissance* (Oxford, 2009).
Collard, F. and Samama, É., ed., *Le corps polychrome: couleurs et santé* (Paris, 2018).
Conrad, L. I., '*Ṭāʿūn* and *Wabāʾ*: Conceptions of Plague and Pestilence in Early Islam', *Journal of the Economic and Social History of the Orient* 25 (1982), 268–307.
Conrad, L. I., 'The Plague in the Early Medieval Near East' (unpublished Ph.D. dissertation, Princeton University, 1981).
Cook, H., 'Physick and Natural History in Seventeenth-Century England', in *Revolution and Continuity: Essays in the History of Philosophy of Early Modern Science*, ed. P. Barker and R. Ariew (Washington, 1991), pp. 63–80.
Crawford, C., 'Legalizing Medicine: Early Modern Legal Systems and the Growth of Medico-legal Knowledge', in *Legal Medicine in History*, ed. M. Clark and C. Crawford (Cambridge, 1994), pp. 89–116.
Crespo, F. A. and M. B. Lawrenz, 'Heterogeneous Immunological Landscape and Medieval Plague: An Invitation to a New Dialogue between Historians and Immunologists', *The Medieval Globe* 1 (2014), 229–57.
Crespo, F. A., J. White, and C. A. Roberts, 'Revisiting the Tuberculosis and Leprosy Cross-Immunity Hypothesis: Expanding the Dialogue between Immunology and Paleopathology', *International Journal of Paleopathology* 26 (2019), 37–47.
Cronica di Giovanni Villani: A miglior lezione ridotta coll'ajuto de'testi a penna, IV, ed. I. Moutier and F. G. Dragomanni (Florence, 1845).
Cui, Y. et al., 'Historical Variations in Mutation Rate in an Epidemic Pathogen, *Yersinia pestis*', *Proceedings of the National Academy of Sciences* 110 (2013), 577–82.
Demaitre, L., *Leprosy in Pre-Modern Medicine: A Malady of the Whole Body* (Baltimore, 2007).
Demaitre, L., 'The Idea of Childhood and Childcare in the Medical Writings of the Middle Ages', *The Journal of Psychohistory* 4 (1977), 461–90.
De Renzi, S., 'Medical Expertise, Bodies, and the Law in Early Modern Courts', *Isis* 98 (2007), 315–22.
De Voragine, J., *The Golden Legend: Readings on the Saints*, trans. W. G. Ryan, 2 vols (Princeton, 1993).
De Vos, P. S., *Compound Remedies: Galenic Pharmacy from the Ancient Mediterranean to New Spain* (Pittsburg, 2021).
Di Giammatteo, L. and J. A. Mendelsohn, 'Reporting for Action: Forms of Writing Between Medicine and Polity in Milan, 1580–1650', in *Civic Medicine: Physician, Polity and Pen in Early Modern Europe*, ed. J. A. Mendelsohn, A. Kinzelbach and R. Schilling (London and New York, 2020), pp. 135–60.
Dols, M., *The Black Death in the Middle East* (Princeton, 1977).
Donoghue, H. D. et al., 'Co-Infection of Mycobacterium Tuberculosis and Mycobacterium Leprae in Human Archaeological Samples: A Possible Explanation for the Historical Decline of Leprosy', *Proceedings of the Royal Society B: Biological Sciences* 272 (2005), 389–94.
Donohue, J. M., 'The Rite for the Commendation of the Dying in the 1983 *Pastoral Care of the Sick: Rites of Anointing and Viaticum*: A Study Through a Comparison with its Counterparts in the 1614 *Rituale Romanum* and in the 1972 *editio typica* of *Ordo unctionis infirmorum eorumque pastoralis curae*' (unpublished Ph.D. dissertation, Catholic University of America, 2000).
Duchêne, S., S. Y. W. Ho, A. G. Carmichael, E. C. Holmes and H. Poinar, 'The Recovery, Interpretation and Use of Ancient Pathogen Genomes', *Current Biology* 30 (2020), R1215–31.
Einbinder, S., *After the Black Death: Plague and Commemoration among Iberian Jews* (Philadelphia, 2018).
Eldem, E., *Death in Istanbul: Death and Its Rituals in Ottoman-Islamic Culture* (Istanbul, 2005).

Ell, S. R., 'Reconstructing the Epidemiology of Medieval Leprosy: Preliminary Efforts with Regard to Scandinavia', *Perspectives in Biology and Medicine* 31 (1988), 496–506.

Evans, J., *Magical Jewels of the Middle Ages and the Renaissance, Particularly in England* (London, 1921).

Fancy, N., 'Verification and Utility: Authorial and Exegetical Practices in the Commentaries on the *Canon of Medicine* of Fakhr al-Dīn al-Rāzī (d. 1210) and Ibn al-Nafīs (d. 1288)', *Journal of the History of Medicine and Allied Sciences* 75 (2020), 361–82.

Fancy, N. and M. H. Green, 'Plague and the Fall of Baghdad (1258)', *Medical History* 65 (2021), 157–77.

Finucane, R. C., *Miracles and Pilgrims: Popular Beliefs in Medieval England* (New York, 1995 [1977]).

Finucane, R. C., *The Rescue of the Innocents: Endangered Children in Medieval Miracles* (New York, 2000).

Flint, V. J., 'The Early Medieval "Medicus", the Saint – and the Enchanter', *The Society for the Social History of Medicine* 2 (1989), 127–45.

Fowler, C. J., *Pharmacopoeia Londinensis 1618 and Its Descendants* (London, 2018).

Geltner, G., 'In the Camp and on the March: Military Manuals as Sources for Studying Premodern Public Health', *Medical History* 63 (2019), 44–60.

Geltner, G., *Roads to Health: Infrastructure and Urban Wellbeing in Later Medieval Italy* (Philadelphia, 2019).

Gilbert, M. T. P. et al., 'Absence of *Yersinia pestis*-Specific DNA in Human Teeth from Five European Excavations of Putative Plague Victims', *Microbiology* 150 (2004), 341–54.

Givens, J. A., K. Reeds and A. Touwaide, ed., *Visualizing Medieval Medicine and Natural History, 1200–1550* (London, 2006).

Goldstein, B. and D. Pingree, 'Levi ben Gerson's Prognostication for the Conjunction of 1345', *The American Philosophical Society* 80 (1990), 1–60.

Goodich, M., *Miracles and Wonders: The Development of the Concept of Miracle, 1150–1350* (Aldershot, 2007).

Green, M. H., 'Documenting Medieval Women's Medical Practice', in *Practical Medicine from Salerno to the Black Death*, ed. L. García-Ballester, R. French, J. Arrizabalaga and A. Cunningham (Cambridge, 1994), pp. 322–52.

Green, M. H., 'Four Black Deaths', *American Historical Review* 125 (2020), 1601–31.

Green, M. H., *Making Women's Medicine Masculine: The Rise of Male Authority in Pre-Modern Gynaecology* (Oxford, 2008).

Green, M. H., ed., *The Medieval Globe*, Special Issue: Pandemic Disease in the Medieval World, 1 (2014).

Hamlin, C., 'Forensic Facts, the Guts of Rights', in *Global Forensic Cultures: Making Fact and Justice in the Modern Era*, ed. I. Burney and C. Hamlin (Baltimore, 2019), pp. 1–33.

Hartnell, J., 'Medicine's Image', in *The Routledge Companion to Medieval Iconography*, ed. C. Hourihane (London, 2016), pp. 322–39.

Hartnell, J., *Medieval Bodies: Life, Death and Art in the Middle Ages* (London, 2018).

Hathaway, J., *The Chief Eunuch of the Ottoman Harem: From African Slave to Power-Broker* (Cambridge, 2018).

Huggest, J. and N. Mikhaila, ed., *The Tudor Child: Clothing and Culture 1485–1625* (Lightwater, 2013).

Isserles, J., 'Bloodletting and Medical Astrology in Hebrew Manuscripts from Medieval Western Europe', *Sudhoffs Archiv* 101 (2017), 2–41.

Jones, L., '"Apostumes, Carbuncles, and Botches": Visualizing the Plague in Late Medieval and Early Modern Medical Treatises', in *Asclepius, the Paintbrush, and the Pen: Representations of*

Disease in Medieval and Early Modern Art and Literature, ed. M. Ciavolella and R. F. Canalis (Turnhout, 2021), pp. 173–200.
Jones, L., *Patterns of Plague: Changing Ideas about Plague in England and France, 1348–1750* (Montreal, 2022).
Jones, L. and R. Nevell, 'Plagued by Doubt and Viral Misinformation: The Need for Evidence-Based Use of Historical Disease Images', *The Lancet Infectious Diseases* 16 (2016), e235–40.
Katajala-Peltomaa, S., *Gender, Miracles and Daily Life. The Evidence of Fourteenth-Century Canonization Processes* (Turnhout, 2009).
Koopmans, R., *Wonderful to Relate: Miracle Stories and Miracle Collecting in High Medieval England* (Philadelphia, 2011).
Kuuliala, J., *Childhood Disability and Social Integration in the Middle Ages: Constructions of Impairments in Thirteenth- and Fourteenth-Century Canonization Processes* (Turnhout, 2016).
Lett, D., *L'enfant des miracles: Enfance et société au Moyen Âge (XIIe–XIIIe siècle)* (Paris, 1997).
Little, L., ed., *Plague and the End of Antiquity: The Pandemic of 541–750* (Cambridge, 2007).
Little, L., 'Plague Historians in Lab Coats', *Past and Present* 213 (2011), 267–90.
Lynteris, C., ed., *Plague Image and Imagination from Medieval to Modern Times* (Cham, 2021).
Magnus, A., *Book of Minerals*, trans. D. Wyckoff (Oxford, 1967).
Manchester, K. and C. A. Roberts, 'The Palaeopathology of Leprosy in Britain: A Review', *World Archaeology* 21 (1989), 265–72.
McDade, T. W., 'The Ecologies of the Human Immune Function', *Annual Review of Anthropology* 34 (2005), 495–521.
McNamer, S., *Affective Meditation and the Invention of Medieval Compassion* (Philadelphia, 2010).
McVaugh, M., 'Arnald of Villanova's *Regimen Almarie* (*Regimen Castra Sequentium*) and Medieval Military Medicine', *Viator* 23 (1992), 201–14.
Metzler, I., *Disability in Medieval Europe: Thinking about Physical Impairment during the High Middle Ages, c.1100–1400* (London, 2006).
Mitchell, A. W., 'The Chant of the Earliest Franciscan Office' (unpublished Ph.D. dissertation, University of Western Ontario, 2003).
Mitchell, P., 'The Spread of Disease with the Crusades', in *Between Text and Patient: The Medical Enterprise in Medieval and Early Modern Europe*, ed. F. E. Glaze and B. Nance (Florence, 2011), pp. 309–30.
Mulhall, J., 'Plague before Pandemics: The Greek Medical Evidence for Bubonic Plague before the Sixth Century', *Bulletin of the History of Medicine* 93 (2019), 151–79.
Murray, A., *Suicide in the Middle Ages: Volume 2: The Curse on Self-Murder* (Oxford, 2010).
Nicoud, M., *Le Prince et les Médecins: Pensée et pratiques médicales à Milan, 1402–1476* (Rome, 2014).
Öberg Strådal, S. M., 'Depictions of Physical Order: Diagrams in Late Medieval English Medical Manuscripts' (unpublished PhD dissertation, University of Glasgow, 2015).
Öberg Strådal, S. M., 'Utility Beyond Function: Practical and Social Uses of Diagrams in Late Medieval English Medical Manuscripts', in *The Diagram Paradigm*, ed. D. Roxburgh, J. Hamburger and L. Safran (Dumbarton Oaks, forthcoming).
Ottosen, K., *The Responsories and Versicles of the Latin Office of the Dead* (Aarhus, Denmark: 1993).
Palmer, R. J., 'Girolamo Mercuriale and the Plague of Venice', in *Girolamo Mercuriale: medicina e cultura nell'europa del cinquecento*, ed. A. Arcangeli and V. Nutton (Florence, 2008), pp. 51–65.
Paxton, F. S., *Christianizing Death: The Creation of a Ritual Process in Early Medieval Europe* (Ithaca and London, 1990).

Paxton, F. S., 'Death by Customary at Eleventh-Century Cluny', in *From Dead of Night to End of Day: The Medieval Customs of Cluny*, ed. S. Boynton and I. Cochelin, Disciplina Monastica 3 (Turnhout, 2005), pp. 297–318.

Paxton, F. S., *The Death Ritual at Cluny in the Central Middle Ages* (Turnhout, 2013).

Peterson, J. L., *Suspect Saints and Holy Heretics: Disputed Sanctity and Communal Identity in Late Medieval Italy* (Ithaca, 2019).

Preto, P., *Peste e società a Venezia nel 1576* (Vicenza, 1978).

Rasmussen, S. et al., 'Early Divergent Strains of *Yersinia pestis* in Eurasia 5,000 Years Ago', *Cell* 163 (2015), 571–82.

Rawcliffe, C., *Leprosy in Medieval England* (Woodbridge, 2006).

Riddle, J. M., ed., *Marbode of Rennes' (1035–1123)* De lapidibus*: Considered as a Medical Treatise with Text, Commentary, and C. W. King's Translation, Together with Text and Translation of Marbode's Minor Works on Stones* (Wiesbaden, 1977).

Ridley, D. S. and W. H. Jopling, 'Classification of Leprosy According to Immunity', *International Journal of Leprosy* 31 (1966), 255–73.

Roberts, C. A., *Leprosy: Past and Present* (Gainsville, FL, 2020).

Rosenwein, B. H., *Emotional Communities in the Early Middle Ages* (Ithaca and London, 2007).

Ruderman, D. B., *Kabbalah, Magic, and Science: The Cultural Universe of a Sixteenth-Century Jewish Physician* (Cambridge, MA, 1988).

Ruderman, D. B., ed. and trans., *A Valley of Vision: The Heavenly Journey of Abraham ben Hananiah Yagel* (Philadelphia, 1990).

Russell, P., *A Treatise of the Plague* (London, 1791).

Saenger, P., *A Catalogue of the Pre-1500 Western Manuscript Books at the Newberry Library* (Chicago, 1989).

Savage-Smith, E., 'Anatomical Illustration in Arabic Manuscripts', in *Arab Painting: Text and Image in Illustrated Arabic Manuscripts*, ed. A. Contadini (Leiden, 2007), pp. 147–60.

Schuenemann, V. J. et al., 'Genome-Wide Comparison of Medieval and Modern Mycobacterium Leprae', *Science* 341 (2013), 179–83.

Sicard, D., *La liturgie de la mort dans l'église latine des origines à la réforme carolingienne* (Münster, 1978).

Singer, M. et al., 'Syndemics and the Biosocial Conception of Health', *The Lancet* 389 (2017), 941–50.

Spyrou, M. A. et al., 'Phylogeography of the Second Plague Pandemic Revealed through Analysis of Historical *Yersinia pestis* Genomes', *Nature Communications* 10 (2019), 4470.

Temkin, O., *The Falling Sickness: A History of Epilepsy from the Greeks to the Beginnings of Modern Neurology* (Baltimore, 1971).

The Final Book of Giovanni Villani's New Chronicle, trans. R. I. Diakité and M. Sneider (Kalamazoo, 2016).

Touati, F. O., 'Contagion and Leprosy: Myth, Ideas and Evolution in Medieval Minds and Societies', in *Contagion: Perspectives from Pre-Modern Societies*, ed. L. I. Conrad and D. Wujastyk (Aldershot, 2000), pp. 179–201.

Van Dijk, S. J. P., 'Some Manuscripts of the Earliest Franciscan Liturgy', *Franciscan Studies* 16 (1956), 60–101.

Van Dijk, S. J. P. and J. Hazelden Walker, *The Origins of the Modern Roman Liturgy: The Liturgy of the Papal Court and the Franciscan Order in the Thirteenth Century* (London, 1960).

Varlık, N., 'From "Bête Noire" to "le Mal de Constantinople": Plagues, Medicine, and the Early Modern Ottoman State', *Journal of World History* 24 (2013), 741–70.

Varlık, N., *Plague and Empire in the Early Modern Mediterranean World: The Ottoman Experience* (New York, 2015).
Vauchez, A., *La sainteté en Occident aux derniers siècles du Moyen Âge: D'après les procès de canonisation et les documents hagiographiques* (Rome, 1988 [1981]).
Vauchez, A., *Sainthood in the Later Middle Ages* (Cambridge, 1997).
Vitiello, J. C., 'Forensic Evidence, Lay Witnesses and Medical Expertise in the Criminal Courts of Late Medieval Italy', in *Medicine and the Law in the Middle Ages*, ed. S. M. Butler and W. Turner (Leiden, 2014), pp. 133–56.
Voigts, L. E. and M. R. McVaugh, 'A Latin Technical Phlebotomy and Its Middle English Translation', *Transactions of the American Philosophical Society* 74 (1984), 1–69.
Wagner, D. M. et al., '*Yersinia pestis* and the Plague of Justinian 541–543 AD: A Genomic Analysis', *Lancet Infectious Diseases* 14 (2014), 319–26.
Ward, B., *Miracles and the Medieval Mind: Theory, Record, and Event, 1000–1215* (Philadelphia, 1982).
Webb, D., 'Friends of the Family: Some Miracles for Children by Italian Friars', in *The Church and Childhood*, ed. D. Wood (Oxford, 1994), pp. 183–95.
Weinstein, D. and R. M. Bell, *Saints and Society: The Two Worlds of Western Christendom, 1000–1700* (Chicago, 1982).
Yagel, A., *Moshi'ah Ḥosim* (Venice, 1587).
Zanella, G., 'La peste del 1348: Italia, Francia, e Germania', in *La Peste Nera: dati di una realta et elementi di una interpretazione: atti del XXX Convegno storico internazionale, Todi, 10–13 ottobre 1993*, pp. 49–60 (Spoleto, 1994).
Ziegler, J., 'Practitioners and Saints: Medical Men in Canonization Processes in the Thirteenth to Fifteenth Centuries', *Social History of Medicine* 12 (1999), 191–225.

Index

Health and Healing in the Middle Ages

1 SAINTS, CURE-SEEKERS AND MIRACULOUS HEALING IN TWELFTH-CENTURY ENGLAND
Ruth J. Salter

2 ETHNICITY IN MEDIEVAL EUROPE, 950–1250
Medicine, Power and Religion
Claire Weeda

3 THE GUILD BOOK OF THE BARBERS AND SURGEONS OF YORK (BRITISH LIBRARY, EGERTON MS 2572)
Study and Edition
Richard D. Wragg